New Trends in Reproductive Medicine

Springer
Berlin
Heidelberg
New York
Barcelona
Budapest
Hong Kong
London
Milan
Paris
Santa Clara
Singapore
Tokyo

K. H. Broer, I. Turanli (Eds.)

New Trends in Reproductive Medicine

With 46 Figures and 50 Tables

Springer

Editors:

Prof. Dr. med. Karl Heinz Broer
Chefarzt Frauenklinik
Krankenhaus Porz am Rhein
Akademisches Lehrkrankenhaus der Universität Köln
Urbacher Weg 19, 51149 Köln
Germany

Dr. med. Ismet Turanli
Frauenarzt
Dürener Straße 209, 50931 Köln
Germany

ISBN-13: 978-3-642-64630-0 **e-ISBN-13: 978-3-642-60961-9**
DOI: 10.1007/ 978-3-642-60961-9

Library of Congress Cataloging-in-Publication Data. New trends in reproductive medicine / K.H. Broer; I. Turanli (eds.). p. cm. Includes bibliographical references. ISBN 978-3-642-64630-0 (alk. paper) 1. Infertility, Female. 2. Human reproductive technology. 3. Infertility, Male. I. Broer, K.H. (Karl Heinz), 1943– II. Turanli, I. (Ismet), 1930– . RG201.N48 1996 616.6′92–dc20 95-44731

Softcover reprint of the hardcover 1st edition 1996

SPIN: 10484442 21/3135 - 5 4 3 2 1 0 – Printed on acid-free paper

Contents

Andrology

Other Specific Topics

In Vitro Fertilization and Related Techniques

Contributors

S. Al-Hasani, Dr. med.
Klinik für Frauenheilkunde und Geburtshilfe,
Medizinische Universität Lübeck,
Ratzeburger Allee 160, 23538 Lübeck, Germany

A. Arici, Prof., M.D.
Department of Obstetrics and Gynecology,
Division of Reproductive Endocrinology,
Yale University School of Medicine,
333 Cedar Street, New Haven, CT 06510, USA

E. Attar, M.D.
Department of Obstetrics and Gynecology,
Division of Reproductive Endocrinology,
Yale University School of Medicine,
333 Cedar Street, New Haven, CT 06510, USA

M.M. Babic, M.D.
Department of Obstetrics and Gynecology,
Medical School University of Zagreb,
Sveti Duh 64, 10000 Zagreb, Croatia

L. Beck, Prof. Dr. med.
ehem. Direktor der Universitätsfrauenklinik Düsseldorf,
Moorenstraße 5, 40225 Düsseldorf, Germany

H.M. Beier, Prof. Dr. med.
Direktor Institut für Anatomie,
RWTH Universität Aachen, Wendlingweg 2,
52076 Aachen, Germany

M. S. Beksac, Prof. Dr. med.
Division of Maternal and Fetal Medicine, Department of Obstetrics and Gynecology, Hacettepe University, 06100 Ankara, Turkey

D. Beyer, Prof. Dr. med.
Radiologische Abteilung,
Akademisches Lehrkrankenhaus der Universität Köln,
Krankenhaus Porz/Rhein,
Urbacher Weg 19, 51149 Köln, Germany

P. Bielfeld, PD Dr. med.
Universitätsfrauenklinik Düsseldorf,
Moorenstraße 5, 40225 Düsseldorf, Germany

H. G. Bohnet, Prof. Dr. med.
Fertility Institute,
Schomburgstraße 120, 22767 Hamburg, Germany

K. H. Broer, Prof. Dr. med.
Frauenklinik,
Akademisches Lehrkrankenhaus der Universität Köln,
Krankenhaus Porz/Rhein,
Urbacher Weg 19, 51149 Köln, Germany

D. Broer-Ahlers, Dr. med.
Frauenärztin, Zytologisches Labor,
Ebertplatz, Köln, Germany

O. Bukulmez, M.D.
Department of Obstetrics and Gynecology,
Division of Reproductive Endocrinology,
Yale University School of Medicine,
333 Cedar Street, New Haven, CT 06510, USA

A. N. Cakar, Prof. Dr. med.
Department of Embryology and Histology,
Hacettepe University,
06100 Ankara, Turkey

C. C. Coddington, M.D.
Department of Obstetrics and Gynecology,
The Howard and Georgeanna Jones Institute for Reproductive Medicine, Eastern Virginia Medical School,
601 Colley Avenue, Norfolk, VA 23507, USA

K. Diedrich, Prof. Dr. med.
Klinik für Frauenheilkunde und Geburtshilfe,
Medizinische Universität Lübeck,
Ratzeburger Allee 160, 23538 Lübeck, Germany

O. Djahanbakhch, M.D., M. Phil, FRCOG, M.D.
Academic Department of Obstetrics and Gynecology,
London Hospital Medical College,
Royal London Hospital,
Whitechapel, London E1 1BB, UK

U. Engelmann, Prof. Dr. med.
Klinik und Poliklinik für Urologie,
Medizinische Einrichtungen der Universität zu Köln,
Joseph-Stelzmann-Straße, 50931 Köln, Germany

A. K. Ertan, M.D.
Department of Obstetrics and Gynecology,
Medical School University of Zagreb,
Sveti Duh 64, 10000 Zagreb, Croatia

H. Frangenheim, Prof. Dr. med.
ehem. Chefarzt der Frauenklinik,
Christoph-Daniel-Schenck-Straße 10,
78464 Konstanz, Germany

D. E. Gagel, Dr. med., Dipl. Psych.
Universitätsklinikum Rudolf Virchow,
Standort Charlottenburg,
Pulsstraße 4, 14059 Berlin, Germany

C. De Geyter, Dr. med.
Klinik und Poliklinik für Frauenheilkunde und Geburtshilfe B, Westfälische Wilhelms-Universität Münster,
Albert-Schweitzer-Straße 33, 48129 Münster, Germany

Ü. B. Gör, Dr. med.
Abteilung Gynäkologische Endokrinologie und Reproduktionsmedizin, Universitätsfrauenklinik Heidelberg,
Voßstraße 9, 69115 Heidelberg, Germany

V. Gomel, Prof. M.D.
Department of Obstetrics and Gynecology,
University of British Columbia,
Vancouver, B.C., Canada

K. Grunwald, Prof. Dr. med.
Abteilung Gynäkologische Endokrinologie und Reproduktionsmedizin, Universitätsfrauenklinik Heidelberg,
Voßstraße 9, 69115 Heidelberg, Germany

T. Gürgan, Prof. Dr. med.
Department of Obstetrics and Gynecology,
Division of Reproductive Endocrinology and Infertility,
Faculty of Medicine, Hacettepe University,
06100 Ankara, Turkey

G. Haidl, Prof. Dr. med.
Klinik und Poliklinik für Haut- und Geschlechtskrankheiten,
Rheinische Friedrich-Wilhelms-Universität,
Sigmund-Freud-Straße 25, 53105 Bonn, Germany

H. Hassa, Prof. M.D.
Department of Obstetrics and Gynecology,
Faculty of Medicine, Osmangazi University,
26130 Eskisehir, Turkey

A. Helvacioglu, M.D., Assoc. Prof.
Department of Obstetrics and Gynecology,
University of South Alabama,
CC/CB, Rm. 324, Mobile, AL 36688, USA

Y. Karaman, M.D.
Hôpital Francais Reine Elisabeth,
Institut Médical Edith-Chavell,
Av. W. Churchill 226, 1180 Brussels, Belgium

H. Kentenich, PD Dr. med.
Universitätsklinikum Rudolf Virchow,
Standort Charlottenburg,
Pulsstraße 4, 14059 Berlin, Germany

A. K. Ertan, M.D.
Department of Obstetrics and Gynecology,
Medical School University of Zagreb,
Sveti Duh 64, 10000 Zagreb, Croatia

S. Kupesic, M.D., Ph.D.
Department of Obstetrics and Gynecology,
Medical School University of Zagreb,
Sveti Duh 64, 10000 Zagreb, Croatia

A. Kurjak, M.D.
Department of Obstetrics and Gynecology,
Medical School University of Zagreb,
Sveti Duh 64, 10000 Zagreb, Croatia

H. Ludwig, Prof. Dr. med.
Wartenbergstraße 9, 4052 Basel, Switzerland

M. Ludwig, Dr. med.
Klinik für Frauenheilkunde und Geburtshilfe,
Medizinische Universität Lübeck,
Ratzeburger Allee 160, 23538 Lübeck, Germany

S. D. Maguiness, M.D. MRCOG
Princess Royal Maternity Hospital,
Saltshouse Road, Hull HU8 9HE, UK

M. J. Mathers, Dr. med.
Klinik und Poliklinik für Urologie,
Medizinische Einrichtungen der Universität zu Köln,
Joseph-Stelzmann-Straße, 50931 Köln, Germany

U. P. Merten, Dr. med.
Institute for Laboratory Medicine,
Lindenthalgürtel, 50931 Köln

V.-S. Pastor, Dipl.-Psych.
Universitätsklinikum Rudolf Virchow,
Standort Charlottenburg,
Pulsstraße 4, 14059 Berlin, Germany

I. Psalti, Ph.D.
Hôpital Francais Reine Elisabeth,
Service de Gynecologie, Unité FIVETE,
Rue Josse Goffin 180, 1080 Brussels, Belgium

T. Rabe, Prof. Dr. med.
Abteilung Gynäkologische Endokrinologie und Reproduktionsmedizin, Universitätsfrauenklinik Heidelberg,
Voßstraße 9, 69115 Heidelberg, Germany

B. Runnebaum, Prof. Dr. med.
Abteilung Gynäkologische Endokrinologie und Reproduktionsmedizin, Universitätsfrauenklinik Heidelberg,
Voßstraße 9, 69115 Heidelberg, Germany

E. Saridogan, M.D.
Academic Department of Obstetrics and Gynecology,
London Hospital Medical College, Royal London Hospital,
Whitechapel, London E1 1BB, UK

S. Schmidt, Dr. med.
Department of Obstetrics and Gynecology,
Medical School University of Zagreb,
Sveti Duh 64, 10000 Zagreb, Croatia

M. Sillem, Dr. med.
Abteilung Gynäkologische Endokrinologie und Reproduktionsmedizin, Universitätsfrauenklinik Heidelberg,
Voßstraße 9, 69115 Heidelberg, Germany

P. J. Taylor, M.D.
Department of Obstetrics and Gynecology,
University of British Columbia,
Vancouver, B.C., Canada

I. Turanli, Dr. med.
Dürener Straße 209, 50931 Köln, Germany

R. Turanli, Dr. med.
Universitäts-Frauenklinik,
50924 Köln, Germany

H. Yarali, M.D.
Division of Reproductive Endocrinology and Infertility,
Department of Obstetrics and Gynecology,
Faculty of Medicine, Hacettepe University,
06100 Ankara, Turkey

M. Yildirim, Prof. Dr. med.
University of Gazi,
Department of Obstetrics and Gynecology,
06100 Ankara, Turkey

J. Zumbé, Dr. med.
Klinik und Poliklinik für Urologie,
Medizinische Einrichtungen der Universität zu Köln,
Joseph-Stelzmann-Straße, 50931 Köln

Foreword

H.M. Beier

Reproductive medicine has emerged from the classical fields of gynecology, obstetrics, andrology, embryology, endocrinology, and genetics. It will therefore always be an area of collaborative effort and teamwork. The goals and strategies of the field of reproductive medicine have been established and clearly defined since the earth-shaking event of the birth of the first in vitro fertilized baby, Louise Brown, during the summer of 1978 at the Oldham District Hospital, near Manchester in England. This event demonstrated to everybody that success in reproductive medicine is truely the result of teamwork, in particular when the pathological obstacles are high and the efforts to overcome these difficulties need to be exceptionally intense. It was the evident collaboration of a basic researcher, Robert G. Edwards, and a gynecologist, Patrick Steptoe, which made those first efforts successful. There were a few essential and extremely busy helpers at each part of the team, nurses, physicians, lab endocrinologists, and technicians, not to forget the late Jean Purdy, who settled the laboratory conditions of what today is called an IVF lab.

Since those days of 1978, it has become an accepted fact in the world of gynecology and andrology that there will be never any progress in reproductive medicine if the lively and fruitful collaboration between clinician and basic researcher does not continue unabated. Such basic research is moving constantly and rapidly, and the progress in cell biology, molecular biology, and molecular genetics is very evident. The methodological spectrum of these fields is expanding in a fascinating manner. Today everyone understands what is meant by polymerase chain reaction, RNA blotting, in situ hybridization, gene targeting, cell transfection etc.

However, with these extraordinary methods and molecular skills, the field of reproductive medicine encounters ethical battle fields in several regard. "*A child, my own baby by all means*", "*A child is a joy at any age.*" Reproductive medicine has created the biggest challenge to its acting professionals by developing methods which seem to surpass nature. The availability of using donor ova with menopausal women as recipients launched the controversy surrounding not only reproduction per se but the age limitation of reproduction independent of the limits drawn by biological conditions.

Although the latest achievement of reproductive medicine, intracytoplasmic sperm injection (ICSI), was just a minor technical improvement of gamete micromanipulation, it was a major step towards overcoming some inevitable hurdles set by nature. The ongoing debate whether such major steps are legitimate advances in the field of reproductive medicine demands intense and critical assessments by the basic researcher, particularly the geneticist, and the clinician.

Any progress in reproductive medicine will only pase a serious achievement, either for an infertile couple or for mankind, if we all feel truly responsible for staying within the ethical framework of our profession.

This book may contribute to defining the goals and strategies of our exciting field. The authors are experts in their disciplines. Their experience and critical assessment may lead the specialists of tomorrow to what is generally agreed to be good medical practice, including responsibility and respect to the human beings most deeply involved in reproductive medicine, the patients.

Preface

K.H. Broer, I. Turanli

Reproductive medicine is concerned with the problems of human reproduction, i.e., sterility and contraception, and is becoming increasingly important on an international scale. It becomes clear just how important this branch of medicine is if one considers that the world's population currently stands at around five billion and the percentage of childless couples who want children is relatively high; for the industrialized countries, it is estimated to be 10%–15%, while for the developing countries the figures vary greatly, ranging somewhere between 5% and 45%. It is this international significance which the authors aim to reflect in the present volume. Renowned scientists and clinicians who are internationally active in particular areas of reproductive medicine present the state of the art in their own fields.

The pace of development in reproductive medicine has been increasingly rapid in the past few years, and research results have swiftly been integrated into clinical practice. This process has by no means come to a standstill, but continues to develop fast and is in need of constant review.

Since the first success was achieved in in vitro fertilization and intratubal gamete transfer, the focus of attention has turned to ICSI microinsemination measures, which have opened up completely new areas of indication and decisively broadened the range of options available for treating sterility problems. In addition, the use of GnRH analogs and other established diagnostic and therapeutic procedures have led to a continual improvement in the overall concept of treating sterile couples.

The aim of this volume is to give clinicians and students a survey of current knowledge and the treatment options available in the field of reproductive medicine. The authors are aware that a complete overview would be impossible within the given framework of this book, and thus have restricted themselves to focusing on important individual aspects, which range from research results to everyday clinical practice. The book is intended as a complementary volume to the up-to-date information provided by specialist congresses, seminars, and other single publications. The editors hope to broaden their readers' knowledge of the subject and to address aspects of treating sterile couples which can be adjusted to give individual attention to the problems of individual couples.

Introduction

Sterility: Diagnosis, Therapeutics, and Monitoring

K.H. Broer and I. Turanli

Sterility

Diagnosis, Therapeutics, and Outpatient Monitoring

In recent years it has become increasingly important and time-consuming to care for sterile couples. Modern techniques now offer medical specialists a number of possibilities in the outpatient care of patients who, only a few years ago, could only be treated in large clinics and special centers. It has become possible to shift a considerable part of sterility diagnosis, therapeutics, and monitoring to the outpatient sector, leaving only a small group of sterility patients for treatment or supervision in a center, such as those requiring surgery. The medical specialist is usually in a position to supervise the entire treatment course of the sterile couple. In the near future it should even be possible to ensure outpatient supervision of in vitro fertilization. About 20% of the gynecologic patients in outpatient surgery are sterility cases, and 10%–15% of all couples in Germany stay childless unintentionally.

The term "sterility" is applied when regular sexual activity without the use of contraception over a period of 1 year has not produced gravidity although there is a strong desire for a child. If fecundation took place, but the fetus was lost, the woman's inability to carry the pregnancy to term is called "infertility."

In consultations with sterile couples a few general factors have to be considered, such as the couple's age and the fact that nearly half of all sterility cases can be attributed to a pathological gynecologic condition. 40% to a pathological andrologic condition, and approximately 10% to a combination of gynecologic and andrologic problems.

Sterility in Women

The reasons for sterility in women vary according to their anatomic localization. Since in most cases (35%–40%) the reasons are ovarian, they involve hormonal disturbances requiring hormonal therapy. Such disturbances represent the most common etiology of sterility out of the wide range of prominent factors, and in these cases the changes of a successful therapeutic outcome are very good.

Approximately 30% of gynecologic sterility cases are caused by tubal deficiencies. The therapy of choice for tubal sterility is usually microsurgery or similar invasive operations which, however, have met with the lowest rates of success. Cervical sterility accounts for approximately 10% of cases; in these diagnosis is not complicated and therapy is generally successful. All other causes of sterility (vaginal, extragenital, psychological) are of secondary importance, and there is little chance of success for the treatment methods currently available. About 10%–15% of the gynecologic causes of sterility are idiopathic, i.e., it is not possible to determine a somatic reason despite modern diagnostic methods such as laparoscopy.

A brief description of the different causes of sterility is given next.

Vaginal Factors in Female Sterility

Inflammations resulting in painful changes on the vaginal epithelium and vaginal wall which are caused by chronic or acute bacterial, viral, or fungal infections require adequate diagnosis and therapeutics, which normally causes no problems. In addition to such inflammations, psychogenic factors may induce changes in the pH value of the vaginal environment (hyperacidity) and may consequently reduce the buffer capacity of the sperm deposit.

Psychogenic factors in vaginismus are frequently due to problems in the partnership and may necessitate psychological assistance by a physician.

Vaginal obstruction to immissio penis may be caused by a cicatrized hymen, a too small orificium hymenis, vaginal asplasia, vaginal duplex, or other anatomic deficiencies. These abnormalities require surgical correction which can easily be performed with high success rates.

Cervical Factors in Female Sterility

1. *Posttraumatic cervical alterations* caused by gynecologic operations such as status after conization or portio amputation, or by laceration or cauterization: depending on the anatomy such alterations on the cervix may result in a partial destruction of the cervical mucus glands and concomitant alterations of the cervical factor. The application of a cap plastic portio is the most common treatment. Local therapy, e.g., administration of estrogen with the aim of reconstructing the cervical gland and the cervical epithelium, are also successful.
2. *Changes in position of the cervix and uterus in cases of severe descensus uteri or upper vaginal stenosis and in* (rarely occurring) *retroflexio uteri:* Today, invasive correction of a retroflexio uteri is a rather rare indication, especially when the retroflexio uteri fixata is caused by cicatricial alterations in the small pelvis.
3. *Disturbed development of cervical factor due to inadequate production of cervical mucus* caused by infections with bacteria, trichomonas, fungi, viruses, or mycoplasms or by insufficient ovarian stimulation and impeded estrogen production: Diagnosis and therapy of the cervical factor are among those tasks of the gynecologist that achieve high success rates since a wide range of treatment schemes may be applied.

Uterine Factors in Female Sterility

1. *Chronic endometritis.* Status after abortions, or after tuberculous endometritis or other acute or chronic inflammations may cause alterations on the endometrial mucosa. For diagnosis and therapy a combination of outpatient treatment and hospitalization is possible.
2. *Changes in uterus size,* e.g., hyper- or hypoplasia. Uterine hypoplasia is often found in endocrinological imbalances and may be treated with estrogens or human menopausal gonadotropin/human chorionic gonadotropin (MG/CG).
3. *Alterations of the endometrium* caused by the absence of transformation during the menstrual cycle. These alterations may easily be diagnosed by an endometrial biopsy.
4. *Uterine amenorrhea* (Ascherman's syndrome) *with formation of intrauterine synechiae.* Causes: curettages or abortions, status after sectio or endometritis. The evaluation of these alterations is supported by hysterosalpingography and hysteroscopy.
5. *Mechanical disturbances of fertility* such as intrauterine polyps, fibroma, myoma, or endometriosis requiring diagnosis in hospital and, in most cases, invasive therapy.
6. *Uterine malformations,* e.g., uterus double bicornuate, uterus arcuate.
7. *Repeated abortions.*

Cervical Factors in Female Sterility

1. *Tubal occlusion* caused by postoperative or postinflammatory alterations such as salpingitis, endometriosis, formation of hydrosalpinx or pyosalpinx, and even tumors: These tubal occulusions require diagnosis by hysterosalpingography or preferably laparoscopy possibly followed by invasive microsurgical therapy.
2. *Adhesions,* both tubal and ovarian, resulting from inflammatory alterations in the small pelvis (causes: appendicitis, salpingitis, or postabortive or puerperal inflammations): These alterations also require diagnosis by laparoscopy, possibly followed by laparoscopic or surgical therapy.
3. *Disturbed tubal motility* or secretion after salpingitis (endometriosis or formation of tumors) requiring endoscopic diagnosis and therapy.

Ovarian Factors in Female Sterility

1. Anovulation
   a) Hypothalamic-pituitary: hyperprolactinemia (prolactinoma; functional, psychogenic, CNS tumors; Scheehan's syndrome)
   b) Ovarian: polycystic ovaries (Stein-Leventhal syndrome), ovarian tumors, dys- or agenesis of the ovaries, climacteric praecox, resistant ovarian syndrome
   c) Extragonadal: hyper- or hypothyroidism, hyper- or hypocorticosteroids, diabetes mellitus, internal systemic diseases, hyper- or hypoalimentation
   d) Psychogenic: acute or chronic stress, anorexia nervsa, anoretic reaction, hysterical pregnancy

2. Corpus luteum insufficiency
   a) Psychogenic factors
   b) Vaginismus, dyspareunia, frigidity, lack of libido, anorgasm, problems in the partnership

Recommendations to Gynecologists for Outpatient Care of Infertility

Patients diagnosis and therapy of infertility should be carried out by the gynecologist on an outpatient basis, freeing the infertile couple from unnecessary visits and time consuming stressful situations. As a first step, less costly and risk-free examination methods such as recording of basal body temperature (BBT), determination of cervicovaginal secretions, postcoital tests, and seminal fluid analysis should be applied. Only then should invasive methods bearing higher risks be undertaken for the evaluation of the cervical factor (pertubation, hydrotubation, salpingography, laparoscopy, and hysterosalpingography).

The following evaluative steps are recommended:

1. Anamnesis and general diagnosis
2. Gynecologic examination
3. Check of ovarian function
4. Postcoital tests and examination of the cervical factor
5. Seminal fluids analysis
6. Evaluation of the cervical factor proper (if necessary, of the uterine cavity)

A detailed presentation of these parameters is provided next.

Anamnesis

At about the age of 20 a woman reaches the peak of her ability to conceive. The chances of fertilization rapidly decline at the age of 30. A decline of fertility in men older than 40 years has been observed. This decline in relation to the couple's age is of importance whenever infertility treatment requires invasive and costly diagnostic or surgical methods.

The time elapsed during which no pregnancy was achieved is of great importance to the chances of conception. The probability of conception is 15% after 2 years of unprotected intercourse without therapeutic modalities, with the chances sinking to almost zero after 7 years.

Despite the high-tech diagnostic methods now available to infertile couples, some cases remain unexplained. About 10%–15% of all cases of infertility are idiopathic, i.e., a reason cannot be found, not even with modern examination methods including immunology.

General Diagnosis

A detailed initial anamnesis may provide essential facts regarding the diagnosis of infertility and the treatment schemes to be applied. It is important to know the couple's age and how long there has been a desire for a child (intentionally unprotected intercourse). The longer there has been such a wish, and the older the partners are, the more the biologic possibilities of conception decline and the smaller the chances of fertilization. Details on acute and chronic stress or psychogenic diseases should be requested as well. The anamnesis of the menstrual cycle reveals the characteristics of ovarian function. Information on the age of menarche is collected; disturbances in the menstrual cycle may imply a labile reproductive system. Abortions, births, surgery, or inflammatory diseases may indicate a mechanical component due to resulting disturbances in the tubal uterine factor. A high degree of psychological sensitivity on the part of the gynecologist is indispensable to correctly interpret the couple's sexual history (sexual activity during the period of ovulation, frequency of intercourse, orgasm).

General Examination

Information on non gynecologic diseases is recorded along with height, weight, extreme adipositas, indicators of hypo- or hyperthyroidism, adrenopathy, hirsuitism, and diabetes mellitus as well as general psychological disturbances, eating habits, or business situations causing excessive stress. Only recently has the considerable influence of obesity and anorexia nervosa become apparent.

Gynecologic Examination

On examination, hypoplastic secondary sex characteristics may indicate genital hypoplasia, and hypertrophy of clitoris or distinct hirsutism may imply increased production of androgens. (Individual characteristics should, however, be considered, as in dark-skinned Mediterranean populations.)

Examination by speculum allows the identification of vaginal causes for sterility, which are quite rare, with relative ease. Anatomic deficiencies (e.g., vagina duplex or septum vaginale) may be corrected by surgical treatment. Alteratiions of the vaginal wall and portio, mainly due to inflammation, may be evaluated by a native preparation and cytological swab diagnosis and treated accordingly. Patients are often aware of vaginal obstructions to immissio, such as intact rigid hymen, a too small vaginal orifice or aplasia, and they consult the gynecologist. Pain during coitus often indicates psychogenic problems or inflammatory processes. Should the native preparation examined under the phase-contrast microscope (trichomonas, candida, bacteria) be impossible to identify quickly, a culture becomes necessary. Hyperacidity of the vaginal secretions can be eliminated by determination of the pH. The pH should not exceed or be inferior to 4.0 since spermatozoa may otherwise be immobilized or their ascension hindered.

Cervical Score

The parameters of the cervix (width of the uterine orifice, amount of secretion, spinnbarkeit, fern phenomena, number of cells, pH of the mucus) should be determined according to the Insler score (see Table, Insler score). Evaluation of the cervical parameters may be completed by measuring the cervicovaginal secretions, which will be described later.

Gynecological Palpation

Gynecological palpation aims to define the location and length of the uterus and ovaries. Ultrasonographically guided examinations offer additional support. Retroflexio uteri can easily be diagnosed but it is hardly ever corrected surgically. Nodular alterations palpated in the Douglas and uterus should be indicators of endometriosis, myoma, or other mechanical hindrances in the small pelvis.

Consultation

The gynecologic consultation certainly represents a most essential factor in the treatment of the infertile couple. The importance of taking a good history cannot be overemphasized. These couples are already in a stress situation since the unsatisfied wish for a child has usually been present for an extended period before their initial visit to the gynecologist. A careful approach to the couple, with due consideration of psychological aspects, is a precondition to success. Detailed information on intercourse during the period of ovulation, recording to the basal body temperature, and aspiration of the cervicovaginal secretions may even result in pregnancies sooner than expected since rather often there is still a lack of information on sexual functions. Each treatment scheme requires adaptation to the couple's individual situation.

Outpatient Diagnosis of Infertility

A special sterility examination should be performed by the gynecologist in a graded series which may be altered according to existing findings, anamnesis, and individual situations. Graded examination patterns are recommended for obtaining rapid, non invasive, and less costly diagnoses that involve a minimum of strain.

Examination of Ovarian Function

A gynecologist can examine ovarian function without difficulty. Since its disturbance is one of the most prominent reasons for involuntary childlessness, ovarian insufficiency should be determined as the first priority.

Recording of the basal body temperature (BBT) curve is the most common method of gaining information on ovarian function. It allows the prediction of both follicular maturation and the active luteal phase, as the progesterone produced during this stage exerts a thermogenetic effect. Basal body temperature should be measured for 5 min rectally or sublingually and noted on a curve. Time-consuming modern recording methods supported by computer are only applied in special cases since the results do not allow further evaluation. BBT curves bear a 20%–30% margin of error as circumstances such as infections, travel, stress, recording mistakes, the irregular sleeping patterns of shift workers, etc. may falsify the curve and interfere with determination of the ovulation day.

Corpus Luteum Insufficiency

A staircase-shaped increase in temperature or a short phase of hyperthermia of less than 12 days in an indicator of insufficient formation of corpus luteum with lack of progesterone production. Such a conclusion drawn from a BBT curve requires determination of the progesterone status or a biopsy of the endometrium.

Anovulation

If the BBT curve or cervicovaginal secretion records show a monophasic development, the following additional examinations are recommended:

1. *Determination of prolactin in plasma..* From 20% to 30% of all hyperprolactinemic patients (with prolactin levels above 20–30 μ/mg) may exhibit corpus luteum insufficiency, anovulation, and amenorrhea. It must be remembered that serum prolactin levels are subject to a rhythm thus requiring repeated evaluations supported by a prolactin stimulation test if necessary. Sometimes these stimulation tests reveal latent hyperprolactinemia in normal basal serum values, and prolactin-inhibiting treatment achieves normalization of the menstrual cycle with ensuing gravidity.
2. *Radiological examination of the sella.* The simultaneous presence of manifest hyperprolactinemia and secondary amenorrhea usually excludes hypophyseal adenomas, which are often associated with hyperprolactinemia. However, if there is no radiological evidence of a macroadenoma, it may nevertheless be possible to visualize a microadenoma by computed tomography.
3. *Determination of testosterone, 17-ketosteroids, and dehydroepiandrosterone sulfate (DHEAS).* Hyperandrogenemia may be the reason for anovulation or hirsutism, and Stein-Leventhal syndrome, amenoblastoma, or suprarenal cortex tumors may be clinically relevant due to ensuing sterility.
4. *Clomiphene test.* The administration of clomiphene citrate starting on the 3rd to 5th day of the menstrual cycle (50 g b.i.el. for 5 days) is aimed at testing the endocrine regulation centers. Monitoring of BBT and cervicovaginal secretions may pinpoint ovulation and demonstrate the increase in BBT normally expected on the 5th to 7th day after the last dose of clomiphene (14th to 18th day of the cycle).
5. *Gestagen test.* Oral administration of gestagens (10 mg/day for 10 days) may provide information about estrogen production and endometrial proliferation followed by hormonal withdrawal bleeding.
6. *Luteinizing hormone releasing hormone (LH-RH) test.* With the administration of releasing hormones (e.g., 225 mg LH-RH i.v.) in a prior. LH/follicle-stimulating hormone (FSH) test, further findings may be anticipated if there is no response to clomiphene. An LH and FSH increase after injection of LH-RH as compared to the serum baseline value is an indicator of hypophyseal function.
7. *Measurement of cervicovaginal secretions.* Another method of supplementing the BBT curve is the measurement of cervicovaginal secretions. By means of a recently developed aspirator (similar to a suction device for aspirating vaginal secretions) the amount of cervical and vaginal secretions

under the influence of estrogen is determined. Estrogens exercising a direct influence on the production of cervical and vaginal mucus are excellent predictors of the adequacy of estrogen production and hte maturing follicle and thus of imminent ovulation. In combination with the BBT curve, the volume curve of vaginal secretions provides further precise information on ovulation induction which can usually only be determined by measuring the follicle diameter by ultrasound or LH testing in urine or serum. Correlations of LH levels, follicular diameter, and progesterone levels have shown very good conformity with cervical secretion volume measurements.

One of the advantages of this method is its uncomplicated application, requiring no special devices or training. Rather, as with BBT, it allows the patient to proceed with record-keeping herself and discuss the results with her gynecologist. Moreover, unlike BBT, this technique allows ovulation to be planned and the day of induced ovulation to be predicted almost exactly, which is of great importance for planned sexual intercourse, insemination therapies, and other fertility stimulation procedures.

Thus the measurement of secretions offers a new kind of menstrual cycle monitoring which can be carried out in the gynecologist's office. Savings can be achieved by eliminating costly diagnoses of hormone levels and follicle size measurements, making this an economical method of supervision.

When measuring cervicovaginal secretions some particularities should be kept in mind to keep errors to a minimum:

a) Secretions should always be measured at the same time of day, either in the morning or the evening.
b) Secretions should not be measured immediately after sexual intercourse; 6 h need to have elapsed to avoid falsification of the volume curve.

There is no chance of fertilization in the cases mentioned. In normogonadotropic women, ovulation-inducing treatment with clomiphene, epimestrol, or cyclophenil as well as with combined doses suppressing prolactin (pravidel) was successful in most cases. Hypogonadotropic disturbances or failure of ovulation-inducing therapy for several months requires treatment by MG/CG. This form of therapy is costly and necessitates a complete work-up of the cervical factor, cervicovaginal volume, ultrasound examinations, and determination of ovary and follicle size as well as testing of estrogen and LH levels in plasma and urine.

The highest ovulation rate achieved by these methods is 70%–80%; however, the aim should be to keep side effects such as formation of cysts and multiple-gestation pregnancies as low as possible by close monitoring.

In cases of hyperandrogenetic anovulation, as in the Stein-Leventhal syndrome or polycystic ovaries, clomiphene therapy or a wedge-shaped excision from both ovaries might be a promising alternative. Suppression of the elevated androgen level by dexamethasone (0.5–1 mg/day) may also lead to ovulation induction.

Examination of Cervical Parameters

The uterine cervix is highly important as the site of the first intensive interaction between spermatozoa and the femal genital tract. The main functions of the uterine cervix in the conception process are morphological, biophysical, and biochemical. These complicated functions are coordinated by a fine-tuned, cyclically alternating system. During the periovulatory period, in the middle of the proliferation phase, the uterine cervix produces abundant thin mucus allowing high sperm penetrability, which reaches a peak the day before and on the day of ovulation. Sperm penetrability normally ends 1 or 2 days post ovulation; it may, however, last even longer.

References

Brinsden R, Rainsburry P (1991) In-vitro fertilization and assisted reproduction. Parthenon, P. Group UK-USA

Broer KH (1981) Diagnostik und Therapie zervikaler Sterilitätsursachen. In: Kaiser R, Schumacher GFB (eds) Menschliche Fortpflanzung. Thieme, Stuttgart

Broer KH (1991) Gift. In: Turanli I, Broer KH (eds) Sterilite ve IVF. Önel, Cologne, p 57

De Cherney AH et al (1990) Steriles Paar. Diesbach, Berlin

Diedrichs K Neue Wege in Diagnostik and Therapie der Sterilität. Enke, Stuttgart

Grudzinska JG (1993) The fallopian tube. Springer, Berlin Heidelberg New York

Insler V, Bettendorf G (1980) Advances in diagnosis and treatment of infertility. Elsevier, Amsterdam

Kaiser R, Schumacher GFB (1981) Menschliche Fortpflanzung. Thieme, Stuttgart

Lunenfeld B, Insler V, Glezermann M (1993) Diagnosis and treatment of functional infertility. Blackwell, Berlin

Krebs D, Schneider HPG (1994) Endokrinologie und Reproduktionsmedizin. Urban and Schwarzenberg, Munich

Mastroianni L, Contifaris C (1990) FIGO manual of human reproduction. Parthenon P. Group UK-USA

Runnebaum B, Rabe T (1994) Fortpflanzungsmedizin. Springer, Berlin Heidelberg New York

Schirren C, Leidenberger F (1995) Unerfüllter Kinderwunsch. Deutscher Ärzte-Verlag, Cologne

Schneider HPG, Lauritzen C, Nieschlag E (1988) Grundlagen und Klinik der menschlichen Fortpflanzung. de Gruyter, Berlin

Turanli I, Broer KH (1991) Sterilite ve IVF. Önel, Cologne

The History of Infertility Treatment

H. Ludwig

The therapeutic means of effectively treating infertile couples which are available at the end of the twentieth century seem altogether to be the result of a long and laborious scientific development. It is justified to date the beginning of this development back to the conceptual foundation of "steroid chemistry" as formulated by Windaus in 1903. It was not until then that biochemistry became the principle scientific basis for future development, itself leading to the crystallization of ovarian hormones that was finally achieved. Progress was fast, but detailed knowledge increased only step by step until the two last decades, when extracorporal fertilization in humans appeared on the scence and gave rise to further rapid expansion of the reproductive technologies, their refinement and extension going hand in hand. A new field, that of reproductive medicine, was born, and no one would have foreseen the course of scientific events and the relative ease of their applicability to infertile women at the beginning of our century. The literature in reproductive medicine which reflects the technological development has grown tremendously since 1980. Nevertheless, three main streams can still be recognized:

1. Gynecologic endocrinology for conservative treatment and for the medical preparation of superovulation before assisted reproduction (Table 1)
2. Microsurgery of the tubes (Table 2)
3. Medically assisted reproduction in a stricter sense with multifold technical variations already existing (Table 3)

Donation of preimplantation embryos, zygotes, and oocytes even offers medical help in patients whose age lies beyond the natural borders of the ability to conceive. The awareness of gynecologists of the ethical implications of these exuberantly prolifertating new techniques is an important and challenging issue (Wilder 1995).

I was asked to write about the historical development of infertility therapy; this task turned out to be a retrospective view of the past 100 years. It will be a retrospective that illustrates part of the history of gynecology itself, which remains the central discipline in the twentieth century. Despite rapid development in one of its subspecialities, gynecology and obstetrics has survived as a single coherent medical discipline. This fact alone can be regarded as an advantage in comparison to other medical disciplines. This chapter will

Table 1 Scientific development of gynecologic endocrinology with special regard to infertility treatment

Year	Author	Place	Concept
1903	Windaus	Göttingen	Steroideal chemistry
1908	Hitschmann and Adler	Berlin	Relation between endometrium and menstruation investigated
1910	Fraenkel	Berlin	Function of corpus luteum perceived
1913	Schröder	Kiel	Cycle of endometrium described
1917	Stockard and Papnicolaou	New York	Histologic criteria for cyclic changes in the vaginal epithelium described
1921	Haberlandt	Berlin	First concept of hormonal sterilization
1923	Allen and Doisy	New York	Pregnancy test using cytologic criteria
1927	Zondek and Aschheim	Berlin	Pituitary hormones and estrogens in the urine of pregnant women
1928	Schröder	Leipzig	Pharallelism of ovary and endometrium described; *Zykluslehre*
1929	Corner and Allen	Rochester	Progesterone is a product of the corpus luteum; endometrium undergoes secretory changes
1929	Butenandt	Göttingen	Crystallization of estrogen
1930	Allen	Rochester	Extraction of corpus luteum hormone
1930	Zondek	Berlin	FSH activity in urine of postmenopausal women
1932	Kaufmann	Berlin	Menstruation after substitution
1934	Hohlweg	Graz	Positive feedback of high estrogen dosage
1935	Stein and Leventhal	Chicago	Amenorrhea associated with sterility and polycystic ovaries
1938	Inhoffen and Hohlweg	Vienna/Berlin	Synthesis of estrogens (ethinyl-estradiol)
1945	Albright	Boston	Estrogene as a means of fertility control?
1951	Pincus	Shrewsbury	Hormonal contraception
1953	Pincus and Chang	Shrewsbury	Progesterone inhibits ovulation, seen in animal experiments
1954	Djerassi	[Syntex]	Synthesis of progestins
1954	Zander	Marburg, Cologne	Progesterone metabolism in ovarian tissues clarified
1955	Saffran and Schally	New Orleans	First releasing hormone detected: "corticotropin"
1958	Gemzell and Diczfalusy	Copenhagen	Clinical effects of FHS and indications for treatment of infertility
1960	Lunenfeld	Geneva	Clinical series with MG in infertility
1964	Bettendorf and Breckwoldt	Hamburg	First series of FSH treatment in Germany and side effects of ovarian stimulation
1971	Schally	New Orleans	LH/FSH-releasing hormone: peptides
1978	Steptoe and Edwards	Cambridge	First successful in vitro fertilization and embryo transfer with living child
1980	Knobil	Pittsburgh	Neuroendocrine control of cycle
1984	Fleming and Kenigsberg		"Medical hypophysectomy" with GnRH agonists

FSH, follicle-stimulating hormone; hMG, human menopausal gonadotropin; LH, luteinizing horme; GnRH, gonadotropin-releasing hormone.

Table 2 A hundred years of fallopian tube surgery

Year	Author	Place	Method
1895	Martin	Berlin	First surgical aperture of obstructed tube (successful in two out of 65 cases)
1950	Palmer	Paris	Laparoscopic procedures in infertility
1959	Frangenheim	Constance	Operative laparoscopy and culdoscopy
1965	Swolin	Göteborg	Electromicrosurgery of the tubes
1967	Steptoe	Cambridge	Gynecological laparoscopy
1975	Semm	Kiel	Minimally invasive surgery by pelviscopy
1977	Winston	London	Microscopic surgery of the tubes
1980	Bruhat	Clermont-Frd	Laparoscopic reconstruction of tubes
1986	Nezhat	Atlanta	Laser laparoscopy in endometriosis
1993	Jansen	Sydney	Transcervical tuboplasty

Table 3 Development of extracorporal fertilization and assisted reproduction

Year	Author	Place	Method
In vitro fertilization (IVF) and related developments			
1973	De Kretzer and Lopata	Melbourne	First embryo transfer in human: abortion
1978	Steptoe and Edwards	Cambridge	First embryo transfer after IVF; birth of a living child
1981	Trotnow	Erlangen	IVF begun in Germany
1982	Craft	London	Oocytes and sperm intrauterine
1983	Trounson	Melbourne	Cryopreservation of embryos
1985	Asch	Irvine	Intratubal gamete transfer (GIFT)
1986	Cruz	N. Brunswick	Intrauterine insemination (IUI)
1986	Forrler	Schiltigheim	Direct intraperitoneal insemination (DIPI)
1987	Sharma	London	Peritoneal oocyte and sperm transfer (POST)/ultrasound
1988	Jansen and Sutherland	Sydney	Nonsurgical intratubal zygote transfer (ZIFT)
Oocyte and embryo donation			
1988	Sauer	Los Angeles	Zygotes by uterine lavage
1988	Borrero	Irvine	GIFT after gamete donation
1989	Abdalla and Studd	London	ZIFT after cryopreservation of zygotes
1990	Rotsztejn	Irvine	Intratubal embryo transfer (TET)
1993	Sauer and Paulson	Los Angeles	IVF: oocyte donation to postmenopausal women
Micromanipulation for male infertility			
1986	Cohen	Atlanta	Embryos after intrazonal injection
1988	Ng and Ratnam	Singapore	Subzonal insemination (SUZI)
1992	Palermo and van Steirteghem	Brussels	Intracytoplasmatic insemination (ICSI)

therefore repeatedly refer to the history of gynecology. As we can see, the subspeciality itself, reproductive medicine, contains parts where either conservative surgical, or technological orientation prevail. This has consequences for postgraduate training skills in the subspeciality: after being trained in general gynecology and obstetrics, a physician studied becomes a reproductive medicine subspecialist onyl if he or she has endocrinology, microsurgery, and/or endoscopic technology, not to forget (transvaginal) ultrasound imaging and psychological counseling of infertile patients.

Surgery of Fallopian Tube

Ludwig Nürnberger, when writing his comprehensive chapter about sterility in 1924, described the beginnings of tubal reconstructive surgery as follows: the occluded tube was punctured and, if clear contents spilled out, an area of approximately 1 cm was excised; the bulging mucosa was then sutured circularly to the tubal serosa for eversion of the mucosal flaps. Following the proposal of Skutsch, this operation was called "salpingostomy." Until 1895, A. Martin carried out this operation 65 times, but he was only successful in two cases with resulting pregnancies. Term pregnancies after this type of salpingostomy were even rarer events in the hands of other surgeons. Modern development in tubal surgery only started when the laparoscopic view enabled gynecologists to survey the internal female genital tract (Palmer, Frangenheim, Semm, Gomel). Swolin (1975) from Sweden was one of the most experienced pioneers in tubal surgery before the age of microscopic surgery.

Among the manipulative procedures presently available, competition arose between open microsurgery using the microscope, minimaly invasive laparoscopic surgery (Semm), and nonsurgical transcervical tubal cannulation (Risquez and Confino 1993). All of these procedures need to be measured against the results of assisted reproduction in bilaterally damaged tubes (Hull and Fleming 1995). Regarding the prognosis for natural conception following surgery, we have learned to differentiate between minor, intermediate, and severe cases, the latter being cases with bilateral severe tubal damage, extensive tubal fibrosis, tubal distension of more than 1.5 cm, abnormal mucosal appearance, and extensively dense adhesions. In patients older than 35 years and those with unfavorable surgical prognosis, primary assisted reproduction is recommended. Reconstruction after tubal sterilization has a slightly better prognosis. Even the results of laparoscopic reconstructive surgery in cases of doubtful prognosis (distal salpingostomy, adhesiolysis) are comparably good if the surgeon is qualified (Canis and Bruhat 1991; Dlugi and Jacobsen 1994; Dubuisson et al. 1994). In cases of infertility due to endometriosis, the use of laser appears to be and advancement (Nezhat et al. 1986).

Traditionally, tubal surgery belonged to the broad spectrum of gynecologic pelvic surgery, and every gynecologist was trained in that field as well as in oncologic surgery during his or her residency. With the advent of the surgical microscope, the situation changed: from then on microsurgery had to be taught in special courses with foregoing and sometimes parallel animal experimentation in order to keep in practice. Conventional pelvic surgery lost its importance for tubal reconstruction. Recently, there has been growing competition from transcervical cannulation (Jansen 1993; Gleicher et al. 1993) and from assisted reproduction, even in cases where the surgical prognosis is quite favorable. It appears as if the area of open microsurgery of the fallopian tubes will prove to have been an episode within the modalities of infertility treatment. However, the learning of manual skills – a strong requirement for microsurgery – is an advantage even for those wo decide to leave surgery to devote their time to a wider variety of reproductive technologies. The classical gynecological endocrinologist will now even be challenged by more surgical and manipulative duties to perform, and he or she must meet this challenge, coher ever possible, in order to serve the patients in the best way, which might be conservative, surgical, or technical-manipulatory. It might be the same in the future as it was in the past: treatment of infertility always involves both sides, conservative medical brain work and manual dexterity.

Development of Basics and Conservative Approach to Infertilitiy: Gynecologic Endocrinology

Between the formulation of the existence of steroid chemistry (Windaus 1903) and the perception that the female cycle is controlled by neuroendocrine impulses (Knobil 1980), only 80 years passed, but what a tremendous scientific development has taken place in those 80 years! Our present insight into the cycle and the role of the pituitary gland and hypothalamus was elaborated during that time, some of us nearly being contemporaries and a few contributing toward laying the foundations for our present knowledge.

Ovary and Endometrium Are Functionally Linked

The first important contribution came from Hitschmann and Adler (1908), who were able to convincingly demonstrate the existing connection between menstruation and endometrium, which before that were not seen as being interdependent. The details of endometrial glandular maturation from early proliferation to secretory ripeness during the cycle were described by Robert Schröder, then in Kiel, according to microscopical criteria (1913). His *Zykluslehre* (1928), a well-formulated theory about the change from proliferation to the secretory state and finally shedding, has retained its validity up to the present. Evaluation of the cycle morphologically using day to day biopsies ("dating" the endometrium) would not have been possible without Schröder's previous descriptions (Noyes, Hertig, Rock 1950).

At the same time as Schröder published his first morphological observations on the endometrium, the first indications that the corpus luteum is a source of endocrine function appeared (Fraenkel 1910). Shortly after that, Stockard and Papanicolaou (1917) designed an experimental test depending on changes in histologic criteria of the vaginal epithelium in the female guinea pig to validate the presence of estrus. Edgar Allan and Edward Doisy (1923) proposed a further cytologic test using the keratinization of vaginal epithelial cells in infantile or castrated mice after exposure to estrogens. For a long time, their test was the classical one worldwide for proving estrogenic activity (Allen-Doisy test). It seems as if the advent of the contraceptive pill was already anticipated by Ludwig Haberlandt (1921), who was able to produce temporary infertility in experimental animals after feeding them extracts from ovaries.

Pituitary Hormones Are Superior to the Gonads

The two, brilliant investigators Bernhard Zondek and Selmar Aschheim (1927), working in the maternity laboratory at the Charité Hospital in Berlin, found that tissue extracted from the pituitary glands of cattle as well as from women and dissolved is able to stimulate the ripening of follicles in the human ovary, giving rise to a corpus luteum. With this observation, the anterior pituitary could be defined as the steering organ for the rhythmic functioning of the ovaries. The investigators named the pituitary hormone prolan. They also found that the urine of pregnant women had follicle-stimulating properties. Erroneously they thought both hormones (from the glands and the urine of pregnant women) were one and the same, but the two hormones were later identified as follicle-stimulating hormone (FSH) or "exogenous" human chorionic gonadotropin (hCG). Nevertheless, an objective test proving the existence of a pregnancy thus became available. Many years later, Wide and Gemzell (1973) described an immunological approach for testing hCG, which became the basis of modern hormonal diagnostics for early pregnancy. Zondek (1930) discovered FSH (later human menopausal gonadotropin, hMG) in the urine of postmenopausal women as well, naming it prolan as before. It was Lunenfeld in Geneva (1960) who made use of the same hormone purified out of the urine of postmenopausal women and commercially manufactured. His attempt to produce superovulation in women suffering infertility due to insufficient ovaries turned out to be successful.

Therapeutic Usefulness of Gonadal Steroids

Estrogens. While the production of gonadotropins still depends on biologic sources, Butenandt's crystallization of an estrogen was a breakthrough (Butenandt 1929). With this biochemical milestone the substitution of gonadal steroids in women appeared to be a nearer possibility. The first clinical scheme with the use of estrogens was published by Kaufmann in 1933; although he did not have either estrogens nor the corpus luteum hormone at that time in an orally administrable form, Kaufmann's scheme of substituting the female cycle by exogenous hormones is still known under his name today. To mimic the full cycle he had to use extracts from luteinized follicles obtained from animals in order to hormonally substitute the second half of the female cycle in amenorrheal women. It was Inhoffen and Hohlweg (1938) who succeeded in the production of an orally effective estrogen.

Progesterone and Progestins. Josef Zander (1954, 1962), pupil and later collaborator of Carl Kaufmann in Marburg and in Cologne, clarified the conditions of the natural source of progesterone production in the ovaries of animals and women. To produce 1 mg progesterone at that time, the ovaries of approximately 2500 pregnant pigs had to be collected. Accordingly, the price was high. Clinical availability also remained low. Like the original crystallized estrogen, progesterone could not be used by the oral route. However, unlike estrogens, where the introduction of an ethinyl group in position 17 transformed the molecule to an enterally absorbable steroid, it took 10 more years to do the same for progestins. In 1939, Russell Marker (Syntex) became convinced that the solution to the problem of obtaining large quantities of steroid hormones was to find plants which contained sufficient amounts of sapogenin, a plant steroid which could be used as a starting point for steroid hormone synthesis. This conviction was strengthened by the discovery that a species of trillium, known locally as Beth's root, was collected in North Carolina and used in the preparation of Lydia Pinkham's Compound, popular at that time to relieve menstrual problems. The active compound in Beth's root was diosgenin, a botanical steroid (Speroff et al. 1978). The synthesis of progesterone was eventually successful in 1942, and some years later cortisone was also extracted and crystallized from the dame phytogenetic origin (Djerassi 1951). The first synthetic progestins were norethindrone, followed by norethinodrel (1951–1954). With 17-hydroxy-progesteron acetate, a second type of orally effective progestin was detected and soon manufactured.

At the beginning of the 1950s, steroid hormones were in principle available for oral administration for the first time. It was only one more step to the pill, a steroid hormonal contraception (Pincus and Chang 1953; Pincus et al. 1956).

Ovarian Stimulation by Gonadotropins

The scientific and clinical investigations to devise a temporary, reversible sterilization by hormones were carried out parallel to the experiments on the conditions for stimulating a defective ovary for ovulation. On the basis of the previous discovery that the urine of postmenopausal women contains large amounts of a stimulating hormone deriving from the anterior lobe of the pituitary gland (Zondek), it was Gemzell's group in Scandinavia (1958) that reported about the potency of FSH. Women with secondary amenorrhea started to menstruate under the influence of FSH, and the small follicles in their ovaries grew. The principle of the dominant follicle was yet to be investigated. As already mentioned, Lunenfeld treated infertile women for the first time with the purified extract from the urine of postmenopausal women and achieved ovulations (1960). It remains his merit to have established this type of stimulation therapy.

In Germany, he was followed by Bettendorf and Breckwoldt (1961–1964), who published the first series of successful treatments with pituitary human gonadotropin. The WHO classification of all known forms of amenorrhea and ovarian insufficiency (classes I–VII) facilitated a stepwise clinical diagnostic procedure, starting with prolactin and the effect of exogenic steroids on menstrual bleeding.

At that time the variety of forms of primary and secondary sterility could be better classified and henceforth the therapeutic approach became more rational than ever before.

Clomiphen, A Useful Derivative for to Ovarian Stimulation. The similarity of the clomiphen structure to stilbenes, themselves phytogenetic substances of estrogenic activity, encouraged experiments with the substance as a fertility pill (Johnson et al. 1966). Clomiphen was shown to be able to interrupt the negative feedback between estradiol and FSH; the estrogen receptors in the hypothalamic center are competitively blocked by clomiphen and send out a kind of signal as if the peripheral estrogens were decreasing, their level being persistently low. Luteinizing hormone (LH) releasing hormones (see below) are then secreted into the portal circulation of the pituitary gland and, as a consequence, FSH and LH are released. Thus, the effectiveness of clomiphen depends on the amount of liberated (and available) FSH. It was soon demonstrated that, in cases of failing ovulation but with the pituitary-ovarian axis remaining intact, clomiphen could be introduced as an effective drug for enhancing gonadotropin secretion.

Without Previous Ovarian Stimulation no Extracorporal Fertilization with Gonadotropins

Treatment with gonadotropins was at the center of all treatment regimens – apart from cases with obvious tubal obstruction – until the first successful extracorporal fertilization was reported (Lopata et al. 1978; Steptoe and Edwards 1978). The rapid development of extracorporal fertilization would not have been possible without the previous investigations on ovarian regulation by the pituitary gland and above all by the hypothalamus.

The criteria for the effective production of more than one ovum (as in the natural cycle) were established long before the in vitro fertilization/embryo transfer (IVF/ET) schemes known today could start. Newer modifications appeared and replaced the classical stimulation concept as soon as the GnRH were found to be peptides (Schally et al. 1971), for which it was easy to construct analogues. Soon, the most effective alteration to the classical scheme proved to be receptor down-regulation with gonadotropin-releasing analogues (see Table 1).

The functional state of the ovaries could soon be assessed by transvaginal ultrasound with clear-cut images, much better than by the abdominal approach. The instant diagnostics of the LH surge by methods using monoclonal antibodies made the surveying of treatment cycles much easier as well. Observation by ultrasound and hormonal assays were as important as the puncture of follicles, in vitro cultivation or embryo transfer. The aim was no longer to surmount one individual couple's infertility and to reestablish the changes of conception to equal those of a natural cycle, but to even overcome the natural age limit for becoming a mother.

Bypassing Nature: The Development of Extracorporal Fertilization

Stimulation of Ovarian Function in Order to Attain Polyovulation

What has been achieved during the past 80 years in understanding the female genital cycle is the gradual unmasking of functional connections between ovary and endometrium, the genital and extragenital functions of ovarian hormones, their ability to being stimulated by pituitary hormones, and the superior steering by neuroendocrine influences originating from the hypothalamus. The invention of extracorporal fertilization was aimed at first at overcoming obstructed the problem of obstructed fallopian tubes only, and solely in cases where microsurgery could not help. The initial positive results were obtained by in vitro fertilization under the condition of a natural cycle (Lenton et al. 1992). Stimulation of ovaries in order to produce superovulation soon afterwards became the rule in preparing extracorporal fertilization. Stimulting regimens with gonadotropins were soon more effective than previous attempts with clomiphen.

Gonadotropin-Releasing Hormone Analogues

From the mid-1980s on, even better results could be expected if the LH surge induced by rising estrogen levels due to stimulation could be minimized or completely avoided. Based on the concept of gonadotropin release by GnRH, a new combined regimen of pretreatment with GnRH analogues (agonists and antagonists) was suggested and became accepted. It functioned in a similar way to medical hypophysectomy, rendering patients temporarily hypogonadotropic (Fleming et al. 1982; Kenigsberg et al. 1984). It was possible to produce polyovulation with FSH and hMG preparations without the endogenous LH level increasing, which had been observed as being disadvantageous to the impregnability of mature oocytes. Today, GnRH analogues are constituents of the most effectively used medication for ovarian stimulation prior to IVF and its modifications (Gordon and Hodgen 1991).

Further Developments Beyond Classical In Vitro Fertilization/Embryo Transfer

The original scheme of in vitro fertilization/embryo transfer (Steptoe and Edwards 1978; Lopata et al. 1978; Trotnow et al. 1981) has undergone considerable extensions by four main scientific developments. The luminal fallopian tube was reinvented as the natural habitat of the early preimplantation embryo; zygotes were transferred instead of multicellular, but mobile embryos; and micromanipulation of oocytes in the presence of spermatozoa marked a reform in the treatment of male infertility. Instead of fresh gametes, cryopreserved oocytes and embryos have been successfully used for fertilization, as have cryopreserved spermatozoa. More than in former times, these developments are accompanied by public sociological, ethical, and even political discussions. Infertility treatment has become an issue of public interest, despite the fact that infertile couples still represent a minority and have a right to privacy.

The important scientific developments were the following:

1. Oocytes are injected in combination with prepared sperm solutions into the uterus in midcycle (Craft 1982); attempts have been made to cryopreserve spare embryos from polyovulations and impregnation of more than only a few fertile eggs in order to avoid serial follicle puncture and reperated stimulative treatment (Trounson 1983).
2. The transferal of gametes to the oviduct tried to keep the natural surrounding for the creation of an embryo, the fallopian tube (GIFT; Asch 1985). The next step was the transfer of already cultivated preimplantation

embryos or zygotes into the fallopian tube (ZIFT; Jansen and Sutherland 1988).

3. Progress in cryopreservation not only of human preimplantation embryos, but also of oocytes (which is the more difficult procedure) made the donation of embryos or oocytes possible to women whose ovarian functions were irreversibly defunct. Extracorporal fertilization with donated embryos or oocytes in postmenopausal women on a large scale in commercial settings rather than in scientifically critical environments (Antinori et al. 1993) has provoked public and professional criticism. This path seems to be leading to prohibition on account of ethical considerations.
4. The longstanding heterologue insemination (with donor semen) in order to help couples with subfertile male partners will be increasingly replaced by micromanipulation, whether by intrazonal injection of homologue spermatozoa via puncturing of the zona pellucida (Cohen 1988), by direct subzonal injection (Ng and Ratnam 1988), or by direct intracytoplasmatic insemination (ICSI; van Steirteghem 1992).

Conclusion

Within less than 20 years, this branch of infertility treatment using new reproductive medical technologies has left behind the original concept of bypassing blocked tubes; it has started to bypass nature. As the extracorporal method, although of very short duration in human prenatal development, exposes the human being to external influences, discussion about the pros and cons of the new technologies is already widespread. The field of infertility treatment was once the center of gynecology. It gave rise to the most intellectual branch of gynecology, gynecologic endocrinology. There are undoubtedly tendencies at present to make reproductive medicine an independent discipline, splitting off from gynecology and obstetrics, with only the core remaining within the field of gynecology, but with the addition of essential constituents from genetics, human biology, andrology, medical ethics, and even sociology and law. Gynecology would tremendously suffer from this loss. The field of reproductive medicine has attracted great interest, far beyond the scope of our gynecologic profession. It should be allowed to develop further in the same way as other fields of medicine flourish, guided by science, conscience, and compassion. The juxtamedical expansion of the field is something that could not have been foreseen 100 years ago.

References

Abdalla HI, Baber RJ, Kirkland A et al (1989) Pregnancy in women with premature ovarian failure using tubal and intrauterine transfer of cryopreserved zygotes. Br J Obstet Gynaecol 96:1076

Alikani M, Cohen J, Palermo GD (1995) Enhancement of fertilization by micromanipulation. Curr Opin Obstet Gynecol 7:182

Allen E, Doisy EA (1923) An ovarian hormone: Preliminary report on its localization, extraction and partial purification, and action in test animals. JAMA 81:819
Allen WM (1930) Physiology of the corpus luteum. VI. The production of progestational proliferation of the endometrium of the immature rabbit by progestin (an extract of the corpus luteum) after preliminary treatment with oestrin. Am J Physiol 92:612
Antinori S, Versaci C, Gholami GH et al (1993) Oocyte donation in menopausal women. Hum Reprod 8:1487
Asch RH, Balmaceda JP, Ellsworth LR, Wong PC (1985) Gamete intrafallopian transfer: a new treatment for infertility. Int J Fertil 30:41
Bettendorf G, Breckwoldt M (1964) Klinisch-experimentelle Untersuchungen mit hypophysärem Human-Gonadotropin. Arch Gynakol 199:423
Borrero C, Remohi J, Ord T et al (1989) A program of oocyte donation and gamete intrafallopian transfer. Hum Reprod 4:275
Bruhat MA, Manhes H, Mage G, Pouly JL (1990) Treatment of ectopic pregnancy by means of laparoscopy. Fertil Steril 33:411
Butenandt A (1929) Über Progynon, ein krystallisiertes weibliches Hormon. Naturwissenschaften 17:879
Canis M, Mage G, Pouly JL et al (1991) Laparoscopic distal tuboplasty: report of 87 cases and a 4-year experience. Fertil Steril 56:616
Cohen J, Nalter H, Wright G et al (1988) Implantation of embryo after partial opening of oocyte zona pellucida to facilitate sperm penetration. [Letter] Lancet 2:162
Corner GW, Allen WM (1929) Physiology of the corpus luteum. II. Production of a special uterine reaction (progestational proliferation) by extracts of the corpus lutuem. Am J Physiol 88:326
Craft I, McLeod F, Green S et al (1982) Human pregnancy following ooctye and sperm transfer to the uterus. Lancet 1:1031
Cruz RI, Kemmann E, Brandeis VT et al (1986) A prospective study of intrauterine insemination of processed sperm from men within oligoasthenospermia in superovulated women. Fertil Steril 46:673
De Kretzer D, Dennis P, Hudson B et al (1973) Transfer of a human zygote. Lancet 2:728
Diepgen P (1937) Geschichte der Frauenheilkunde. I. Die Frauenheilkunde der Alten Welt. In: Stoeckel W (ed) Handbuch der Gynäkologie. Bergmann, Munich, Bd. XII/1
Diepgen P (1942) Die Kulturgeschichte der Frau und die Frauenheilkunde. Arch Gynakol 173:12
Djerassi C, Miracontes G, Rosencrancz G, Sontheimer F (1954) Synthesis of 19-nor-17-ethinyl-testosteron and 19-nor-17-methyl-testosteron. J Am Chem Soc 76:4092
Dlugi AM, Reddy S, Saleh WA et al (1994) Pregnancy rates after operative endoscopic treatment of total (neosalpingostomy) or near total salpingostomy) distal tubal occlusion. Fertil Steril 62:616
Dorini P, Puzzoli D, Montezemolo R (1964) Purification of human gonadotrophin from human menopause urine. Acta Endocrinol 45:321
Dubuisson JP, Chapron C, Morice P et al (1994) Laparoscopic salpingostomy: fertility results according to the tubal mucosa appearance. Hum Reprod 9:334
Engle ET (1938) Gonadotrope Stoffe im Blut, Harn und in anderen Körperflüssigkeiten. Arch Gynakol 166:131
Eskes TKAB, Longo LD (eds) (1994) Classics of obstetrics and gynecology. Parthenon, Carnforth
Fischer I (1924) Geschichte der Gynäkologie. In: Halban J, Seitz L (eds) Biologie und Pathologie des Weibes. Urban and Schwarzenberg, Berlin Bd. I
Fleming R, Adam AH, Barlow DH et al (1982) A new systematic treatment for infertile women with abnormal hormone profiles. Br J Obstet Gynaecol 89:80
Fleming R, Haxon MJ, Hamilton MPR et al (1985) Successful treatment of infertile women with oligomenorrhoea using a combination of an LHRH agonist and exogenous gonadotropins. Br J Obstet Gynaecol 92:369
Forrier A, Dellenbach P, Nisand I et al (1986) Direct intraperitoneal insemination in unexplained and cervical infertility. Lancet 1:916
Fraenkel L (1903) Die Funktion des Corpus luteum. Arch Gynakol 68:438
Fraenkel L (1910) Neue Experimente zur Funktion des Corpus luteum. Arch Gynakol 91:705
Frangenheim H (1959) Die Laparoskopie und die Kuldoskopie in der Gynäkologie. Thieme, Stuttgart

Gemzell CA, Diczfalusy F, Tillinger G (1958) Clinical effect of the human pituitary follicle stimulating hormones (FSH). Clin Endocrinol (Oxf) 18:1333
Gleicher N, Confino E, Corfman R et al (1993) The multicenter transcervical balloon tuboplasty study: conclusions and comparison to alternative technologies. Hum Reprod 8:1264
Gomel V (1977) Reconstructive surgery of the oviduct. J Reprod Med 18:181
Gordon K, Hodgen GD (1992) GnRH agonists and antagonists in assisted reproduction. Baillières Clin Obstet Gynaecol 6:247
Hafez ESE (1980) Human reproduction, 2nd edn, Harper and Row, Hagerstown pp 1–31
Hitschmann F, Adler L (1908) Der Bau der Uterusschleimhaut des geschlechtsreifen Weibes unter besonderer Berücksichtigung der Menstruation. Mschr Geburtsh Gynakol 27:1
Hohlweg W (1934) Veränderungen des Hypophysenvorderlappens und des Ovariums nach Behandlung mit grossen Dosen von Follikelhormon. Klin Wschr 13:92
Hull MGR, Fleming CF (1995) Tubal surgery versus assisted reproduction: assessing their role in infertility therapy. Curr Opin Obstet Gynecol 7:160
Inhoffen HH, Hohlweg W (1938) New female glandular derivatives active per os: 17-ethinyl-estradiol and pregnenein-3-one-17-06. Naturwissenschaften 26:96
Jansen RPS, Anderson JC, Sutherland PD (1988) Nonoperative embryo transfer to the fallopian tube. N Engl J Med 319:288
Janssen RPS (1993) Medicine and surgery inside the Fallopian tube. Med J Aust 158:799
Kaufmann C (1933) Echte Menstruation bei einer kastrierten Frau durch Zufuhr von Ovarialhormone. Zentralbl Gynakol 57:42
Kaufmann C (1938) Die Behandlung der Eierstockinsuffizienz durch Keimdrüsenhormone. Arch Gynakol 166:113
Kenigsberg D, Littman BA, Hodgen GD (1984a) Medical hypophysectomy. I. Dose response using a gonadotropin-releasing hormone antagonist. Fertil Steril 42:112
Kenigsberg D, Littman BA, Williams RF, Hodgen GD (1984b) Medical hypophysectomy: II. Variability of ovarian response to gonadotropin therapy. Fertil Steril 42:116
Kanus H (1929) Ueber den Zeitpunkt der Konzeptionsfähigkeit des Weibes im Intermenstruum. Münchn Med Wschr 76:1157
Knobil E (1980) The neuroendocrine control of the menstrual cycle. Recent Prog Horm Res 36:53
Lenton E, Cooke ID, Hooper M et al (1992) In vitro fertilization in the natural cycle. Baillières Clin Obstet Gynecol 6:229
Lopata A, Brown JB, Leeton JF, Talbot JM, Wood EC (1978) In vitro fertilization of preovulatory oocytes and embryo transfer in infertile patients treatet with clomiphen and human chorionic gonadotrophin. Fertil Steril 30:27
Lunenfeld B, Menzi A, Volet B (1960) Clinical effects of human postmenopausal gonadotropin. 1st Int Cong Endocrinol (Copenh) 587
Mandelstamm A, Tschaikowsky WK (1932) Zur hormonalen Sterilisierung des Weibes. Untersuchungen über die Wirkungen des Prolans auf die Eierstöcke. Arch Gynakol 151:686
Martin A (1895) Die Krankheiten der Eileiter. Leipzig
Nezhat C, Crowgey SR, Garrison CP (1986) Surgical treatment of endometriosis via laser laparoscopy. Fertil Steril 45:778
Ng S, Bongso A, Ratnam SS et al (1988) Pregnancy after transfer of sperm under zona [Letter]. Lancet 2:790
Noyes RW, Hertig AT, Rock J (1950) Dating the endometrial biopsy. Fertil Steril 1:3
Nürnberger L (1924) Sterilität. In: Halban J, Seitz L (eds) Biologie und Pathologie des Weibes. Bd. III, Urban and Schwarzenberg, Berlin, 689
Palermo G, Joris H, Devroey P, van Steirteghem AC (1992) Pregnancies after intracytoplasmatic injection of single spermatozoa into an oocyte. Lancet 340:17
Palmer R (1950) La stérilité involuntaire. Masson, Paris
Pincus G, Chang MC (1953) The effects of progesterone and related compounds on ovulation and early development in the rabbit. Acta Physiol Latinoam 3:177
Pincus G, Chang MC, Hafez ESE et al (1956) Effects of certain 19-nor-steroids on reproductive process in animals. Science 124:890
Risques F, Confino E (1993) Transcervical tubal cannulation: past, present, and future. Fertil Steril 60:211

Rotsztejn DA, Remohi J, Weckstein LN et al (1990) Results of tubal embryo transfer in premature ovarian failure. Fertil Steril 54:348
Saffran M, Schally AV, Benfey BG (1955) Stimulation of the release of corticotropin from the adenohypophysis by a neurohypophyseal factor. Endocrinology 57:439
Sauer MV, Bustillo M, Gorrill MJ et al (1988) An instrument for the recovery of preimplantation uterine ova. Obstet Gynecol 71:804
Sauer MV, Paulson RJ, Lobo RA (1990) A preliminary report on oocyte donation extending reproductive potential to women over 40. N Engl J Med 323:1157
Schally AV, Baba Y, Arimura A, Redding TW, White WF (1971) Evidence of peptide nature of LH- and FSH-releasing hormones. Biochem Biophys Res Commun 42:50
Schröder R (1913) Der normale mensuelle Zyklus der Uterusschleimhaut. Hirschwald, Berlin
Schröder R (1928) Der mensuelle Genitalzyklus des Weibes und seine Störungen. In: Stoeckel W (ed) Handbuch der Gynäkologie, Bd. I/2 Bergmann, München
Semm K (1987) Operative manual for endoscopic abdominal surgery. Year Book, Chicago
Sharma V, Mason B, Pinker G et al (1987) Ultrasound guided peritoneal oocyte and sperm transfer. J in Vitro Fertil Embryo Transfer 4:89
Simmer HH (1987) Zur Geschichte der Endokrinologie der Fortpflanzung. In: Käser O et al (eds) Gynäkologie und Geburtshilfe, 2nd edn, Bd. I/1, p 4
Speroff L, Glass RH, Kase NG (1983) Clinical gynecologic endocrinology and infertility. Williams and Wilkins, Baltimore, 3rd edn, pp 414–415
Steptoe PC (1967) Laparoscopy and Gynaecology. Livingstone, London
Steptoe PC, Edwards RG (1978) Birth after the reimplantation of a human embryo. Lancet 2:366
Stockard CR, Papanicolaou GN (1917) A rhythmical "heat period" in the guinea pig. Science 46:42
Swolin K (1975) Electromicrosurgery and salpingostomy: long term results. Am J Obstet Gynecol 121:418
Stein IF, Leventhal ML (1935) Amenorrhea associated with bilateral polycystic ovaries. Am J Obstet Gynecol 29:181–191
Trounson A, Mohr L (1983) Human pregnancy following cryopreservation, thawing and transfer of an eight-cell embryo. Nature 305:707
Trotnow S (1987) In-vitro-Fertilisierung und Embryotransfer. In: Runnebaum B, Rabe T (eds) Gynäkologische Endokrinologie. Springer, Berlin Heidelberg New York, p 397
Trotnow S, Kniewald T, Al-Hasani S, Becker H (1981) Follikelpunktion. In-vitro-Fertilisierung, Embryotransfer und eingetretene Schwangerschaften in Dyneric/HCG-stimulierten Zyklen. Geburtsh Frauenheilk 41:835
Tucker MJ, Morton PC, Sweitzer CL, Wrigth G (1995) Cryopreservation of human embryos and oocytes. Curr Op in Obstet Gynecol 7:188
WHO Scientific Group Report (1976) Agents stimulating gonadotropin function in the human. World Health Organization, Technical Reports, Series N 514:WHO consultation on the diagnosis and treatment of endocrine forms of female infertility
Wilder BL (1995) Ethical issues related to the new reproductive technologies. Curr Opin Obstet Gynecol 7:199
Wide L, Nillius SJ, Gemzell C, Roos P (1973) Radioimmunosorbent assay of fillicle-stimulating hormone and luteinizing hormone in serum and urine from men and women. Acta Endocrinol [Suppl] 174
Winston RML (1980) Microsurgery of the Fallopian tube: from fantasy to reality. Fertil Steril 34:521
Zander J (1954) Progesterone in human blood and tissues. Nature 174:406
Zander J, Wiest WG, Ober KG (1962) Klinische, histologische und biochemische Beobachtungen bei polycystischen Ovarien mit gleichzeitiger adenomatöser, atypischer Hyperplasie des Endometriums. Umwandlung von Progesteron-4-C14 im Ovarial-Gewebe. Arch Gynakol 196:481
Zondek B (1930) Hypophysenvorderlappen. Arch Gynakol 144:133
Zondek B, Aschheim S (1927) Das Hormon des Hypophysenvorderlappens. Klin Wschr 6:248

Anatomy, Histology and Cytology

Endometrial Receptivity

A. Arici and E. Attar

Introduction

In recent years, due to the development of in vitro fertilization-embryo transfer (IVF-ET), significant basic and clinical research has been focused on human reproductive processes occurring from the latter stages of gametogenesis through fertilization and implantation. Particular attention is now being paid to the role of endometrial receptivity because it is apparent that successful implantation is one of the remaining blocks to higher pregnancy rates. The true incidence of failed implantation as a cause of infertility is unknown but most clinics report 30% of couples with "unexplained" infertility, of whom a significant number are likely to have this problem. It seems that early pregnancy losses may also arise from disorders of implantation.

Strictly speaking, the term "implantation" should only be applied to cases in which an embryo is actually embedded inside the wall of the uterus. However, the term is now broadly applied to any attachment of the embryonic membranes to the wall of uterus. The less widely used term "nidation" is reserved for blastocysts embedded into the wall of the uterus. The implantation process can be divided into three stages: adhesion of the blastocyst to the surface epithelium, then penetration of the trophectoderm cells between epithelial cells, and lastly intrusion of the trophoblasts in the subepithelial zone.

Embryos enter the uterine cavity at the morula stage, approximately 2–3 days following fertilization. Attachment of the trophoblast begins several days later, on about the 6th–7th day after fertilization, with the embryonic pole of the blastocyst aligned with the endometrium (Fig. 1). Although we have some knowledge about the adhesion of blastocyst to the uterine epithelium, the real mechanisms of this process are still a dilemma. The adhesion phenomenon is probably dependent on an enzymatic molecular rearrangement at the surface of both cell types. There is a reduction in the electronegative charge in the endometrial epithelium surface during the implantation window [1]. The presence of fucose, galactose and acetylgalactosaminyl residues at the epithelial cell level appears to play a role in the reduction of the negative charge. Primitive trophoblast is essentially coated with galactose residues.

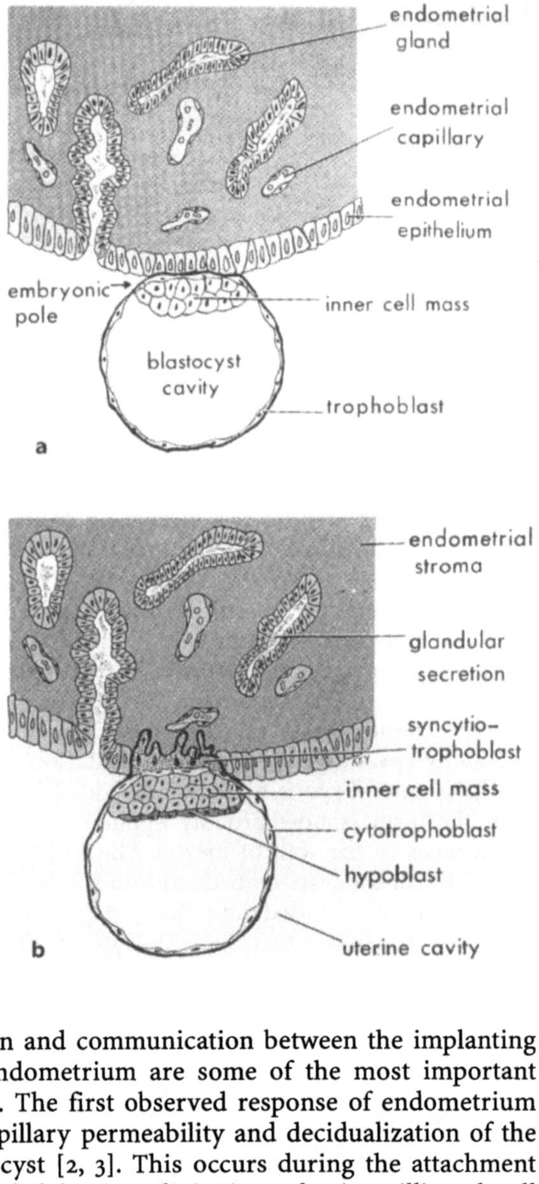

Fig. 1a–d. Stages of implantation. **a** Adhesion of the blastocyst to the surface epithelium. **b** Penetration of the trophectoderm cells between epithelial cells. **c** Intrusion of the trophoblasts in the subepithelial zone. **d** Implantation process completed. (Reprinted with permission from Moore KL (1993) (ed) The developing human, 5th edn. Saunders

The first stages of interaction and communication between the implanting blastocyst and the maternal endometrium are some of the most important but least understood processes. The first observed response of endometrium to implantation is increased capillary permeability and decidualization of the stromal cells adjacent to blastocyst [2, 3]. This occurs during the attachment of the blastocyst and is preceded by interdigitation of microvilli and cell membrane apposition between blastocyst trophectoderm and uterine epithelium [4, 5]. Following adhesion, the penetration events begin. Early embryos are fully capable of producing collagenase enzyme that degrades basement membrane [6]. This degradation, together with the local edema induced by prostaglandin activation, allows invasive cells such as trophoblasts to enter the endometrial stroma completely. Trophoblasts send long protrusions between epithelial cells and there is an obvious rupture of lateral tight junc-

Fig. 1 c, d

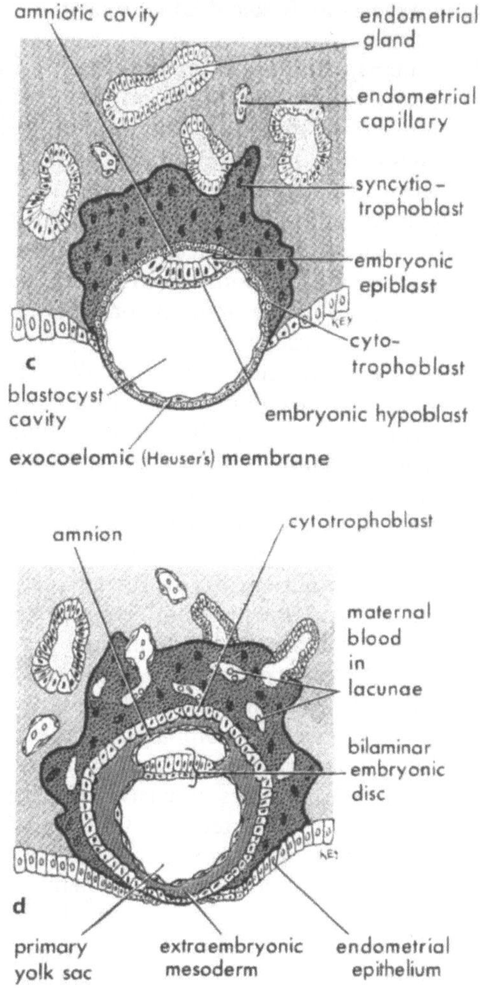

tions. Immediately afterwards, the contact between primary trophoblast and the subepithelial zone is established. The earliest phenomenon is a displacement of epithelial cells by trophoblast. Strong evidence exists that trophectoderm attaches preferentially to laminin and/or fibronectin [7, 8], hence to basement membrane components surrounding decidual cells [9]. It has also been shown that throphoblast expresses proteolytic activities [10]. Various protease inhibitors have been simultaneously demonstrated in both extravillous trophoblast and endometrial cells [11, 12]. A true possibility exists that the depth of trophoblast penetration is regulated, at least partly, by state of equilibrium between trophoblastic proteases and decidual protease inhibitors.

Basic Aspects of Endometrial Receptivity

In humans, the period during which a blastocyst can implant is limited and is almost totally dependent on the establishment of an equilibrium between the hormonal milieu of the woman and the degree of development of the blastocyst together with the signals it sends to the maternal organism.

Estrogen-dependent cell proliferation of the surface epithelium, gland, stroma, and blood vessels in the superficial layers (zona functionalis) [13, 14] and a concurrent enhancement of the activity of various metabolic enzymes characterize the endometrium during the follicular phase of the cycle. Under the influence of the preovulatory elevation in circulating estradiol, the endometrium increases in thickness 2–3 times as a result of cell hyperplasia and moderate tissue edema [15–17]. With the onset of progesterone production from the corpus luteum, the proliferative effect of estradiol is neutralized and endometrial growth ceases. The first obvious effect of progesterone on the endometrium is a marked change in the glandular epithelium. Endometrium becomes secretory, with the appearance of secretory vacuoles in the cytoplasm of the cells that line the endometrial glands. These vacuoles are located initially under the nucleus in the deeper portion of the cell. Four days after ovulation, the secretory vacuoles move toward the superficial part of the cell and are progressively excreted into the lumina of the glands; thus secretory cells become exhausted by 7–8 days after ovulation. Progesterone also affects the stromal cells of the endometrium. The most dramatic stromal response in a normal luteal phase is the initiation of a predecidual reaction, which is delayed as compared to the relatively rapid changes that occur in the glandular epithelium. During the normal menstrual cycle the human endometrium undergoes extensive changes in the vascularization, including the spiral arteries, the arterioles, the capillaries, the venous lakes, and veins. One of the earliest modifications of the endometrium in response to signals produced by the blastocyst is a tremendous increase in the vascular permeability. There is some evidence that platelet activating factor (PAF) is one such signal with unique vasodilating properties [18]. It is not clear, however, whether PAF acts alone or also triggers the local production of prostaglandins by the endometrial epithelial cells [19]. Under the influence of progesterone, the endometrial arterioles become thickened and increasingly coiled [20, 21]. These vascular changes play an important role in the penetration phase of the implantation process, causing stromal edema which offers a loose interstitium for trophoblast and also allows the volume expansion of the decidual cells. In addition, increased permeability of the endothelial cells permits complexes of serum proteins to cross the blood vessel walls. Finally, the contact between trophoblast cells and the subepithelial capillaries develops into the formation of the hemochorial placentation, which will assure the continued survival and development of the embryo.

In the late luteal phase, small fibroblast-like stromal cells enlarge and become rounded and epithelioid in appearance. Decidualization begins around the spiral arterioles and spreads to the cells beneath the surface [22, 23]. During the final days of the cycle, the stroma in more superficial portions of the

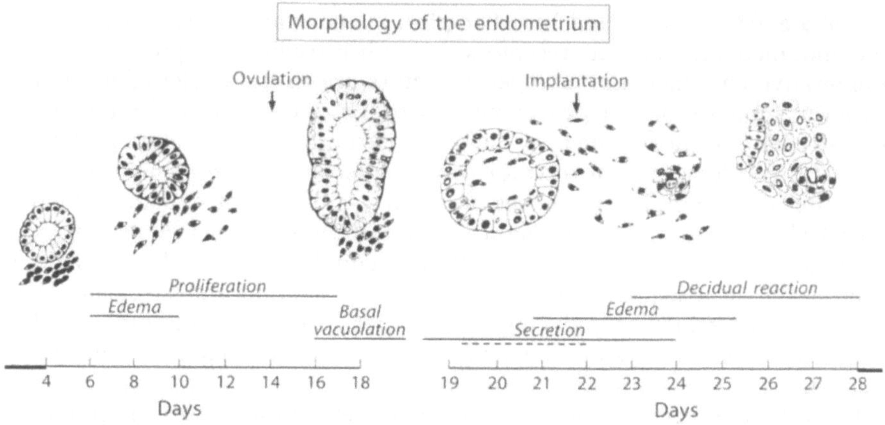

Fig. 2. Schematic representation of the major morphologic changes that occur in the glandular epithelium and stroma of the superficial endometrium (functionalis) during an ideal 28-day cycle. (Reprinted with permission from Seminars in Reproductive Endocrinology (1989), 6:115–128. Thieme Medical

endometrium often appears to consist of a solid mass of decidualized cells [15]. The decidualization process is associated with a remodeling of the matrix fibrillar network, and allows free transfer of molecules via the interstitial route and of trophectoderm (Fig. 2).

After ovulation, there is a short period, "a window," during which endometrial receptivity is maximal. During this window, a blastocyst travelling to the uterine cavity can establish a physical contact with the maternal organism and eventually implant. The ideal implantation window is situated between the 5th and 7th postovulatory days (after the luteinizing hormone surge). In addition to the receptive state it has also been postulated that the uterus passes through "implantation natural" and "implantation hostile" states. During the neutral phase the embryo can survive in the uterus but will not implant, while during the hostile phase the embryo will be actively destroyed. How the uterus effects these receptive, neutral, and hostile states remains unclear, although embryotoxic compounds have been demonstrated in uterine flushings from rats and mice taken at times other than when implantation normally occurs. Endometrial surface epithelium may prevent implantation outside of the window period because in unprimed mouse uterus the embryo is only able to implant if the surface epithelium has been removed.

The appearance of the endometrium during the implantation window is fairly characteristic. Mucosal thickness is 2.5–4.0 mm. Glands are widened, tortuous, and lined by simple epithelium. Cytoplasmic vacuoles are no longer present but there is a copious secretion in the gland lumen.

Role of Steroid Hormones and Their Receptors in Endometrial Receptivity

The endometrium contains receptors for both estradiol and progesterone. In proliferative endometrium estrogen receptors are in the nuclei of most cells. However, progesterone or exogenous progestins cause a marked reduction in the estrogen receptor content of the endometrium. Immunostaining of endometrial tissue for estrogen receptor reveals intense nuclear staining up to 1–3 days after ovulation, but in tissues obtained 4–5 days after ovulation, there is a marked decrease in the staining. In the luteal phase tissues (6–14 days post-ovulation), most of the cells in the functionalis layer either do not stain or stain weakly. Consequently, progesterone exerts a rapid antiestrogenic effect on the endometrium by reducing the number of estrogen receptors binding to nuclear acceptor sites and by suppressing estrogen receptor replenishment [24, 25].

Progesterone receptor content of the endometrium increases in the follicular phase of the cycle, presumably owing to estrogen-induced receptor synthesis [26–30]. Data from several studies that examined endometrium obtained from women [26, 27, 29] indicate that the concentrations of nuclear, cytosolic, and total progesterone receptors decrease significantly during the luteal phase of nonpregnant cycles. This has been attributed to a negative effect of progesterone on the synthesis of its own receptor and to the antiestrogenic effects of progesterone that inhibit estrogen-stimulated steroid receptor synthesis.

The circulating levels, as well as the ratio of estrogen to progesterone, can be important in controlling the receptivity of the endometrium. However, the available data suggest that the absolute amounts of both hormones may be of greater importance in inducing a normal secretory endometrium than the ra-

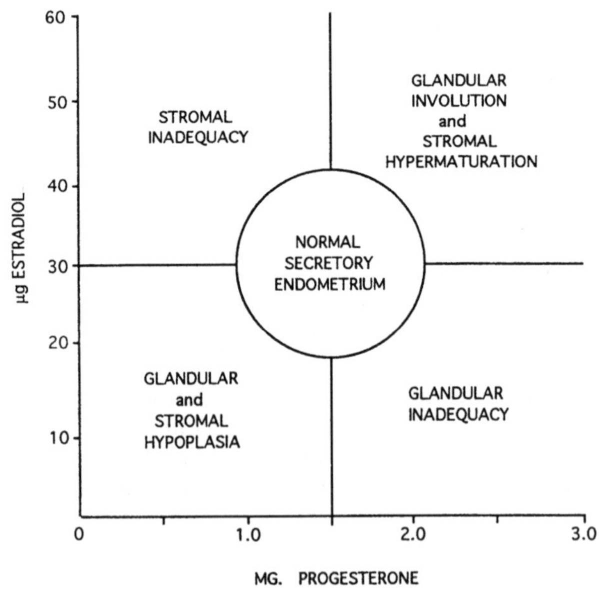

Fig. 3. Relationship between the morphology of the endometrium and various doses of estrogen and progesterone replacement in ovariectomized rhesus macaques. (From Good RG, Moyer DL (1968). Estrogen-progesterone relationships in the development of secretory endometrium. Fertil Steril 19:37–49. Reproduced with permission of the publisher. The American Fertility Society)

tio between the two (Fig. 3). Insufficient progesterone production during the luteal phase may result in poorly synchronized or incompletely developed endometrium and in infertility, failed implantation, or early pregnancy loss that can, in some cases, be corrected by exogenous progesterone [31, 32]. A deficiency in progesterone receptors in the endometrium is also associated with inadequate differentiation of the secretory endometrium; however, the resulting infertility is resistant to progesterone therapy [33, 34]. The role of estrogen on implantation is less clear; estrogen may influence the timing of different aspects of the endometrial response to progesterone. As has been mentioned above, implantation can occur only during a brief period, a window of endometrial receptivity, the duration of which depends upon and is strictly limited by the prevailing hormonal milieu. Retrospective analysis of serum steroid concentration in women who become pregnant during spontaneous cycles [35] or after IVF-ET during gonadotropin-stimulated cycles [36, 37] indicates that viable pregnancies occur most frequently when progesterone is relatively high and estradiol is relatively low during the early luteal phase of the cycle. Elevated levels of estradiol in the preimplantation period, resulting in a high estrogen and progesterone ratio, were associated with failure and pregnancy loss. However, high serum estrogen concentrations are not incompatible with pregnancy when progesterone levels are also elevated. When superovulation is induced in women by treatment with exogenous gonadotropins, serum steroid levels are often elevated [38], yet many of these patients become pregnant in spite of the fact that high concentrations of steroid hormones must exert a significant effect on the endometrium. Studies to address this paradox have shown that high progesterone levels cause early maturation of endometrium and that pregnancies most often occur in patients in whom estimation of serum progesterone levels indicates the endometrium to be "advanced" by 1–4 days. This could be the result of a wider window for endometrial acceptance and/or the advanced endometrium may be conducive to maintenance of a conceptus regardless of its growth stage, given that a four-cell embryo can be transferred into an endometrium which was prepared to receive a blastocyst.

Endometrial Leukocytes Relevant to Implantation

In addition to the vascular elements, fibroblasts, and fibroblast-like cells, endometrial stroma also contains a variety of lymphocytes (10%–15% of the total cells in the endometrium) that is characteristic of an immunologically active tissue. Lymphoid aggregates with germinal centers and dendritic cells are localized basally, and lymphocytes and macrophages are distributed diffusely throughout the stroma. However, organization of the endometrial lymphoid system is atypical in several respects: no intraepithelial B cells are present and only a few B cells are identified in the stroma, no plasma cells are found in normal endometrium, and an unusually large proportion of T cells are identified as suppressor/cytotoxic ($T8^+$) cells. The endometrial granulocytes, also called granular endometrial stromal cells, which may belong to the lymphoid cell population [39, 40], are found in the stroma and accumulate in increasing numbers during the luteal phase of the cycle. These large granular lymphocytes are also present in the decidua during the first trimester of pregnancy. The role of these cells in nonpregnant endometrium is uncertain. However, they may be involved in the production of cytokines which may have a role in immunosuppression or placental growth regulation. In addition they may have a critical role in implantation and maintenance of the conceptus as a semi-allograph.

Recently, data indicating that progesterone results in an increased leukocyte and T-cell concentration in human endometrium have been presented [40a].

Paracrine Factors Relevant to Implantation

Growth factors comprise a group of polypeptides that interact with specific cell membrane receptors, initiating cellular signaling pathways that affect cellular proliferation and differentiation [41, 42]. Growth factors and cytokines can act via autocrine, paracrine, or endocrine mechanisms. The role of growth factors and cytokines in implantation may be divided into three sections. First, they may mediate the actions of steroids in preparing the endometrial receptivity. Second, maternal growth factors expressed in the fallopian tubal epithelial cells and endometrial cells may have a direct action on the embryo, improving the implantation. Finally, the decidual changes that accommodate the embryo and control the trophoblast invasion may be mediated by cytokines or growth factors. To improve implantation rates in women the factors that are related to their expression should be well understood.

A number of proteins have been isolated from the human endometrium and decidua. Some of these proteins are relevant to the implantation period. *Progesterone-associated endometrial protein* (PEP) is also known as pregnancy-associated endometrial a_2 globulin (a_2-PEG), endometrial protein 15 (EP15), placental protein 14 (PP14), and lactoglobulin. PEP is the major secretory product of the glandular endometrium during the implantation period of the menstrual cycle. Its secretion dramatically increases from postovulatory days 5–7 and reaches peak serum levels during the last 2 or 3 days of the cycle. It has been suggested that it transports retinol to the embryo, thereby promoting cell growth and differentiation, and may play a role in the immunoprotection of the embryo [43].

Pregnancy-associated endometrial a_1 globulin (a_1-PEG) is also called embryonal protein 14 and placental protein 12 (PP12). It is secreted in small amounts in the late luteal phase and maximally produced during the first trimester. This protein is similar to insulin-like growth factor binding protein-1 (IGFBP-1) and inhibits as well as augments insulin-like growth factor (IGF) action. It may modulate IGF action on trophoblasts, possibly by binding to IGF receptors which regulate trophoblast proliferation.

IGFs or somatomedins are polypeptides that are similar in structure to proinsulin and insulin [44] and exist in two forms, IGF-I (somatomedin A) and IGF-II (somatomedin B). There is a preferential expression of IGF-I during the proliferative phase and of IGF-II in the secretory phase in human endometrium [45]. One characteristic function of IGFs is that binding proteins,

IGFBPs, modulate their functions. In humans, the IGFBP-1 (α_1-PEG) is localized to the stromal cells, and increased immunoreactivity of this protein is found in the secretory phase as well as in gestational endometrium [46, 47].

Colony-stimulating factors (CSFs), a group of regulatory glycoproteins, may also play an important role in placental growth [48]. They stimulate placental lactogen and hCG synthesis by cultured trophoblasts [49]. Because CSF-1 is produced by glandular epithelium and its receptor is present in this cell type, it is postulated that CSF-1 may be involved in cyclic differentiation of the endometrial epithelium, acting as an autocrine factor.

Leukemia inhibitory factor (LIF) is a glycoprotein with a remarkable range of biological actions in different tissue systems. It has recently been showed that well-timed expression of LIF in the endometrium of mice is crucial for successful implantation of the embryo [50]. We have found that LIF is also expressed in human endometrium, that its level is modulated by cytokines and growth factors, and that the highest levels of LIF mRNA are present around the expected time of blastocyst invasion of the endometrium. We have obtained evidence that LIF may shift trophoblast differentiation toward the anchoring-invading phenotype. Thus, the regulation of the expression of LIF may play an important role in the regulation of trophoblast differentiation and may prove critical for successful implantation.

Epidermal growth factor (EGF) is a potential mediator of estradiol (E_2) action in the uterus [51, 52]. E_2 treatment enhances the expression of uterine EGF [53], EGF receptor mRNAs, and proteins [53, 54]. EGF increases glandular epithelial cell numbers and stimulates stromal cell differentiation. It seems that EGF acts synergistically with other growth factors and steroid hormones in its stimulation of endometrial cell proliferation and differentiation [42, 55].

Platelet-derived growth factor (PDGF) is also a potent mitogen that consists of two subunits, A and B, connected by interchain disulfide bonds [56, 57]. These subunits can be combined, giving rise to three dimeric forms of PDGF (PDGF-AA,-AB,-BB). In human endometrium PDGF-BB is expressed. It has been shown that it is mitogenic to cultured endometrial stromal cells, an effect in which steroids do not act synergistically [58, 59]. On the other hand PDGF and EGF enhance each other's action.

Transforming growth factor-β (TGF-β) consists of three isoforms in mammals. It modulates cell differentiation, proliferation, and morphogenesis and is also a potent immunomodulating agent [73–75]. A recent study has shown that TGF-β is expressed in mouse endometrial epithelium during the preimplantation period and in the mouse decidua [76]. TGF-β has been shown to be present in endometrium/decidua at the maternal-fetal interface in early human implantation sites, suggesting that it may function in the controlled invasion of the uterine decidua during implantation [76a].

Angiogenesis, characterized by new capillary growth [60], is a major process in promoting proliferative endometrium [61]. Endothelins and fibroblast growth factor (FGF) induce endometrial angiogenesis and thus may play an indirect role in the endometrial receptivity.

Interleukin-1 (IL-1), which is involved in the regulation of cell proliferation, differentiation, and programmed cell death in many cell types [66], is produced by the endometrial cells. We have recently shown that IL-1 enhances LIF levels in the endometrial stromal cells in culture, thereby playing a role in implantation. In mice, the blockade of the type 1 IL-1 receptor was found to prevent implantation of blastocyst [66a].

Interferon-γ (IFN-γ) is secreted by human endometrium explants in culture [45]. IFN-γ receptors are present in endometrial epithelium and do not change during the menstrual cell cycle [68]. IFN-γ induces HLA-DR molecules on endometrial epithelium, and expression of these molecules is highest on epithelium adjacent to lymphoid aggregates, supporting a role for IFN-γ in inducing lymphoepithelial interactions [69, 70]. Because activated T cells in lymphoid aggregates are adjacent to the basalis glands and secrete IFN-γ, it has been proposed that the low proliferative activity of the basal epithelium may be due to the paracrine action of this cytokine [45]. Thus, this cytokine may be involved in the regulation of epithelial proliferation as well as epithelial-lymphocyte interactions.

Tumor necrosis factor-α (TNF-α) is expressed in endometrial epithelium in the proliferative phase [71, 72]. A number of roles for TNF-α in endometrial development and function have been proposed, including being a chemotactic factor for granulocytes and macrophages, cellular mitosis, and maintenance of hemostasis [71]. We have also recently shown that it modulates LIF levels in vitro.

It is now widely accepted that prostaglandins (PGs) play a significant role in the vasodilatation reaction [78]. Indomethacin, a prostaglandin synthetase inhibitor, delays or inhibits implantation in rodents. This effect can be reversed by intrauterine or systemic administration of exogenous PG. Both PGE_2 and $PGF_{2\alpha}$ appear to be effective. Since only PGE_2 receptors have been isolated from the rat endometrium, it is hypothesized that $PGF_{2\alpha}$ is activated by conversion into PGE_2.

Decidualization yields an important product, prolactin, the function of which has not been totally elucidated; however, it seems that it acts in a paracrine manner and IGF-1 may exert a positive control on decidual prolactin production together with relaxin [79].

Clinical Aspects of Endometrial Receptivity

The assessment of endometrial function in physiological conditions is one of the most controversial areas in reproduction and the situation is further complicated in human assisted reproduction by the multitude of variables associated with any form of treatment. Endometrial receptivity for adequate implantation may potentially be altered by different degrees of intervention which are intended to overcome an identified or even an unidentified factor in the reproductive failure. Regarding endometrial receptivity, assisted reproduction is associated with certain problems including ovarian hyperstimulation and correct timing of the blastocyst implantation. The stimulated cycle may affect the production of various growth factors from the endometrium, which may cause an unfavourable implantation window. Another important aspect regarding the endometrial environment is the different timing of arrival of embryos in the uterine cavity and the different developmental stage of the embryo at that time. Embryos which are placed in the uterus too early may not have the capacity to induce some of the implantation characteristics of the endometrium. In spontaneous conception, and we suppose that the same situation exists after the replacement of embryos and gametes into the tubes, a morula or an early blastocyst will arrive in the uterine cavity 5–6 days after fertilization. Because the embryos would enter a supposedly more receptive uterus at this time, techniques such as gamete intrafallopian transfer (GIFT) or zygote intrafallopian transfer (ZIFT) may have a theoretical superiority over IVF-ET, where embryos at the blastomere stage are usually replaced in the uterine cavity 48 h after oocyte retrieval. The results of the 1990 United States registry shows that the live delivery rate for IVF treatment is 12%, for GIFT 21% and for ZIFT 20%.

Clinical Importance of the Implantation Window

With modern assisted reproductive technologies, ovulatory agents, and laboratory techniques, high rates of oocyte retrieval may be achieved (86%). However, as has been mentioned above, pregnancy rates are still disappointingly low. Endometrial receptivity plays an important role in pregnancy rates, as does the quality of the embryo. Therefore, it is critical to recognize the time for embryo transfer (ET) that would best correspond with the implantation window.

Although controversies still exist, embryo quality may be evaluated morphologically; however, endometrial receptivity can only be assessed circumstantially. There are still no accepted criteria for evaluating endometrial receptivity in standard IVF. Because it is possible to control the embryo quality with ovum donation, the role of endometrial receptivity alone can be evaluated. In oocyte donation, where endogenous hormonal activity is absent, the accepted time point for uterine ET is between 2 and 3 days after fertilization. This is true both after suppression by GnRH analogues in eugonadal women and in agonadal ovum recipients. Such treatments have proved to be quite successful despite the fact that normally blastocyst apposition begins about LH day +6 and is complete by LH day +10 [79]. Davies et al. [80] have reported that in 21 ET cycles resulting from oocyte donation, patients who conceived had a significantly better endometrial response than who did not. Five of seven patients (71%) conceived when the endometrium was "in phase" (a less than 2-day delay). Endometrial maturation had been determined in a previous mock cycle of hormone replacement therapy. They concluded that endometrial receptivity is a key factor in conception. The width of the implantation window has been found to be different for patients receiving donor oocytes, the duration of the window being extended from 1 to 6 luteal days [81, 82].

Therapeutic Maturation of the Endometrium and Endometrial Receptivity

As has been mentioned earlier in this chapter, human endometrium is highly compliant to a wide range of E_2 and P stimulation. Various doses of estrogen, with either oral, transdermal, or vaginal routes of administration, are capable of producing morphologically and ultrastructurally normal endometrium. Natural P is superior to synthetic progestins for induction of receptive secretory endometrium. Because morphological adequacy is accompanied by normal function, namely, the ability to sustain embryo implantation.

The Role of Ovarian Stimulation on Endometrial Receptivity. Ovarian stimulation, widely employed as a part of IVF treatment, frequently adversely affects the process of endometrial maturation, resulting in significant endometrial imbalance. The specific reason for aberrant endometrial development is as yet unknown. It might be the result of a direct effect of the regimen on endometrium and/or higher circulating E_2 and P levels. Various kinds of hormonal supplementations used in clomiphene citrate (CC)- and/or human menopausal gonadotropin-stimulated cycles have not improved treatment outcome. It has been shown that CC has a negative impact on endometrial development. The negative influence of CC on the endometrium has been linked to its antiestrogenic effect. It is known that CC acts as a competitive inhibitor at the estrogen receptor site. Human chorionic gonadotropin (hCG) or natural P supplementation administered after controlled ovarian stimulation with GnRH and hMG effectively corrects the luteal phase defect and results in an improved conception rate.

Artificial Endometrial Cycle in IVF Treatment with Donated Oocytes. Higher pregnancy rates have been achieved with ovum donation compared with standard IVF [80, 83], GIFT [84] and frozen-thawed embryos [85]. These higher rates can be attributed to some extent to ovum quality but mainly to better endometrial receptivity [86]. In standard IVF, controlled hyperstimulation results in high levels of E_2, which is known to have an interceptive effect on the endometrium [87, 88]. In oocyte donor programs, simple hormonal replacement therapy creates a more favourable endometrium. Paulson compared embryo implantation rates in IVF stimulated and donor oocyte replacement cycles and concluded that the implantation rates per embryo were only one-third as high in the former [89]. There was also a doubling of the pregnancy rate in the non-stimulated recipients of the donor eggs. The embryo factor can be excluded as the stimulated cycle has a lower success rate with comparable embryos.

Influence of Ovarian Status. Recently, patients with normal menstrual cycles who have repeatedly failed in IVF, patients who do not respond to ovulation induction, or patients with a genetic trait precluding use of their own oocytes have been included in ovum donation programs. Unlike the patients with ovarian failure, the endometrium in these patients is subject to the influence of endogenous ovarian hormones. Thus a comparison between such patients and those with ovarian failure allows for assessment of endometrial receptivity with regard to influence of ovarian status.

Edwards et al. found the conception rate to be higher in previously amenorrheic women than in cycling women, irrespective of age (48.4% versus 20.3% respectively) [90]; similarly, Yaron et al. found the conception rate to be higher in women with ovarian failure (29.7%) than in cycling patients undergoing egg donation (19.6%; $P<0.02$) [91]. The reduced pregnancy rates in eugonadal ovum recipients may be the result of adverse effects of endogenous ovarian hormones on the endometrium in cycling patients and/or better timing of the ET in artificially induced cycles. Moreover, the endometrium of agonadal women is highly amenable to hormonal manipulation. Most of the reported treatment protocols produced satisfactory endometrial maturation. If, indeed, patients with nonfunctioning ovaries fare better in egg donation programs, then perhaps pretreatment with a GnRH analogue to create medical hypophysectomy will improve success rates in eugonadal patients receiving donated oocytes [92] or frozen-thawed embryos. GnRH analogue has been claimed to be associated with embryos of poor potential for development in standard IVF. Its efficacy in IVF has therefore been attributed to an improvement in endometrial receptivity [93].

Age and Endometrial Receptivity

Endometrial receptivity also decreases with age. In animal studies it has been shown that there are marked age-related changes in the endometrium, including decreased blood flow [94], increased collagen content and reduced number of stromal cells [95], increased mast cell content in the endometrium and myometrium [96], fewer E_2 receptors on endometrial cell surfaces [97], and impaired ability to form decidual tissue [98]. However, in humans there has been no conclusive evidence of age-related changes, except delayed secretory maturation [99]. Nevertheless, the conception rate also declines with increasing recipient age in ovum donation programs [100, 101]. It has been speculated that the abnormal endometrial receptivity is due to the decreased levels of P_2 receptors promoted by the low levels of E_2 receptors [101].

Clinical Assessment of Endometrial Receptivity by Ultrasound and Doppler

Attempts have been made to correlate ultrasonographic parameters and endometrial receptivity. However, it has been concluded that ultrasonographic parameters such as thickness and reflectivity are not helpful in evaluating endometrial receptivity [102]. Nevertheless, Doppler measurements using transvaginal ultrasonography have shown that there is a correlation between lower vascular resistance of the uterine artery and pregnancy rates: vascular resistance was significantly lower on the day of follicular aspiration in patients who became pregnant [103]. In another study, were blood flow impedance, expressed by the pulsatility index, was measured by transvaginal Doppler immediately before ET, patients in the medium pulsatility index group achieved higher pregnancy rates than those in the low pulsatility index group [104]. There were no pregnancies in the high pulsatility index group. These data suggest that endometrial receptivity is correlated with uterine blood flow as measured by Doppler velocimetry; such an approach could be used (a) to increase the implantation rate by identifying cases in which embryos should be cryopreserved until the uterus is more receptive and (b) to reduce the multiple pregnancy rate by allowing the number of embryos transferred to be reduced, given that transfer will take place when the uterus is at its most receptive.

Conclusion

With the modern assisted reproductive technologies, ovulatory agents and laboratory techniques, high rates of oocyte retrieval and ET may be achieved. However, pregnancy rates are still disappointingly low. It seems that this frustrating shortfall in implantation is mainly the result of poor endometrial receptivity. Therefore, understanding of endometrial receptivity is important for achieving high pregnancy rates, as well as for future contraceptive methods. On the other hand, future studies of endometrial receptivity may yield a scientific explanation for the apparent success of immunotherapy in women with recurrent pregnancy loss.

References

1. Jansen RPS, Turner M, Johannison E, Landgren BM, Diczfalusy E (1985) Cyclic changes in human endometrial surface glycoproteins: a quantiative histochemical study. Fertil Steril 44:85–91
2. Betteridge KJ, Eaglesome ND, Randall GCB, Mitchell D, Lugden EA (1978) Maternal progesterone levels as evidence of luteotrophic or antiluteolytic effects on embryos transferred to heifers 12–17 days after estrus. Theriogenology 9:86–93
3. Northey DL, French LR (1980) The effect of embryo removal and intrauterine infusion of embryonic homogenates on the lifespan of bovine corpus luteum. J Anim Sci 50:298–302
4. Heyman Y, Camous S, Fevre J, Mezious W, Martal J (1984) Maintenance of the corpus luteum after uterine transfer of trophoblastic vesicles to cyclic cows and ewes. J Reprod Fertil 70:533–540
5. Knickerbocker JJ, Thatcher WW, Bazer FW, Drost M, Barron DH, Fincher KB, Roberts RM (1984) Proteins secreted by day-16 to -18 bovine conceptuses extend corpus luteum function in cows. J Reprod Fertil 70:533–540
6. Puistola V, Roonberg L, Martikainen H, Turpeeniemi-Hujanen T (1989) The human embryo produced basement membrane collagen (type IV collagen)-degrading protease activity. Hum Reprod 4:309–311
7. Loke YW, Gardner L, Burland K, King A (1989) Laminin in human trophoblast decidua interaction. Hum Reprod 4:453, 457
8. Earl U, Estlin C, Bulmer JN (1990) Fibronectin and laminin in the early human placenta. Placenta 11:223–231
9. Aplin JD (1989) Cellular biochemistry of the endometrium. In: Wynn RM, Jollie WP (eds) Biology of the uterus, 2nd edn. Plenum, New York, pp 89–119
10. Queenan JT Jr, Kao LC, Arbeolda CE, Uloa-Aguirre A, Golos TG, Cines DB, Strauss JF III (1987) Regulation of urokinase type plasminogen activator production by cultured human cytotrophoblasts. J Biol Chem 262:1093–1096
11. Marshall RJ, Braye SG (1987) Immunohistochemical demonstration of α-1-antitrypsin and α-1-antichymotrypsin in normal human endometrium. Int J Gynecol Pathol 6:49–54

12. Feinberg RF, Kao LC, Haimowitz JE, Queenan JT Jr, Wun TC, Strauss JF III, Kliman HJ (1989) Plasminogen activator inhibitor types 1 and 2 in human trophoblasts. Lab Invest 61:20–26
13. Boutselis JG (1963) Histochemical and cytologic observations in the normal human endometrium. Obstet Gynecol 21:423–434
14. Vanells A, Campisi A, Custorella A et al (1986) Ornithine decarboxylase and transglutaminase activities in human endometrium during the menstrual cycle. IRCS Med Sci 14:448–449
15. Noyes RW, Hertig AT, Rock J (1950) Dating the endometrial biopsy. Fertil Steril 1:3–25
16. Bartelmez GW (1957) The phases of the menstrual cycle and their interpretation in terms of pregnancy cycle. Am J Obstet Gynecol 74:931–955
17. Feichtinger W, Kemeter P (1985) Uterine ultrasound. In: Edwards RG, Pudy JM, Steptoe PC (eds) Implantation of the human embryo. Academic, New York, pp 335–349
18. Alecozay AA, Casslen BG, Riehl RM et al (1989) Platelet activating factor in human luteal phase endometrium. Biol Reprod 41:578–586
19. Kennedy TG (1983) Embryonic signals and the initiation of blastocyst implantation. Aust J Biol Sci 36:531–543
20. Christiaens GCML, Sixma JJ, Haspels AA (1982) Hemostasis in menstrual endometrium a review. Obstet Gynecol Surv 37:281–303
21. Abel MH (1985) Prostoglandins and menstruation. In: Baird DT, Michie EA (eds) Mechanism of menstrual bleeding. Serono symposia, vol 25. Raven, New York, pp 139–156
22. Wienke Jr E, Cavazos F, Hall DG et al (1968) Ultrastructure of the human endometrial stromal cell during the menstrual cycle. Am Obstet Gynecol 102:65–77
23. Faber M, Wewer UM, Berthelsen JG et al (1986) Laminin production by human endometrial cells relates to the cyclic and pathologic state of endometrium. Am J Pathol 124:384–398
24. Klatzenellenborgen BS (1980) Dynamics of steroid hormone receptor action. Annu Rev Physiol 42:17–35
25. Leavitt WW, Takeda A, MacDonald RG (1986) Progesterone regulation of protein synthesis and steroid receptor levels in decidual cells. Ann NY Acad Sci 476–157
26. Bayard F, Damilano S, Robel P et al (1978) Cyctoplasmic and nuclear estradiol and progesterone receptors in human endometrium. J Clin Endocrinol Metab 46:635–648
27. Levy C, Robel P, Gautray JP et al (1980) Estradiol and progesterone receptors in human endometrium: normal and abnormal menstrual cycles and early pregnancy. Am J Obstet Gynecol 136:646–651
28. King RJB, Towsend PT, Siddle N et al (1982) Regulation of estrogen and progesterone receptor levels in epithelium and stroma from pre-and postmenapozal endometria. J Steroid Biochem 16:21–29
29. Pollow K, Inthraphuvasak J, Manz B et al (1981) A comparison of cytoplasmic and nuclear estradiol and progesterone receptors in human fallopian tube and endometrial tissue. Fertil Steril 36:615–622
30. Healy DL, Hodgen GD (1983) The endocrinology of human endometrium. Obstet Gynecol Surv 38:509–530
31. DiZerega GS, Hodgen GD (1982) Luteal phase dysfunction infertility: a sequel to aberrant folliculogenesis. In: Wallach EE, Kempers RD (eds) Modern trends in infertility and conception control, vol 2. Harper and Row, Philadelphia, pp 12–22
32. Written BI, Martin SA (1985) The endometrial biopsy as a guide to the management of luteal phase defect. Fertil Steril 44:460–465
33. Keller DW, Wiest WG, Askin FB et al (1979) Pseudocorpus luteum insufficiency: a local defect of progesterone action on endometrial stroma. J Clin Endocrinol Metab 48:127–132
34. Maynard PV, Symonds EM, Johnson J et al (1983) Nuclear progesterone uptake by endometrial tissue in cases of subfertility. Lancet 2:310–312
35. Lenton EA, Sulaiman R, Sobowale O et al (1982) The human menstral cycle: plasma concentrations of prolactin, LH, FSH, oestradiol and progesterone in conceiving and non-conceiving women. J Reprod Fertil 65:131–139
36. Lejeune B, Dehou MF, Leroy F (1976) Tentative extrapolation of animal data to human implantation. Ann NY Acad Sci 476:63–74

37. Gidley Baird AA, O'Neill C, Sinosich MJ et al (1986) Failure of implantation in human in vitro fertilisation and embryo transfer patients: the effects of altered progesterone/estrogen ratios in humans and mice. Fertil Steril 45:69–74
38. Jones GS (1985) The role of luteal support in a programme for in vitro fertilisation. In: Edwards RG, Prudy JM, Steptoe PC (eds) Implantation of the human embryo. Academic, New York, pp 285–302
39. Bulmer JN, Sunderland CA (1983) Bone-marrow origin of endometrial granulocytes in the early human placental bed. J Reprod Immunol 5:383–387
40. Bulmer JN, Sunderland CA (1984) Immunohistological characterization of lymphoid cell populations in the early human placental bed. Immunology 52:349–357
40a. Booker SS, Jayanetti C, Karalak S, Hsiu J-G, Archer DF (1994) The effect of progesterone on the accumulation of leukocytes in the human endometrium. Am J Obstet Gynecol 171:139–142
41. Carpenter G, Cohen S (1979) Epidermal growth factor. Annu Rev Biochem 1:3–25
42. Carpenter G (1987) Receptor for epidermal growth factor and other polypeptide mitogens. Annu Rev Biochem 56:881–914
43. Nicole B, Fournet (1991) Current concepts of ovum implantation. Postgrad Obstet Gynecol 11:1–6
44. Rinderknecht E, Humble RE (1978) The amino acid sequence of human insulin like growth factor-I and its structural homology with proinsulin. J Biol Chem 253:2769
45. Tabibzadeh S (1991) Human endometrium: an active site of cytokine production and action. Endocr Rev 12:272–290
45b. Giudice LC (1994) Growth factors and growth modulators in human uterine endometrium: their potential relevancce to reproductive medicine. Fertil Steril 61:1–17
46. Bell SC, Bohn H (1986) Immunochemical and biochemical relationship between human pregnancy-associated secreted endometrial $\alpha 1$- and $\alpha 2$-globulins ($\alpha 1$- and $\alpha 2$-PEG) and the soluble placental proteins 12 and 14 (PP12 and PP14). Placenta 7:283
47. Waites GT, James RFL, Bell SC (1988) Immunohistochemical localisation of human endometrial secretory protein pregnancy associated endometrial secretory α-1 globulin, an insulin like growth factor binding protein during the menstural cycle. J Clin Endocrinol Metab 67:1100
48. Wegman TG, Athanassakis I, Guilbert L, Branch D, Dy M, Menn E, Chaoulat G (1989) The role of M-CSF and GM-CSF in fostering placental growth, fetal growth and survival. Transplant Proc 21:566
49. Guilbert LJ, Athanassaki I, Branch DR et al (1991) The placenta as an immune-endocrine interface: placental cells as targets to lymphohematopoietic cytokine stimulation. In: Wegmann TG, Gill TJ, Nisbet Brown E (eds) Molecular and cellular immunobiology of the maternal-fetal interface. Oxford University Press, Oxford 1:261–276
50. Stewart CL, Kaspar P, Brunet LJ (1992) Blastocyst implantation depends on maternal expression of leukaemia inhibitory factor. Nature 359:76–79
51. Murphy LJ, Murphy LC, Friesen HG (1987) A role for the insulin like growth factors as estromedins in the rat uterus. Trans Assoc Am Physicians 99:204–214
52. Nelson KG, Takahashi T, Bossert NL, Walmer DK, McLachan JA (1991) Epidermal growth factor replaces estrogen in the stimulation of female genital-tract growth and differentiation. Proc Natl Acad Sci USA 88:1–5
53. Mukku VR, Stancel GM (1985) Regulation of epidermal growth factor by estrogen. J Biol Chem 260:9820–9824
54. Lingham RB, Stancel GM, Loose-Mitchell DS (1988) Estrogen regulation of epidermal growth factor receptor mRNA. Mol Endocrinol 2:230–235
55. Ishihara S, Taketani Y, Mizuno M (1991) EGF rapidly stimulates tyrosine phosphorylation in cultured endometrial cells. Asia Oceania J Obstet Gynaecol 17:363–367
56. Heldin CH, Wateson A, Westermark B (1985) Platelet-derived growth factor. Mol Cell Endocrinol 39:169–187
57. Ross R, Raines EW, Bowen-Pope DF (1986) Biology of platelet derived growth factor. Cell 46:155–169
58. Chegini N, Rossi MJ, Masterson BJ (1992) Platelet-derived growth factor (PDGF), epidermal growth factor (EGF), and EGF and PDGF-β receptors in human endometrial tissue: localization and in vitro action. Endocrinology 130:2373–2385

59. Surrey ES, Halme J (1991) Effect of platelet derived growth factor on endometrial stromal cell proliferation in vitro: a model for endometriosis? Fertil Steril 56:672–679
60. Findley JK (1986) Angiogenesis in reproductive tissues. J Endocrinol 111:357–366
61. Noyes RW, Hertig AT, Rock J (1950) Dating endometrial biopsy. Fertil Steril 1:3–25
62. Economos K, MacDonald PC, Casey ML (1992) Endothelin-1 gene expression and protein biosynthesis in human endometrium: potential modulator of endometrial blood flow. J Clin Endocrinol Metab 74:14–79
63. Gospodarowicz D, Ferrara N, Schweigerer L, Neufeld G (1987) Structural characterization and biological functions of fibroblast growth factor. Endocrinol Rev 8:686–692
64. Terranova VP, DiFlorio R, Lyall RM et al (1985) Human endothelial cells are chemotactic to endothelial cell growth factor and heparin. J Cell Biol 101:2330–2334
65. Montesano R, Vassali JD, Baird A, Guillemin R, Orchi L (1986) Basic fibroblast growth factor induces angiogenesis in vitro. Proc Natl Acad Sci USA 83:7297–7301
66. Arai K-I, Lee F, Miyajiima A, Miatake S, Arai N, Yokota T (1990) Cytokines: coordination of immune inflammatory responses. Annu Rev Biochem 59:783–793
66a. Simon C, Frances A, Piquette GN, Danasouir IE, Zurawski G, Dang W, Polan ML (1994) Embryonic implantation in mice is blocked by interleukin-1 receptor antagonist (IL-1ra). Endocrinology 134:521–528
67. Tabibzadeh SS, Kaffka KL, Satyaswaroop PG, Kilian PL (1990) IL-1 regulation of human endometrium functions: Presence of IL-1 receptor correlates with IL-1 stimulated PGE2 production. J Clin Endocrinol Metab 70:1000–1005
68. Tabibzadeh SS (1990) Evidence of T cell activation and potential cytokine activation in human endometrium. J Clin Endocrinol Metab 71:645–653
69. Tabibzadeh SS, Bettica A, Gerber MA (1990) Variable expression of la antigens in human endometrium and in chronic endometritis. Am J Pathol 86:153–160
70. Tabibzadeh SS, Satyaswaroop PG (1989) Differential expression of HLA-DR, HLA-DP, and HLA-DQ antigen determinants of the major histocompatibility complex in human endometrium. Am J Reprod Immunol Microbiol 18:124–130
71. MacMaster MT, De SK, Dey SK, Andrews GK (1992) Cell specific metallothionein gene expression in mouse decidua and placenta. In: Lavia LA (ed) Cellular signals controlling uterine function. Plenum, New York
72. Hunt JS, Chien H-L, Hu X-L, Tabibzadeh SS (1992) Tumor necrosis factor α, messenger ribonucleic acid and protein in human endometrium. Biol Reprod 47:141–147
73. Sporn MB, Roberts AB (1990) The transforming growth factor-betas: past, present and future. Ann NY Acad Sci 593:1
74. Miller DA, Pelton RQ, Derynck R, Moses HL (1990) Transforming growth factor-β. A family of growth regulatory peptides. Ann NY Acad Sci 593:208
75. Ailenberg M, Tung PS, Fritz IB (1990) Transforming growth factor-β elicits shape changes and increases contractility of testicular pertibular cells. Biol Reprod 42:499
76. Tamada H, McMaster MT, Flanders KC, Andrew GK, Dey SK (1990) Cell type-specific expression of transforming growth factor-$\beta 1$ in the mouse uterus during preimplantation period. Mol Endocrinol 4:965
76a. Selick CE, Horowitz GM, Gratch M, Scott RT Jr, Navot D, Hofmann GE (1994) Immunohistochemical localization of transforming growth factor-β in human implantation sites. J Clin Endocrinol Metab 78:592–596
77. Akhurst RJ, Lehnert SA, Gatherer D, Duffie E (1990) The role of TGF-β in mouse development. Ann NY Acad Sci 593:259
78. Kennedy TG, Squires PM, Yee GM (1989) Mediators involved in decidualization. In: Yoshinaga K (ed) Blastocyst implantation, Serono symposia USA, Randolph, MA, p 135
79. Davies MC, Anderson MC, Mason BA, Jacobs HS (1990) Oocyte donation: the role of endometrial receptivity. Hum Reprod 5:862–869
80. Sauer MV, Paulson RJ, Macaso TM, Francis MM, Lobo RA (1991) Oocyte and pre-embryo donation to women with ovarian failure: an extended clinical trial. Fertil Steril 55:39–43
81. Navot D, Scott RT, Droesch K, Veek LL, Liu H-C, Rosenwaks Z (1992) The window of embryo transfer and the efficiency of human contraception in vitro. Fertil Steril 57:362–365

82. Navot D, Bergh PA, Williams M, Garissi GJ, Guzman I, Sandler B et al (1991) An insight into early reproductive processes through the in vivo model of ovum donation. J Clin Endocrinol Metab 72:408–414
83. Navot D, Laufer N, Kopolovic J, Rabinowitz R, Birkenfeld A, Lewin A et al (1986) Artifically induced endometrial cycles and establishment of pregnancies in the absence of ovaries. N Engl J Med 314:806–811
84. Asch RH, Balmaceda JP, Ord T, Borrero C, Cefalu E, Gastaldi C et al (1988) Oocyte donation and gamete intrafallopian transfer in premature ovarian failure. Fertil Steril 49:263–267
85. deZiegler D, Frydman R (1990) Different implantation rates after transfers of cryopreserved embryos originating from donated oocytes or from regular in vitro fertilization. Fertil Steril 54:682–688
86. Talbert LM (1992) Oocyte donation. Curr Opin Obstet Gynecol 4:732–735
87. Gidley-Baitd AA, O'Neill C, Sinosich MJ, Porter RN, Pike IL, Saunders DM (1986) Failure of implantation in human in vitro fertilization and embryo transfer patients: the effects of altered progesterone/estrogen ratios in humans and mice. Fertil Steril 45:69–74
88. Fossum GT, Davidson A, Paulson RJ (1989) Ovarian hyperstimulation inhibits embryo implantation in the mouse. J In Vitro Fert Embryo Transfer 6:7–10
89. Paulson RJ, Sauer MV, Lobo RA (1990) Embryo implantation after human in vitro fertilization: importance of endometrial receptivity. Fertil Steril 4:678–681
90. Edwards RG, Morcos S, Macnamee M, Balamaceda JP, Walters DE, Asch R (1991) High fecundity of ameuorrhoeic patient women in embryo-transfer programmes. Lancet 338:292–294
91. Yaron Y, Botchan A, Amit A, Kogosowski A, Yovel I, Lessing JB (1993) Endometrial receptivity: the age-related decline in pregnancy rates and the effect of ovarian function. Fertil Steril 60:314–318
92. Meldrum DR, Wisot A, Hamilton F, Gutlay-Yeo AL, Marr B, Huynh D (1989) Artificial agonadism and hormone replacement for oocyte donation. Fertil Steril 52:509–511
93. Tesart J, Forman R, Belaisch-Allart J, Volante M, Hazout A, Strubb N et al (1989) Embryo quality and uterine receptivity in in vitro fertilisation cycles with or without agonists of gonadotropin releasing hormone. Hum Reprod 4:198–201
94. Gosawamy RK, Williams G, Steptoe PC (1988) Decreased uterine perfusion: a cause of infertility. Hum Reprod 3:955–959
95. Craig SS, Jollie WP (1985) Age changes in density of endometrial stromal cells of the rat. Exp Gerontol 20:93–97
96. Gosden RG (1979) Effects of age and parity on the breeding potential of mice with one or two ovaries. J Reprod Fert 57:477–478
97. Han Z, Kokkonen GC, Roth GS (1989) Effect of aging on population of estrogen receptor-containing cells in the rat uterus. Exp Cell Res 180:234–242
98. Shapiro M, Talbert GB (1974) The effect of maternal age on decidualisation in the mouse. J Gerontol 29:145–148
99. Sterzik K, Dallenbach C, Schneider V, Sasse V, Ballenbach-Hellweg G (1988) In vitro fertilization: the degree of endometrial insufficiency varies with the type of ovarian stimulation. Fertil Steril 50:457–462
100. Levran D, Ben-Sholmol, Dor J, Ben-Rafael Z, Nebel L, Mashiach S (1991) Aging of endometrium and oocytes: observation of conception and abortion rates in an egg donation model. Fertil Steril 56:1091–1094
101. Meldrum DR (1993) Female reproductive aging-ovarian and uterine factors. Fertil Steril 59:1–5
102. Sterzik K, Grab D, Rosenbusch B, Hamers S, Dallenbach-Hellweg G (1991) Receptivity of the endometrium. Comparison of ultrasound and histologic findings after hormonal stimulation. Geburtshilfe Frauenheilkd 51:554–558
103. Sterzik K, Grab D, Sasse V, Hutter W, Rosenbusch B, Terinde R (1989) Doppler sonographic findings and their correlation with implantation in an in vitro fertilization program. Fertil Steril 52:825–828
104. Steer CV, Campbell S, Tan SL, Crayford T, Mills C, Mason BA et al (1992) The use of transvaginal color flow imaging after in vitro fertilization to identify optimum uterine conditions before embryo transfer. Fertil Steril 57:372–376

The Importance of Cytology in Menstrual Cycle Diagnosis in Women

D. BROER-AHLERS and K.H. BROER

In the course of cyclic hormonal fluctuation cytological changes in the vaginal and cervical epithelium can be correlated with the stages of the menstrual cycle. Cytology has been applied for many years in the diagnosis of hormonal status in women. Hormonal alterations occurring in pathological cycles may also be identified by other cytological procedures. Although modern diagnostic methods such as determination of hormonal status are more precise and allow an evaluation of cyclic fluctuations closer to the actual ovulation date and with in a shorter testing period, the importance of cytological changes occurring in the vagina should not be neglected. The therapeutic impact of drugs on the cycle can also be assessed via cytology.

Cytology as such is not only of historical importance it also enables the gynecologist to gain insights into the hormonal changes resulting in natural alterations of the vaginal flora, especially in pathological conditions caused by inflammations or tumorous processes. Ever since the Papanicolaou smear came into widespread use a distinction has been made between four different groups of cells in the vaginal epithelium: (1) basic, (2) parabasic, (3) intermediate, and (4) superficial cells. These cells represent the degrees of differentiation of the tessellated epithelium. The cell size increases from the bottom to the top layer, and the germ size declines (relation of caryoplasm). The ripe cells in the superficial layer turn eosinophilic, i.e., pink to light red according to Papanicolaou. All other cells are cyanophilic, i.e., light blue to a shade of green or violet. No strict distinctions can be made. The determination of the degree of proliferation follows the criteria established by Schmitt.

During the ovulatory cycle the cytological pattern of the vaginal epithelium undergoes characteristic alterations known as the follicular and euteal phases. The early fellicular phase (5th–8th day) is characterized by large and small intermediate cells which are predominantly cyanophilic and partly grouped in series. The medium follicular phase 9th–11th day) is dominated by cells gaining in size; the small intermediate cells disappear, the folding of the cells declines, they spread wider, and the eosinophil index rises. The late follicular phase (12th–14th day), i.e., the ovulatory phase, is dominated by large intermediate and superficial cells. In most cases the eosinophil index exceeds the 50% limit. Cells are large with almost no folding, and are lying separately. The early luteal phase (5th–19th day) or the postovulatory phase causes a loss of turgor in which the edges of the cells roll up within 24 h after ovulation. The karyopyknotic index declines, and the eosinophil index eventually increases. On the 2nd and 3rd postovulatory day, typical alterations of the luteal phase begin to show: the rolling up and folding of cell edges, the cell agglomeration, and the formation of groups. Both karyopyknotic and eosinophil indexes decline. The medium luteal phase (25th–28th day) as well as the the late luteal phase leading to the premenstrual phase are characterized by the growth of small intermediate cells and leucocytes. The karyopyknotic and eosinophil indexes hardly ever exceed 10%. During menstruation the cell configuration is strewed with erythrocytes. There are large and small intermediate cells which are mainly cyanophilic and endometrial cells, leucocytes, and histiocytes.

Cytological Aspects of Cycle Diagnosis

If the karyopyknotic and eosinophil indexes of the differentiated tessellated epithelium cells during a cycle are plotted on a curve, a typical course of the hormonal fluctuation can be traced showing a peak between the 14th and 15th days and almost coinciding with the estrogen peak. The latter peak, however, precedes that of cytological indexes by 1–2 days, and individual fluctuations of the menstrual cycle must be taken into consideration. By means of cytology it is also possible to determine the date of ovulation. As a supplement to daily evaluations of hormonal and sonographic parameters, cytodiagnosis is a rather simple yet reliable method of determining ovulation by taking serial swabs.

Similarly to the estrogen peak the beginning of the preovulatory period is marked by a short and rapid increase in the karyopyknotic and eosinophil indexes. With relative predictability, ovulation can be expected to occur within 2–3, or at the latest 4 days. Ovulation is presumed to have taken place 12–24 h before the typical regressive indicators of the postovulatory phase become apparent. On the 1 day the karyopyknotic index remains unchanged while the eosinophil index may perhaps reach its peak. Over the next few days the characteristics of the luteal phase begin to develop.

There is a strong parallel between the cytological pattern and the alterions in the cervical mucus ("spinnbarkeit", which capacity refers to its capacity to be drawn into thererads, the ferning phenomenon, and the volume of cervical secretion), i.e., the maximum spinnbarkeit coincides with the highest differentiation of the vaginal epithelium. In case of persistence of the follicle, the karyopyknotic and eosinophil indexes remain unchanged.

A comparison between the basal body temperature curve and the cytological pattern reveals an increase on the last day of the preovulatory period (or occasionally even 4–6 days later). The temporal limits of the ovulation period can be defined as follows: a simultaneous decline of preovulatory alterations of the vaginal epithelium and of the cervical mucus leads to the assumption that ovulation took place within the last 24 h.

Cytological Alterations of the Vaginal Epithelium Induced by Exogenous Administration of Hormones and Other Drugs

The effects of the administration of sex hormone are evidenced either by increased cell proliferation and differentiation (the estrogen effect) or by a reduction in the degree of proliferation and differentiation of epithelium built up before (the gestagen effect). The latter is intensified, for example, by clomiphene treatment due to the ensuing increased desquamation of cells, loss of turgor, and a tendency of cell folding and agglomeration.

The typical cytological pattern of a smear preparation featuring the full impact of estrogen administration shows a maximum of superficial cells and a peak on the eosinophil and karyopyknotic indexes. Even with a significant increase in the administration of hormones the epithelium does not change. The vaginal epithelium produces similar reactions to androgenic agents such as gestagens.

Cytological Vaginal Alterations Caused by Ovulation-Inducing Medication

When ovulation is induced by clomiphene, hMG/hCG, or LH-RH, typical cytological alterations are found. During medication with clomiphene the antiestrogenic effect is observed on the 2nd and 3rd day of medication (development of small intermediate and parabasal cells). In 75% of all cases the preovulatory period commences after 5 to 8 days. Occurrence of ovulation is confirmed by the gestagen phase that follows immediately. Gonadotropin-induced ovulation (hMG/hCG) does not have a direct impact on the vaginal epithelium. The performance of the stimulated ovary indirectly determines the therapeutic success. If small intermediate and parabasal cells prevail, a hypogonadotropic release may have occurred, whereas under hypergonadotropic conditions, smears are atrophic. At the beginning of gonadotropic treatment, large intermediate cells are present 2–4 days after administration of hMG (increase of the maturation index). Daily examinations on alterations of the vaginal epithelium may facilitate determination of the doses required. If no reaction has set in after 5–7 days the average dose of 2 ampullae hMG will be increased, while a reduction may be necessary in cases of too rapid or intese proliferation of the epithelium.

During the preovulatory phase a rapid and significant increase of the karyopyknotic and eosinophil indexes is observed within 7–8 days of treatment, provided optimum doses are administered. Ovulation can be induced by additional injection of hCG. It is highly important to verify if other preovulatory changes such as the decline of the cellular folding and the tendency of differentiation are present. If these indicators (which may signify overstimulation) are observed, a gradual increase of the dosage is recommended. During the postovulatory phase the typical cytological gestagen effects is generated. High doses of LH-RH analogues may inhibit hyphophyseal gonadotropin secretion with subsequent suppression of estrogen production, resulting in atrophy of the vaginal epithelium.

The cyclic parameters in normal, pathological, and stimulated cycles are monitored by modern methods of hormonal analysis and ultrasound. Cytological follow-up of hormonal alterations of the vagina and examinations of the vaginal epithelium are a relatively simple and effective method for cycle diagnosis which is especially applicable as an alternative to expensive examinations by laboratories. Cytological determination of the ovulation date is considered a valuable complement to clinical and diagnostic evaluations by apparatus.

References

Bardin CW, Lipsett MB (1967) Testosterone and andostendione blood production rates in normal women and women with idiopathic hirsutism or polycystic ovaries. J Clin Invest 46:891
Bercovici B, Gron S, Pisanty S (1985) Vaginal and oral cytology of the menopause. Acta Cytol 29:805
Bettendorf G (1966) Ovarian stimulation in hyposectomized patients by human gonadotropins. Proceedings of the 5th world congress on fertility and sterility. International Congress Series 133, Excerpta Medica Foundation, Amsterdam, p 46
Bettendorf G, Breckwoldt M, Nörr K, Stegner HE (1964) Gravidität nach Hypophysensektomie und Behandlung mit hypohysärem Humangonadotropin. Dtsch Med Wochenschr 89:1952
Bettendorf G, Breckwoldt M, Czygan PJ (1965) Klinisch experimentelle Untersuchungen mit Clomiphen. Geburtsh Frauenheilkd 25:673
Bibbo M, Wied GL (1972) Hormonal cytology. In: Wied GL, Koss G, Reagan JW, Zajicek J (eds) Compendium on diagnostic cytology. International Academy of Cytology, Chicago, p 73
Boquoi E, Hammerstein J (1967) Vergleichende vaginalzytologische und hormonanalytische Untersuchungen bei zyklusgestörten Frauen unter ovulationsauslösender Behandlung. 3. Tagung der Deutschen Gesellschaft für angewandte Zytologie, Mannheim 1967
Boquoi E, Hammerstein J (1969) Discrepancies between colpocytologic and urinary steroid hormone excretion in women treated with clomiphen citrate or gonadotropins for anovulatory sterility. Acta Cytol 13:332
Dallenbach-Hellweg G (1969) Endometrium. Springer, Berlin Heidelberg New York
Dapunt O, Födisch HJ (1968) Die Wirkung von Östriol auf Uterus und Vagina der Frau. Geburtshilfe Frauenheilkd 28:1142
Diczfalusy E, Goebelsmann U, Johannisson E, Tillinger KG, Wide L (1969) Pituitary and ovarian function in women on continuous low dose progestagens; effect of chloermadinone acetate and norethisterone. Acta Endocrinol (Copenh) 62:679
Geiger W (1976) Hormonalalytik bei Zyklusstörungen. Diagnostik 9:470
Gitsch E, Seibert E (1954) Die glanduläre Hyperplasie des Endometriums im Spiegel der Cytologie des Scheidenepithels. Z Geburtsh Gynakol 140:266
Goldzieher JW, Green JA (1962) The polycystc ovar I. Clinical and histological features. J Clin Endocrinol 22:325
Grumbach M, van Wyck MJJ (1974) Disorders of sex differentiation. In: Williams RH (ed) Textbook of endocrinology. Saunders, Philadelphia
Hackelöer BJ, Fleming F, Robinson HP, Adam AH, Couts JRT (1979) Correlation of ultrasonic and endocrinologic assessment of human follicular development. Am J Obstet Gynecol 135:122
Haller U (1986) Die Steuerung des Menstruationszyklus. Gynakol Rundsch [Suppl] 1
Kaiser R (1969) Amenorrhoe. Gynakologe I:104
Kaiser R (1975) Hormonale Behandlung von Zyklusstörungen, 5th edn. Thieme, Stuttgart
Keller E, Dahlen HG, Friedrich E, Bohnet HG, Richter R, Joel EW, Schubring G, Klemt W, Staemmler HJ, Wyss HJ, Schnidler AE, Schneider HPG (1975) Human pituitary gonadotropin index. I. Standardized LRH-test. Criteria for evaluation of functional amenorrhea. J Clin Endocrinol 40:959

Kühndel K, Schürer G, Ebenroth G (1971) Wertigkeit der Farnteste, der Spinnbarkeit des Zervixsekretes und der Basaltemperatur zur Festlegung des Ovulationstermines. Berichte aus gynäkologischen Gesellschaften. Zentralbl Gynakol 93:976
Labhart A (1978) Klinik der inneren Sekretion. Springer, Berlin Heidelberg New York
Lauritzen C (1986) Die Behandlung der klimakterischen Beschwerden durch vaginale, rektale und transdermale Östrogensubstitution. Gynakologe 19:248
Lauritzen C (1987) Normale Entwicklung von der Kindheit zur Pubertät. In: Käser O, Friedberg V, Ober KG, Thomsen K, Zander J (eds) Gynäkologie und Geburtshilfe, vol I/1, 2nd edn. Thieme, Stuttgart
Loch EG, Tenhaeff D, Lohmeyer H (1970) Die zytohormonale Diagnostik bei verschiedenen oralen Kontrazeptiva. Geburtshilfe Gynakol 172:261
Marshall WA, Tanno JM (1969) Variations in pattern of pubertal changes in girls. Arch Dis Child 44:291
Nielsen J (1979) Anomalien der Geschlechtschromosomen. Dtsch Arztebl 13:865
Ober KG (1952) Aufwachtemperatur und Ovarialfunktion. Klin Wochenschr 30:357
Rjosk HK, von Werder K, Fahlbusch R (1976) Hyperprolaktinämische Amenorrhoe. Geburtshilfe Frauenheilkd 36:575
Roth OA (1953) Symposion cytologic. Heidelberg, cited in: Stoll P, Jaeger J (1954) In: Gynäkologische Zytologie, Symposium Heidelberg, 28 Febr und 1 March 1953. Steinkopf, Dresden
Schneider HPG, Bohnet HG (1977) Hyperprolaktinämische Amenorrhoe und Anovulation. Gynakologe 10:84
Vanderkerckhove D, Dhont M, van Eyck J (1975) Diagnostik value of the LH-releasing hormone stimulation test in functional amenorrhea. Acta Endocrinol (Copenh) 78:625
Wied GL (1953) Erfahrungen bei der Behandlung von Klimakterikerinnen mit Östrogen-Androgen-Gemischen. Arztl Wochenschr 8:712
Wied GL (1953) Der zytologische Ausstrichtyp der Patientinnen mit klimakterischen Ausfallbeschwerden. Zentralbl Gynakol 75:75
Wied GL, Bibbo M (1972) Hormonale Zytologie. 1. Fortbildungstagung für klinische Zytologie, Munich
Wied GL, Keebler CM (1967) Vaginal cytology of female children. Ann Ny Acad Sci 142:646
Yen SSC (1978) Chronic anovulation. In: Yen SSC, Jaffe RB (eds) Reproductive endocrinology. Saunders, Philadelphia
Zinser H-K (1957) Die Cytodiagnostik in der Gynäkologie. 2nd edn. VEB Fischer, Jena

Diagnosis and Treatment of Cervical Causes of Sterility

K. H. Broer

Possible cervical causes of sterility are:

- Functional dysregulation
- Morphological changes due to cervical laceration, cervical stenoses, polyps, conizations or cauterization
- Infection
- Effects of medication and toxins
- Local antigen-antibody reactions

Figures as to the proportion of cases of sterility with a cervical cause vary between 3% and 30%.

Diagnosis of Cervical Causes of Sterility

Since the cervix uteri is easily examined and its secretion easy to obtain, the primary examination of the cervix in the context of consulation for sterility should be undertaken by the patient's usual gynecologist; only after this is it appropriate for a more extensive examination to be carried out at the sterility centre.

Functional Dysregulation

The parameters that make up the diagnostic criteria of the "cervix factor" are assessed using various scores and recorded in a table. Of the methods introduced so far, Insler's Cervix Score has come to be the most widely used. This index is made up from the observation and semiquantitative evaluation of four parameters:

1. Arborization
2. Spinnbarkeit (a measure of viscosity)
3. Volume of cervical mucus
4. Cervical size

Each of these receives a score from 0 to 3 (Table 1). These scores are added together to give the cervix index, the maximun number of points (12) being found in the periovulatory phase. A special viscosity test may be added, as may measurement of the pH in the vaginal and cervical environment. Great-

Table 1 Insler's Cervix Score system

	Score 0	1	2	3
Mucus production	–	Slight	Moderate	Plentiful
Spinnbarkeit	–	Low, 1/4 length of vagina	Distinct, 1/2 length of vagina	Extreme, length of whole vagina
Arborization	–	Small signs in a few places	Marked and contiguous, branches beginning to form	Complete picture with branching in all areas
Cervical canal	Closed	Closed	Partly open	Wide open

Sum of scores = cervix indes (0–12)
Scoring of cervical function: 0–3, insufficient; 4–6 restricted; 7–9, good; 10–12, very good.

est reliability in the assessment of the preovulatory phase is achieved by combining cervical examinations with hormone analysis and cytological and phase contrast microscopic studies. For routine diagnostic purposes, however, the combination of basal temperature measurements and determination of the cervix index is usually sufficient. Scoring of the cervix factor is also important in the stimulation of ovulation. It is also of prime importance in treatment by homologous or heterologous insemination.
Jr

Technique for Determination of the Cervix Factor

First the width of the external orifice of the uterus is assessed. With the droplet of cervical secretion acting as a lens, it may be possible to see into the area of the internal orifice. During the speculum examination, under optimal preovulatory conditions, the drops of cervical secretion will also be seen cascading out of the cervix.

A tuberculin syringe should be used to take a sample of the cervical secretion. This is placed without a needle in the area of the external orifice, after the cervix has been cleaned with a cottonwool swab, and the secretion drawn off. Special aspiration syringes with rounded tips are also suitable, as are pipettes, polyethylene catheters, and special forceps. The cervical mucus forceps or else a narrow anatomical forceps allows material to be taken out of the external and internal area of the cervix under good visual control, without injury to the cervix, after which its "spinnbarkeit" can be estimated or measured with a ruler.

Many examiners take the mucus with a tuberculin syringe or similar aspiration instrument and measure the spinnbarkeit by drawing it out into a thread between two slides. Since the length of the thread depends on the method of measurement and the size of the drop of mucus, it is important always to use the same method. Spinnbarkeit values obtained by different examiners should be compared only if the examiners used the same method.

Instruments for automatic determination of the viscoelasticity of the cervical mucus are under development. These instruments measure the cohesive strength of the cervical mucus between two glass plates. A measurement value for the viscoelastic properties of the thread of mucus can be read off as a relative number directly on the apparatus.

Interactions Between Cervical Mucus and Spermatozoa

The next main stage in the cervical sterility diagnostics program is the interaction between cervical mucus and spermatozoa. Various in vivo and in vitro examination methods are available.

Postcoital Test (Sims-Huhner Test). The first study of postcoital cervical mucus was described by Sims, and in 1913 Huhner introduced the postcoital test (PCT) as a routine procedure in the diagnosis of sterility.

The PCT is an important test in the diagnosis of sterility for the following reasons:

- The cervical mucus together with the spermatozoa it contains are easily removed from the cervical area, and the morphology of the vagina and cervix can be assessed at the same time.
- The cervical index can be calculated within a short time of sampling and be compared with the basal temperature curve and, if carried out, the results of hormone analysis, particularly in patients undergoing medical stimulation treatment.
- Assessment of the spermatozoa that have penetrated into the cervical canal gives an indication of the quality of the ejaculate.
- The presence of spermatozoa in the cervical mucus gives evidence of successful coital or artificial insemination.
- The test gives an indication of the interaction between spermatozoa and mucus in the female genital tract.
- If other possible causes of sterility are ruled out, the PCT can give some diagnostic indication of the chances of fertility on the basis of the receptivity of the mucus towards the spermatozoa during the periovulatory phase of the cycle.

Technique of the PCT. The test should be carried out within 24 h after intercourse – ideally after 2 h. A positive result is quite often possible up to 48 h after. If the test is negative, repeats are essential until there are signs that ovulation has taken place. After material has been taken from the lower and upper parts of the cervical canal (the so-called fractionated PCT), the mucus is smeared onto a slide and examined for motile spermatozoa under the phase contrast microscope. The PCT is usually judged to be positive if more than 5–10 motile spermatozoa are shown per field of view at 400× magnification in preovulatory cervical mucus. Additional data relate to morphological characteristics, motility, and whether the spermatozoa have any tendency to agglutinate. If the PCT is repeatedly negative or inadequate, various authors recommend a homologous penetration test in vivo, with insemination either by means of a portio cap (cap test) or by intracervical deposition.

Practical Implications of PCT Results

- If motile spermatozoa are shown to be present in the cervical mucus, a normal insemination or coital technique may be assumed. This largely rules out psychogenic factors such as vaginismus, impotentia coeundi, etc., as causes of the sterility.
- Conception is more frequent when the cervix factor and PCT are good.
- An insufficient or negative PCT does not necessarily mean that there is no chance at all of conception.
- In many cases, merely the timing, the reflux counseling, and the regeneration of the vaginal fluor, resulting from the physician's encouragement of sexual intercourse, are enough to lead to successful pregnancy.
- The result of the PCT is closely linked to the gynecological and andrological parameters.
- Patients with a negative PCT have pathological cervix factor more than twice as often as those with a positive PCT. There is a clear correlation with the individual factors of the spermiogram. In couples with a negative PCT, oligospermia of the male partner is more frequently seen, which agrees with the greater number of spermatozoa that are morphologically abnormal or have impaired motility. However, the PCT cannot replace a spermiogram.
- The PCT can give an insight into interactions between the sperm and the cervical mucus, i.e. as regards immobilization and agglutination.
- Pregnancies after a negative PCT carry a significantly higher abortion rate than those after a positive PCT. This can mainly be explained by the greater frequency of pathological spermiograms. Whether a correlation exists between teratospermia and an increased rate of genetically related abortions is a subject under discussion.

Intrauterine PCT. The Sims-Huhner test can be extended to include material aspirated from the uterine cavity. The uterine secretion is aspirated postcoitally with a thin plastic probe and examined for motile spermatozoa. Owing to the filtering capacity of the cervical mucus, the uterine secretion may contain more progressively motile spermatozoa than the cervical mucus. In general, however, the prognostic value of the simple PCT is not greatly increased by this more complicated method.

Postcoital Douglas Test. Another fairly conclusive assessment of penetration ability is given by Douglas puncture. This test is regarded as positive if spermatozoa can be shown to be present in the peritoneal fluid. However, the time and effort involved in the test, the risk of injuring the patient, and its possible painfulness all militate against its suitability as a routine technique. If a laparotomy is being performed to investigate the tube factor, a Douglas lavage can be carried out with a portio cap in place and the aspirate be examined for motile spermatozoa. This procedure should also only be employed if the purpose of the laparotomy is to assess the tube factor.

In Vitro Penetration Test. If the Sims-Huhner test is repeatedly negative, a practicable in vitro penetration test is indicated. The following may be used:

Miller-Kurzrok Test (Slide Test). A drop of cervical mucus and a drop of ejaculate are placed alongside each other on a slide; they should not touch until the cover slip has been put on. Within a few minutes, finger-like phalanges develop from the seminal fluid into the mucus. These channels are filled with spermatozoa, which penetrate the mucus through the tips of the "fingers". At first only a few spermatozoa enter the mucus, then the mass follow, until they meet resistance from cell particles, leukocytes, etc. This finger-like formation is not specific to the sperm-mucus interaction, but is a general physical phenomenon observed when two biological media of differing viscosity meet. If plenty of spermatozoa penetrate clear mucus that has a high spinnbarkeit and a low cell content, and if they have not lost motility or shown any tendency to agglutination after 15–20 min, the test is judged to be normal.

Crossover Penetration Test. If the simple Miller-Kurzrok test is negative, it can be performed as a "crossover" test using material from two fertile donors to interact with that from the couple being examined. That is, the woman's mucus is tested with fertile donor sperm and her partner's sperm with preovulatory mucus from a fertile female donor. This shows whether the insufficient penetration and interaction are due to the mucus or to the sperm.

This test can also be taken further with the spermcervical mucus contact test. For this, one drop of seminal fluid is carefully placed on one of cervical mucus (or vice versa) and the two mixed together. With normally fertile ejaculate and good preovulatory mucus, the progressive motility is reduced by at the most 30%. The migration speed of the spermatozoa should be unchanged even after half an hour. By contrast, according to Kremer, in the presence of agglutinins 80% of the spermatozoa display a shaking movement (the shaking phenomenon) without any progressive migration. Evidently the antibodies to the spermatozoa cause the latter to adhere to the glycoprotein micelles of the cervical mucus. This test is indicated if an immunological cause of the sterility is suspected, in either the man or the woman. The results correlate well with the serum antispermatozoa antibody titre in both partners and with capillary migration tests.

Kramer's In Vitro Capillary Penetration Test. Kramer's capillary test allows the speed and depth of penetration of the spermatozoa into the cervical mucus to be quantitatively and qualitatively assessed with a fairly high degree of accuracy.

To perform the test, the cervical mucus is drawn up into a round or flat glass capillary tube and examined simultaneously for quantity, spinnbarkeit, pH value, microscopic and macroscopic dirt, arborization, and any bacterial contamination. The capillary tube is then dipped into a glass container filled with ejaculate, and after 1 h incubation at 22°C the depth of penetration is measured under the microscope against a rule.

After a 1-h penetration period, plenty of motile spermatozoa are found in the mucus in a 7-cm length of the capillary. Smears taken at various distances up the tube can be assessed comparatively and in regard to cell morphology. The test is a useful adjunct to the spermiogram in giving an objective measure of motility and progressive penetration capacity. Good penetration means at the same time that the cervical mucus is of good quality. In addition, the filtering effect of the mucus can be evaluated from the percentage of morphologically normal versus pathological spermatozoa before and after the test (Broer 1976, Insler 1977).

A crossover version of this test is also possible, like that of the slide test, to give an indication of whether the cause of the cervical sterility is andrological or gynecological. Overall, the in vitro penetration test has an important place in the diagnosis of cervical sterility.

Other Diagnostic Techniques

Morphological changes of the cervix are normally diagnosed on the basis of the results of examination with the speculum or a cervical probe. Infections are diagnosed by examining the secretion for pathogenic germs, if necessary with additional culture. Reactions to medication or toxins usually also impair the penetration ability of the spermatozoa; the tests described above for determination of functional dysregulation can give a probable indication of whether this has occurred. Diagnostic tests for local antigen-antibody reactions are undertaken if the penetration tests described have not already identified the immunological factor.

Treatment of Cervical Causes of Sterility

The causes of cervical sterility are various and require treatment that is tailored correspondingly. It may be asssumed that the numerically most important cause of pathological interaction between spermatozoa and the cervical mucus lies in the wide spectrum of andrological disorders. This means that the primary target of treatment is usually andrological. One important treatment option in cases of abnormal transport of spermatozoa through the cervix is homologous insemination, i.e. transfer of the male partner's sperm. The indications from the andrological point of view are discussed in Chap. 22, D. 247. Homologous insemination is also a possible method of treatment for cervical sterility, especially for couples with repeatedly pathological PCT results.

The chances that the woman will achieve fertilization with her partner's ejaculate by homologous insemination vary according to the degree of disorder shown by the pathological in vivo or in vitro penetration test. Among cases where the reasons for homologous insemination were purely andrological, success rates between 20% and 40% have been cited. Where the reasons were gynecological, success rates have been between 12% and 20%. Exact comparisons of success rates are difficult, since in many cases the reasons for the procedure are a multifactorial combination of andrological and gynecological causes.

Treatment of a Pathological Functional Cervix Factor

A pathological cervix factor in the preovulatory phase is caused either by impaired follicle maturation or impaired reactivity of the receptive target organs to the effects of estrogen. Treatment is with oral ovulation stimulators, oral estrogens, and gonadotropins in the form of HMG-HCG therapy.

In cases of impaired reactivity, systemic or local estrogen treatment can improve the cervical mucus. Various estrogens may be used with success:

- Ethinylestradiol
- Mestranol
- Conjugated estrogens
- Estriol

Local application of estrogen-containing ovula or ointments intravaginally and in front of the portio has proved an effective treatment. For oral treatment, low doses of 10–20 µg ethinylestradiol (Progynon C) can be given on the 5th–12th days of the cycle (assuming a typical 28-day cycle) to begin with. If monitoring of the cervix factor within a cycle during treatment does not show adequate improvement, higher doses may be given. Administration of 1 or 2 mg estriol (Ovestin) may also improve the cervix factor. This treatment is also appropriate for patients undergoing oral ovulation stimulation with clomifen, for treatment of a poor cervix score caused by anti-estrogenic side effects of the clomifen treatment.

Mechanical or Operative Treatment

In patients with cervical laceration that has resulted in a poor cervix factor, Emmet's operation may be successful. In treatment of an ectopic portio, care should be taken that the removal of glandular area does not result in large-scale destruction of the secreting areas of the cervix. For cervical stenosis, dilatation with Hegar dilators or *Laminaria* stems is the usual treatment. Treatment with laser coagulation has also been described as successful. Overall, portioplastic procedures as treatment for cervical sterility carry varying prospects of success. A pathological cervix factor is seen after conization in about 25% of cases. In young women of child-bearing age who wish to have children, care should therefore be taken to make the conization shallow and not too high, to avoid a negative effect on the cervix factor. Generally, caution should be exercised in the use of electrocoagulation or conization to treat refractory cervical fluor in women who wish to have children.

Treatment of Infections

Contamination of the cervical secretion by pathogens such as bacteria, fungi, viruses, or *Trichomonas* causes a change in sperm migration due to the contaminated barrier of cervical mucus. Our own in vitro penetration tests have shown that contamination of the cervical secretion with *E. coli* and other bacteria results in a reduction of spermatozoic migration that correlates with the density of the contamination. Insler (1977) also found a reduction of spermatozoic migration in the presence of contamination of the cervical secretion by infectious pathogens. The impairment of spermatozoic migration is therefore due more to the mechanical obstacle of the density of the bacteria than to the bacterial toxins as such (Broer et al. 1977a). Treatment of infection-related disorders of spermatozoic migration in the uterine cervix should be tailored on the basis of an assessment of the secretion and testing out in the antibiogram. Local antibiotics, fungistatics, and trichomonacides have all been used successfully. In refractory cases, oral or parenteral treatment is indicated.

Elimination of Noxious Substances

The literature yields numerous indications based on experience that the cervix factor can be affected by medications and noxious substances. For this season, excessive use of various substances such as alcohol or high cigarette consumption should be avoided by patients with a pathological cervix factor.

Closing Remarks

The diagnosis and treatment of the cervix factor is of central importance in sterility counseling. Treatment of a pathological cervix factor has a relatively good prospect of success and gives a better prognosis than treatment of cases where the disease or disorder is purely andrological. Because the cervix is accessible and easy to examine, treatment of the cervix factor is a rewarding task for the gynecologist engaged in sterility counseling.

References

Alexander N (1981) Evaluation of male infertility with an in vitro cervical mucus penetrations test. Fertil Steril 36:201

Asch RH et al (1985) A modern treatment for infertile couples: gift. Am Fert Soc Progr Suppl 18

Broer KH (1981) Diagnostik und Therapie zervikaler Sterilitätsursachen. In: Kaiser R, Schumacher GFB (eds) Menschliche Fortpflanzung. Thieme, Stuttgart

Broer KH (1978) Improvement of motility and morphology of human spermatozoa by filtration assay. In: Emperaire JC, Audebert A (eds) 1st International Symposium on Artificial Insemination: Homologous and Male Subfertility. Bordeaux, p. 188

Broer KH, Winkhaus I (1978) Die Bedeutung des Postcoitaltestes in der Sterilitätsberatung. Fortschr Med 96:351

Broer KH, Hirschhäuser C, Kaiser R (1975a) Morphology of human spermatozoa before and after migration through cervical mucus in vitro. IRCS Med Sci 3:145

Broer KH, Hirschhäuser C, Kaiser R (1976) Filterfunktion der Cervix uteri. Fortschr Fertilitätsforsch 3:36

Broer KH, Dauber U, Kaiser R (1977a) A filtering method of cleaning up spermatozoa in cases of asthenospermia. Fertil Steril 28:335

Broer KH, Schaal P, Siepel G (1977b) In vitro investigations about influence of bacterial infection upon spermatozoa migration through cervical mucus. Fertil Steril 18:397

Broer KH, Knieps U, Kaiser R (1978) Verbesserung der Spermatozoenmotilität und Reproduzierbarkeit im in vitro-Penetrationstest. Fortschr Sterilitätsforsch

Broer KH, Teepe W, Kaiser R (1975b) Untersuchungen zur Filterfunktion der Cervix uteri. Geburtsh Frauenheilkd 35:697

Davajan V, Kulinitake M (1969) Fractional in vivo and in vitro examination of postcoital cervical mucus in the human. Fertil Steril 20:197

Davajan V, Nakamura R, Kharma K (1970) Spermatozoan transport in cervical mucus. Obstet Gynec Surv 25:1

Eggert-Kruse W, Runnebaum B (1989) Clinical significance of crossed in vitro sperm-cervical mucus penetration test in infertility investigation. Fertil Steril 6:1032

Giner J, Merino G, Luna J, Aznar R (1974) Evaluation of the Sims-Huhner postcoital test in fertile couples. Fertil Steril 25:145

Glass RG, Mrouheh A (1967) The postcoital test and semen analysis. Fertil Steril 18:314

Herwitt JJ, Steptoe PC (1985) Treatment of idiopathic infertility, cervical mucus hostality and male infertility. Fertil Steril 44:350

Insler V (1977) Evaluation and treatment of cervical mucus diseases leading to infertility. In: Mucus in health and disease 1977. p. 477

Insler V, Melmed H, Eichenbrenner I, Serr D, Lunenfeld B (1972) The cervical score. Int J Gynec Obstet 10:223

Kaiser R (1977) Anatomie and Physiologie der Fortpflanzung. In: Martius G (ed) Lehrbuch der Geburtshilfe. Thieme, Stuttgart

Kremer J (1965) A simple sperm penetration test. Int H Fertil 10:201

Kremer J, Jager S (1992) The significance of antisperm antibodies for sperm cervical mucus interaction. Hum Repr 7:781

Miller EG Jr, Kurzrok R (1932) Biochemical studies of human semen III. Factors effecting migration of sperm through the cervix. Am J Obstet Gynec 24:19

Moghissi KS (1976) Postcoital test: physiologic basis, technique, and interpretation Fertil Steril 27:2

Moghissi KS, Darich D, Lebine J et al (1964) Mechanism of spermigration. Fertil Steril 15:15

Perloff WH, Steinberger E (1973) In vivo penetration of cervical musus bei spermatozoa. Fertil Steril 14:231

Rabe T, Runnebaum B (1994) Funktionsteste und Untersuchungsmethoden in der gynäkologischen Endokrinologie und Fortpflanzungsmedizin. In: Runnebaum B, Rabe T (eds) Fortpflanzungsmedizin. Springer, Berlin Heidelberg New York, p 29

Scott JZ, Nakamura RM, Mutch J, Davajan V (1977) The cervical factor in fertility: diagnosis and treatment. Fertil Steril 28:12

Semm K (1967) A new instrument for artifical insemination. Excerpta Medica, New York p 593 (International Congress Series, vol 33)

Sims JM (1968) Illustrations of the value of the microscope in the treatment of the sterile condition. Br Med J II:465

Tresway D (1976) Interpretations and significance of the fractional postcoital test. Am J Obstet Gynec 124:352

van der Veen H, Al-Hasani S, Diedrich K (1990) Neue Aspekte der Inseminationsbehandlung. In: Diedrich K (ed) Neue Wege in der Diagnostik und Therapie der Sterilität. Bücherei des Frauenarztes, vol 25. Enke, Stuttgart

Whitelaw MJ (1950) Use of the cervical cap to increase fertility in cases of oligospermy. Fertil Steril 1:33

World Health Organisation (1992) WHO laboratory manual for the examination of human semen and sperm-cervical mucus interaction, 3rd edn. Cambridge University, Press Syndicate, Cambridge

Fallopian Tube Physiology and Its Clinical Implications

E. SARIDOGAN, S.D. MAGUINESS and O. DJAHANBAKHCH

The fallopian tube has many active roles in the process of reproduction, which include ovum pick-up, transportation of both sets of gametes to the site of fertilisation within well-defined time limits, providing an environment in which final gamete maturation and fertilisation take place, and maintenance of the gametes and the pre-embryo, which is delivered to the uterine cavity at a time when conditions are optimal for nidation. Furthermore, the sperm and pre-embryo, which differ antigenically from the mother, are not attacked by the immune system, which differentiates between them and pathogens. The mechanisms by which all these complex processes are controlled are not all well understood, and currently the principial means of assessing tubal function is to observe tubal patency and normal morphological characteristics at endoscopy (Maguiness et al. 1992a).

Physiological study of the fallopian tube has been hampered by its relative inaccessibility. Our knowledge of the fallopian tube physiology comes from several sources:

1. Animal studies
2. Studies on human fallopian tube specimens removed at operation
3. Studies of the tubal fluid obtained by tubal cannulation
4. In vitro short-term explant system or epithelial cell culture of the fallopian tube
5. Endoscopic, electrophysiologic and telemetric studies on the fallopian tube

All these methods have their inherent advantages and disadvantages; therefore, when the data from these studies are analysed, limitations of the methodology have to be kept in mind.

Morphological Changes in the Fallopian Tube

Evidence of changes in the morphology of the tubal eptihelium during the ovarian cycle suggests that there may be an alteration in the tubal environment in response to ovarian steroids. This idea is supported by the recent observation of variation in the endoscopic appearance in human tubal lumen during ovarian cycle and changes in tubal protein secretion and fluid content during the ovarian cycle in both animal and human studies.

Age-Related Changes in Morphology

The fallopian tube has oestrogen receptors, so macroscopic changes with age tend to be associated with alteration in the circulating level of oestrogens (Robertson and Landgren 1975). The event of the menopause is associated with a reduction of circulating levels of 17β-oestradiol. Changes in the tube tend to parallel those in the uterus, with an overall reduction in both the tubal length and diameter (Soriero 1978). The first reported studies on mucosal changes were those of Voinant (1900), who observed that cilia were absent during early foetal life, appearing in small numbers just before birth. Further light and electron microscopy studies have subsequently revealed that there are very few fully developed epithelial cells in the foetal oviduct in the first trimester of pregnancy. Both ciliated and non-ciliated cells have been recognised. Postmenopausally, Voinot (1900) reported the epithelium to be flat and atrophic, buth with cilia still present. Further studies have failed to agree on the rate and extent of these changes (Edman 1983; Gaddum-Rosse et al. 1975; Soriero 1978; Voet 1983; Patek et al. 1972b). Patek et al. (1972b) report little change in the epithelial cells for the first 15 years after the menopause. Thirty years postmenopausally, they report that there are still numerous ciliated cells in the distal portion of the tube, but that they are much reduced in the isthmus. At this stage, secretory cells are flat and atrophic, the villi are small and there is no evidence of secretion. It has been suggested that sufficient oestrogen production may be present postmenopausally to maintain ciliated cells and that oestrogen therapy may prevent or even reverse deciliation (Donnez et al. 1983).

Alterations in the tubal musculature are similar to those of myometrium, with growth during puberty associated wit the increase in circulating levels of oestrogen. After the menopause, secondary to the reduction of circulating oestrogens, there is muscular atrophy. This results in the decrease of average length and diameter of the tube. Contractile activity in the fallopian tube has been reported at birth (Stegner 1961). Changes in the character of both electrical and mechanical activity reflect the hormonal status during the menstrual cycle (Talo and Pulkkinen 1982). After the menopause, Talo and Pulkkinen (1984) report that electrical activity ceases first either in the isthmus near the uterus or at the ampullary-isthmic junction.

Changes in Morphology During the Ovarian Cycle

The mucosa of the oviduct is extremely sensitive to circulating levels of ovarian steroids. In the late follicular phase of the oestrus or menstrual cycle, the tissues of the mucosa become greatly distended as a result of the indirect effect of oestrogens on mucosal lymphatics. This phenomenon is particularly prominent in the lower isthmus and uterotubal junction just before ovulation (Anderson 1972, 1928; Lee 1928).

Patek et al. (1972a) reported ciliated cells of the human tubal mucosa to be reduced in height during the menstrual phase. The height is increased in the proliferative phase when the ciliated cells were covered by well-shaped, regularly distributed microvilli. The maximum height was reached in the periovulatory period, with the cells becoming broader and lower during the luteal phase. There is disagreement about the occurrence of specific ultrastructural changes in ciliated cells during the menstrual cycle. However, there may be an increase in the number and size of cytoplasmic granules and mitochondria as the cycle progresses (Fredricks 1986).

In the human oviduct, there is never complete shedding and regeneration of cilia as seen in the infundibulum of the rhesus monkey oviduct (Brenner 1969). Verhage et al. (1979) have reported cyclical changes in the cilia of ampullary and fimbrial cells of the human tube. They report deciliation of 12%–14% of cells during the luteal phase, with regeneration in the early follicular phase of the next cycle. During the menstrual phase the cilia appear "droopy." In the follicular phase, the cilia become erect and vigorous. The rate of beat of the cilia is greatest at, or just after, ovulation. This suggests it is related to circulating levels of ovarian steroids. At this time of the ovarian cycle, the strokes of the cilia in the fimbrial portion of the tube are synchronised and oriented in the direction of the ostium (Borell et al. 1957; Blandau 1969), while cilia in the ampulla beat towards the ampullary-isthmic junction (Blandau and Verdugo 1976).

In humans, secretory cells of the tubal epithelium generally appear low during the menstrual phase. However, some appear in clusters, are round or sphere-shaped and bulge into the tubal lumen (Patek et al. 1972a). These features are retained from the late luteal phase of the previous menstrual cycle. During the follicular phase, secretory cells increase in height and are covered with tall, well-shaped, regularly distributed, microvilli. In the periovulatory period, the microvilli become swollen and adhere to each other, forming tuft-like formations. The luteal phase is associated with the tall secretory cells bulging into the tubal lumen, creating an irregular epithelial border. The microvilli of these cells are less evenly distributed on their surface (Patek et al. 1972a).

These changes are associated with ultrastructural alterations which reflect changing secretory activity (Ludwig and Metzer 1976; Pauerstein and Eddy 1979b). At the onset of the proliferative phase, the Golgi apparatus is compact, the endoplasmic reticulum limited and the mitochondria diminished. These structures become more prominent during the follicular phase and about cycle day 10 granules of ribonucleoprotein (Palade granules) become numerous. By the end of the follicular phase, secretory granules appear beneath the cell membrane adjacent to the lumen. In the luteal phase, the endoplasmic reticulum dilates and secretory droplets and granules appear, while the Golgi apparatus expands and the mitochondria decrease in number. Some secretory cells rupture and release their contents during the midluteal phase. Liposomes appear in increased numbers in the luteal phase. Secretory activity during the menstrual cycle is more prominent in the isthmus than in the ampulla (Ludwig and Metzer 1976; Pauerstein and Eddy 1979b).

The presence of intercalary cells has been noted more often in the luteal phase of the cycle, supporting the idea that they are exhausted secretory cells (Fredricks 1986).

There is no information available on changes in basal cells during the ovarian cycle. The contractile activity of the lamina muscularis has been reported to have cyclic variation (Seckinger and Snyder 1926; Breiphohl 1938).

The highest frequency of contractions is reported to occur in the proliferative and periovulatory phases. These cyclic changes have been correlated with sex steroid levels (Erb 1969; Lindblom et al. 1980; Helm et al. 1982b). The direction of spread of electrical and mechanical activity has been studied in humans (Talo and Pulkkinen 1982). The probability of spread towards the uterus has been seen to vary both with the location along the tube and the day of the menstrual cycle.

Vascular Supply

It has been reported, from observation on the reproductive tracts of pigs, sheep and dogs at laparotomy, that the capillary bed and larger blood vessels of the fimbria and ampulla become highly engorged near the time of ovulation (Hunter 1988a). In humans, we have demonstrated changes in the blood vessels of the mucosal folds at salpingoscopy. Patients in the periovulatory phase of the menstrual cycle had highly reflective blood vessels in the mucosal folds (Figs. 1, 2). This phenomenon could be due to alteration of the secretion of the ovarian steroids at the periovulatory phase (Maguiness and Djahanbakhch 1992).

In the follicular phase, the mucosal arterioles begin to become coiled. This process continues to progress through the luteal phase, becoming maximal at the time of menstruation (Koritké et al. 1968a b; Gillet and Leissner 1967; Gillet and Koritké (1967). These changes are most pronounced in the fimbria (Koritké et al. 1968 a, b). The mucosal venules become markedly dilated at midcycle and maximally dilated at menstruation (Koritke e al. 1968 a, b; Gillet and Leissner 1967).

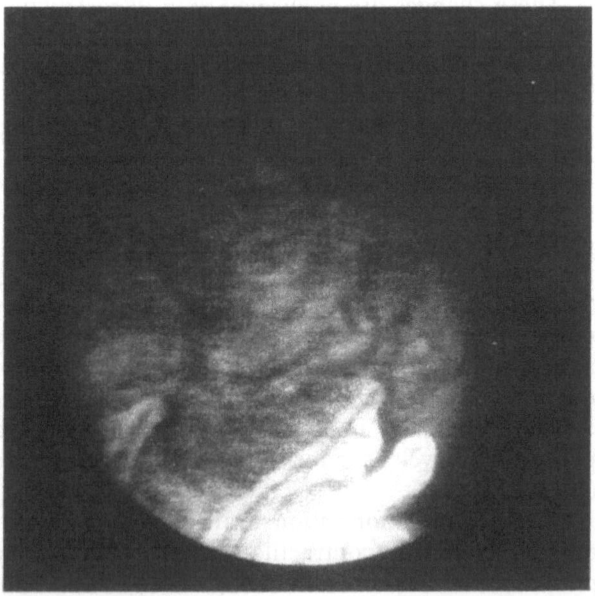

Fig. 1. Brightly reflective blood vessel walls seen in the mucosal folds during the late follicular phase. ×40

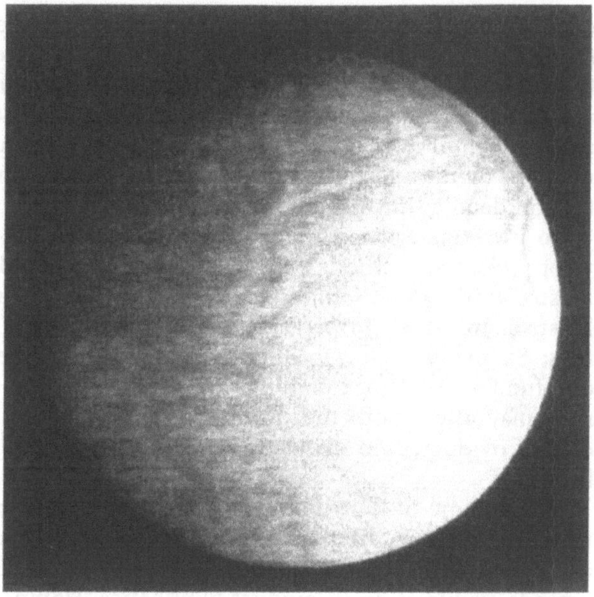

Fig. 2. Mucosal blood vessels. ×40

Lymphatic Drainage

Changes in the lymphatic system during the oestrus cycle were studied by Anderson (1927b), who reported that, in the pig oviduct, lymphatic vessels adjacent to the tube were largest in the follicular phase, while those at the uterotubal junction and proximal uterine horn were dilated in the luteal phase.

Innervation

Oestrogen and progesterone appear to influence the way in which the tubal musculature, via the adrenoceptors, responds to the sympathetic neurotransmitter, and they can also directly affect the function of adrenergic nerves (Helm et al. 1982a). α-Adrenergic receptors in the smooth muscle cells of the fallopian tube are potentiated under the influence of oestrogen, while β-adrenergic receptors are potentiated by increasing levels of progesterone (Hunter 1977).

Environment of the Oviduct Lumen

Fluid can be detected in the oviduct lumen throughout the reproductive years. The volume and composition of the fluid varies according to the levels of circulating gonadal steroids. At a molecular level, production of oviductal fluid depends on a selective flux of molecules which occurs from the mucosal and serosal surfaces of the epithelium to the adjacent fluids and vice versa (Leese 1988). Contributions to the composition of oviduct fluid may also come from the contents of graafian follicles released at ovulation, peritoneal fluid, reflux of fluid from the uterine cavity (Hunter 1988b) and the embryo (Nieder et al. 1987). Oviduct fluid provides an environment in which gametes are transported, undergo final maturation, fertilisation takes place and the resulting embryo is transported to the uterus. The role of the various components of oviduct fluid in these processes has become the subject of systematic and detailed investigation.

To investigate the oviduct environment, various workers have tried to develop effective methods of collecting oviduct fluid (Bishop 1956; Clewe and Mastroianni 1960; Hamner and Williams 1965; Mastroianni and Jones 1965; Mastroianni et al. 1970; Feigelson and Kay 1972; Lippes et al. 1972; Riddick 1975; Shams et al. 1977; Oliphant 1986). All of the collection methods have one fundamental shortcoming; the presence of the cannula in the oviduct lumen may affect both the production and constitution of secretions. All studies of oviduct fluid using this methodology should be interpreted with this in mind.

The volume of fluid in the oviduct lumen has been studied in many mammalian species in different hormonal states. The largest volumes of fluid are associated with high circulating levels of oestrogens and are correlated with periods of dilatation in oviduct lymphatics. Hamner (1973) demonstrated that in ovariectomised rabbits there was a 75% decrease in oviductal fluid production. He also demonstrated that when progesterone and oestrogen were administered to these rabbits, the volume of fluid produced was less than those receiving oestrogen treatment alone (Hamner and Fox 1969). This suggests that oestrogen has a positive effect on oviductal fluid production, while progesterone has a negative effect. Lippes et al. 1972; Lippes 1979) reported that during the menstrual cycle in humans the largest volumes of fluid were obtained in the periovulatory phase, with an average of 3.9 ml/24 h.

In mammalian species without an ovarian bursa, most oviductal fluid flow is from the ampulla into the peritoneal cavity. Hamner (1973) reported that this accounted for 90% of flow in rabbits, sheep and cows. At the time of embryo transport from the fallopian tube through the uterotubal junction to the uterus, Belve and McDonald (1969) reported that most of the reduced volume of oviduct fluid was moving into the uterine cavity.

Factors involved in determining the direction of flow include the currents created by epithelial ciliary movements, muscular stricture of the isthmus and uterotubal junction and oedema of the isthmic mucosa, all of which are regulated by gonadal steroid hormones. Oedema of the isthmic mucosa is considered to be the principal factor (Hunter 1988b). The oedema arises in response to oestradiol and decreases after ovulation in association with increasing circulating levels of progesterone. Hunter (1988b) also restates the possibility of a microflow system close to the epithelium and within the groves between the mucosal folds, where the direction of flow may differ from the bulk of the flow.

It is generally reported that sodium, magnesium and phosphate have concentrations in human tubal fluid similar to those found, in blood plasma (Borland et al. 1977, 1980; Lippes et al. 1972). However, Lippes (1979) has reported lower values for magnesium and phosphate in tubal fluid. The calcium concentration of tubal fluid is less than that of serum in both rhesus monkeys and humans, but its level increases after ovulation (Mastroianni et al. 1973; Lippes et al. 1972; Lippes 1979).

Both potassium and chloride have higher concentrations in human tubal fluid (Borland et al. 1980). Maas et al. (1977) reported that bicarbonate levels were above those of serum and showed an increase from 35 m*M* to 90 m*M* between the proliferative and luteal phases of the menstrual cycle. The measured pH rose suddenly from 7.1–7.3 during the proliferative phase to 7.5–7.8 at ovulation and remained at this level during the luteal phase. In rhesus monkeys, Maas et al. (1976) have reported much lower oxygen tensions (<10 mmHg) during the proliferative phase, with a rise to blood levels at ovulation persisting through the luteal phase.

Steroid Receptors

The fallopian tube is able to concentrate oestradiol and progesterone to levels several times those found in circulating plasma, indicating that high-affinity tissue-binding proteins or receptors are present (Batra et al. 1980; Devoto et al. 1980).

The fallopian tube is considered to be under the influence of steroids acting through specific receptors which are comparable with those in other parts of the genital tract. During the menstrual cycle, there are changes in the ratio of the concentrations of total cytoplasmic oestradiol and progesterone receptors to nuclear oestradiol and progesterone receptors in the human oviduct (Pollow et al. 1981). Early in the follicular phase oestradiol receptor concentrations are high, mostly in the cytoplasm and untranslocated. Late in the follicular phase, when the plasma oestradiol rises prior to ovulation, the proportion of oestradiol receptors translocated to the nucleus rises (Punnonen and Lukola 1981; Pollow et al. 1982; Pino et al. 1982). At the same time there s a high concentration of progesterone receptors in the cytoplasm. After ovulation, the plasma progesterone rises while both oestradiol and progesterone receptors fall, and the concentration of receptors is higher in the nucleus than in the cytoplasm (Pollow et al. 1981).

There is asymmetry of oestrogen receptor concentration at the fimbrial end of the oviducts after ovulation, being much lower on the side of the corpus luteum (Flickinger et al. 1977). The same workers could not show a statistically significant difference in receptor concentrations in other sections of the oviduct. They also noted that the discrepancy between fimbrial and ampullary oestrogen receptor concentrations was greater in ovulatory cycles as opposed to those controlled by oral contraceptives, where the source of progesterone is systemic rather than local.

The changes in distribution of nuclear and cytoplasmic receptors in the oviduct during the ovarian cycle happen in advance of those in the uterus (Pollow et al. 1981). This may represent different responsiveness by uterus and oviduct or a different steroid influence, as suggested by evidence for the effects of ovarian hormones in peritoneal fluid.

Fallopian Tube Proteins

In animal studies granules with staining characteristics of acidic mucopolysaccarides or mucoproteins appear to be under the influence of exogenous oestrogen and are released when progesterone is administered (Greenwald 1958; Brower and Anderson 1969; Lambert et al. 1973). Using immunohistochemical localisation and radioimmunoassay, evidence has been reported for the presence of pregnancy-associated placental protein A (PAPP-A; Sjöberg et al. 1986) and placental protein-5 (Butzow 1989) in the fallopian tube. This method, refined by the use of gel filtration, has also identified the presence of placental protein-10 (Tiitinen et al. 1986) and a major secretory protein of the endometrium, placental protein-14 (PP14; also called endometrial protein-15, pregnancy-associated endometrial a_2-globulin and progesterone-associated endometrial protein, PEP; Julkunen et al. 1986), which is reported to have immunological properties (Bolton et al. 1987; Pockley et al. 1988). The presence of PP14 has also been reported using monoclonal antibodies and immunohistochemical localisation (Waites et al. 1990). All of these proteins are present in serum and may reach the tubal secretions from that compartment. Major studies on the proteins of the fallopian tube have been reviewed by us (Maguiness and Djahanbakhch 1992).

During the ovarian cycle, tissue content of both PAPP-A and PP14 is reported to vary. PAPP-A content was higher in the follicular phase (Sjöberg et al. 1986). PP14 protein tissue content was found to be higher in the luteal phase of the menstrual cycle, but this difference only reached statistical significance in the fimbrial region of the tube (Julkunen et al. 1986). However, we (Maguiness et al. 1993a) recently demonstrated that PP14 synthesis and secretion did not show any significant difference during the ovarian cycle.

In a study concurrently comparing de novo synthesis of proteins by different anatomical sections of the fallopian tube and endometrium, we noted two proteins with molecular masses of 17 and 25 kDa, synthesised by each section of the fallopian tube, but not by endometrium form the same source or controls (Maguiness et al. 1993b). In studies of fallopian tube mucosa from postmenopausal women, the 17-kDa protein was absent, suggesting that its synthesis may have some dependence on ovarian function.

Gamete Transport in the Fallopian Tube

The human ovum, released when the follicle ruptures, is surrounded by granulosa cells, which are exposed to the cilia of the fimbrial epithelium. The activity of cilia depends on the hormonal environment and is greatest just after ovulation (Borell et al. 1957; Blandau 1973), when the direction of cilial beat is towards the isthmic-ampullary junction (Blandau and Gaddum-Rosse

1974). The majority of tubal fluid flows in the direction of the peritoneal cavity during the periovulatory period (Hammer 1973), so it would seem that the ability to "grip" the ovum and the direction of ciliary beat are important. However, patients with Kartagener's syndrome become pregnant, and this suggests that the actions of the cilia are not a functional necessity (Pauerstein and Eddy 1979a). The time taken for the ovum to reach the isthmic-ampullary junction is more than 30 h in humans (Croxatto and Oritz 1975; Pauerstein 1975; Eddy et al. 1976), while it is only a few minutes in most other mammalian species (Harper 1961; Blandau 1969).

The time taken for sperm to travel from the vagina to the fallopian tube may be a few minutes or hours (Thibault 1973; Overstreet and Katz 1977; Hunter et al. 1983). Once in the oviduct, sperm move towards the ampullary-isthmic junction, possibly assisted by a combination of ciliary activity and oviduct muscle contractions, which in the periovulatory period are directed towards this region (Blandau and Goddum-Rosse 1974).

After fertilisation at the isthmic-ampullary junction, the embryo is transported across the isthmus to the uterine cavity. The duration of time spent at the isthmic-ampullary junction and the rate of transport across the isthmic region is species specific and may reflect requirements for species survival and different endocrine environments in the proliferative phase of the ovarian cycle. Human embryos are reported to remain in the ampulla for up to 72 h after fertilisation, followed by rapid transport across the isthmus to the uterine cavity (Croxatto and Ortiz 1975), arriving approximately 80 h after ovulation (Pauerstein and Eddy 1979a).

Conclusion

In this chapter, we review in brief the physiological events in the fallopian tube. These dynamic alterations occurring in morphology, lymphatics, muscle, vessels receptors, tubal environment and tubal secretions are influenced by ovarian steroids. These effects become silent and inefficient with cessation of ovarian function. Similarly, one would expect alterations and disturbances following tubal disorders. Parallel studies in both normal and fallopian tubes are necessary in order to increase our knowledge and understanding of fallopian tube function and for discovery of tubal markers to assess the functional capacity of the fallopian tube.

References

Anderson DH (1927a) The rate of passage of the mammalian ovum through various portions of the Fallopian tube. Am J Physiol 82:557–569
Anderson DH (1927b) Lmyphatics of the Fallopian tube of the sow. Contrib Embryol Carneg Inst 19:135–148
Anderson DH (1928) Comparative anatomy of the utero-tubal junction. Histology and physiology in the sow. Am J Anat 42:255–305

Batra S, Helm G, Owman C, Sjoberg NO, Wales B (1980) Female sex steroid concentrations in the ampullary and isthmic regions of the human fallopian tube and their relationship to plasma concentration during the menstrual cycle. Am J Obstet Gynecol 136:986–991
Bishop DW (1956) Active secretion in ther rabbit oviduct. Am J Physiol 187:347–352
Belve AR, McDonald MF (1968) Directional flow of fallopian tube secretion in the Romney ewe. J Reprod Fertil 6:275
Blandau RJ (1969) Gamete transport – comparative aspects. In: Hafez ESE, Blandau RJ (eds) The mammalian oviduct. University of Chicago Press, Chicago, pp 129–162
Blandau RJ (1973) Gamete transport in the female mammal. In: Greep RO, Astwood EB (eds) Handbook of physiology, section 7, endocrinology II. American Physiology Society, Washington, pp 153–163
Blandau RJ, Gaddum-Rosse P (1974) Mechanism of sperm transport in pig oviducts. Fertil Steril 25:61–67
Blandau RJ, Verdugo P (1976) An overview of gamete transport – comparative aspects. In: Harper MJK, Pauerstein CJ et al (eds) Symposium on ovum transport and fertility regulation. Scriptor, Copenhagen, pp 138–156
Bolton AE, Clough KJ, Stocker RJ, Pockley AG, Mowles EA, Westwood OMR, Chapman MG (1987) Identification of placental protein 14 as an immunosuppressive factor in human in reproduction. Lancet 1:593–595
Borell U, Nilsson O, Westman A (1957) Ciliary activity in the rabbit fallopian tube during oestrus and copulation. Acta Obstet Gynaecol Scand 36:22–28
Borland RM, Hazra S, Biggers JD, Lechene CP (1977) The elemental composition of the environments of the gametes and preimplantation embryo during the initiation of pregnancy. Biol Reprod 16:147–157
Borland RM, Biggers JD, Lechene CP, Taymor ML (1980) Elemental composition of the fluid in the human fallopian tube. J Reprod Fertil 58:479–482
Breihpol W (1938) Experimentelle Untersuchungen über Bewegungen menschlicher Eileiter in den verschiedenen Phasen des Zyklus und der Schwangerschaft. Geburtsh Gynakol 118:1–27
Brenner RM (1969) Renewal of oviduct cilia during the menstrual cycle in the rhesus monkey. Fertil Steril 20:599–611
Brower LK, Anderson E (1969) Cytological events associated with the secretory process in the rabbit oviduct. Biol Reprod 1:130–148
Butzow R (1989) The human fallopian tube contains placental protein 5. Hum Reprod 4:17–20
Clewe TH, Mastroianni L (1960) A method for continuous volumetric collection of oviduct secretions. J Reprod Fertil 1:146–150
Croxatto HB, Ortiz ME (1975) Egg transport in the fallopian tube. Gynaecol Obstet Invest 6:215–225
Devoto L, Soto E, Magofke AM, Sierralta W (1980) Unconjugated steroids in the fallopian tube and peripheral blood during the normal menstrual cycle. Fertil Steril 33:613–617
Donnez J, Casanas-Roux F, Ferin J, Thomas K (1983) Changes in ciliation and cell height in human tubal epithelium in the fertile and post-fertile years. Maturitas 5:39–45
Eddy CA, Garcia RG, Kraemer DC, Pauerstein CJ (1976) Ovum transport in non-human primates. In: Harper MJK, Pauerstein CJ, Adams CE, Coutinho EM, Croxatto HB, Paton DM (eds) Symposium on ovum transport and fertility regulation. Scriptor, Copenhagen, pp 447–453
Edman (1983) The climacteric. In: Buchsbaum HJ (ed) The menopause. Springer, Berlin Heidelberg New York, pp 23–33
Erb H (1969) Zur hormonalen Regulation der Tubenmotilität. In-vitro-Versuche an menschlichen Tuben. Bibl Gynakol 51:1–87
Feigelson M, Kay E (1972) Protein patters of rabbit oviductal fluid. Biol Reprod 6:244–252
Flickinger GL, Elsner C, Illingworth DV, Muechler EK, Mikhail G (1977) Estrogen and progesterone receptors in the female genital tract of humans and monkeys. Ann N Y Acad Sci 286:180–189
Fredricks CM (1986) Morphological and functional aspects of the oviduct epithelium. In: Siegler AM (ed) The fallopian tube: basic studies and clinical contributions. Futura, New York, pp 67–80

Gaddum-Rosse P, Rumery RE, Blandau RJ, Thiersch JB (1975) Studies on the mucosa of post-menopausal oviducts: surface appearance, ciliary activity and the effect of oestrogen treatment. Fertil Steril 26:951–969
Gillet GY, Koritké JG (1967) Les artérioles spiralées de la trompe utérine chez la femme. Acta Anat 68:609
Gillet GY, Leissner P (1967) Les variations de la microvascularisation de la trompe utérine au cours du cycle ovarien chez la femme. Acta Anat 68:608
Greenwald GS (1958) Endocrine regulation of the mucin in the tubal epithelium of the rabbit. Anat Rec 130:477–495
Hamner CE (1973) Oviductal fluid – composition and physiology. In: Greep RO, Astwood EB (eds) Handbook of physiology, section 7, endocrinology. American Physiological Society, Washington DC, pp 141–151
Hamner CE, Fox SB (1969) Biochemistry of oviducatal secretions. In: Hafez ESE, Blandau RJ (eds) The mammalian oviduct. University of Chicago Press, Chicago, pp 333-355
Hamner CE, Williams W (1965) Composition of rabbit oviductal secretions. Fertil Steril 16:170–176
Harper MJK (1961) The mechanisms involved in the movement of newly ovulated eggs through the ampulla of the rabbit Fallopian tube. J Reprod Fertil 2:522–524
Helm G, Owman C, Rosengren E, Sjoberg N-O (1982a) Regional and cyclic variations in catecholamine concentration of the human fallopian tube. Biol Reprod 26:553–558
Helm G, Owman C, Rosengren E, Sjoberg N-O, Walles B (1982b) Motor activity of the human fallopian tube in vitro in relation to plasma concentration of estradiol and progesterone
Hunter RHF (1977) Function and multifunction of the Fallopian tubes in relation to gametes, embryos and hormones. Eur J Obstet Gynecol Reprod Biol 7:267–283
Hunter RHF (1988a) The fallopian tubes: their role in fertility and infertility. Springer, Berlin Heidelberg New York, pp 12-29
Hunter RHF (1988b) The fallopian tubes: their role in fertility and infertility. Spinger, Berlin Heidelberg New York, pp 30–52
Hunter RHF, Cook B, Poyser NL (1983) Regulation of oviduct function in pigs by local transfer of ovarian steroids and prostaglandins: a mechanism to influence sperm transport. Eur J Obstet Gynecol Reprod Biol 14:225–232
Julkunen M, Walström T, Seppälä M (1986) Human fallopian tube contains placental protein 14. Am J Obstet Gynecol 154:1076–1079
Koritké JG, Gillet JY, Leissner P (1968a) La microvascularisation de la muqueuse tubaire et ses variations au cours du cycle ovarien chez la femme. Z Zellforsch 88:48–56
Kortiké JG, Muller PG, Gillet JY (1968b) LA vascularisation de la trompe utérine chez la femme. Bull Fed Soc Gynaecol Obstet 20:405–407
Lambert JC, Hammer Ce, Gemmill CL (1973) Ultrastructural study of secretion in the rabbit oviduct under different hormonal influences. Fed Proc 32:13 (abstract)
Lee FC (1928) the utero-tubal junction in various animals. Bull Johns Hopkins Hosp 42:335–357
Leese HK (1988) The formation and function of oviduct fluid, J Reprod Fertil 82:843–856
Lindblom B, Hamberger L, Ljung B (1980) Contractile patterns of isolated oviductal smooth muscle under different hormonal conditions. Fertil Steril 33:283–287
Lippes J (1979) Analysis of human oviductal fluid for low molecular weight compounds. In: Beller FK, Schumacher GFB (eds) The biology of the fluids in the female genital tract. Elsevier, North Holland, pp 373-387
Lippes J, Enders RG, Pragay DA, Bartholomew WR (1972) The collection and analysis of human fallopian tube fluid. Contraception 5:85–103
Lippes J, Krasner J. Alfonso LA, Dacalos ED, Lucero R (1981) Human oviductal fluid proteins. Fertil Steril 36:623–629
Ludwig H, Metzer H (1976) The human reproductive tract. A scanning electron microscopic atlas. Springer, Berlin Heidelberg New York, pp 79–105
Maas DHA, Storey BT, Mastroianni L (1976) Oxygen tension in the oviduct of the rhesus monkey (Macaca mullata). Fertil Steril 27:!312–1317
Maguiness SD, Djahanbakhch O (1992) Salpingoscopic findings in women undergoing sterilization. Hum Reprod 7:269–273

Maguiness SD, Shrimanker K, Djahanbakhch O, Grudzinskas JG (1992a) Oviduct proteins. Contemp Rev Obstet Gynaecol 4:42–50
Maguiness SD, Djahanbakhch O, Grudzinskas JG (1992b) Assessment of the fallopian tube. Obstet Gynaecol Surg 47:587–603
Maguiness SD, Shrimanker K, Djahanbakhch O, Deeks J, Teisner B, Grudzinskas JG (1993a) In-vitro synthesis of total protein and placental protein 14 by the fallopian tube mucosa: variation in relation to anatomical site, the ovairan cycle and the menopause. Hum Reprod 7:269–273
Maguiness SD, Shirmanker K, Djahanbakhch O, Teisner B, Grudzinskas JG (1993b) Evidence for the in-vitro de-novo synthesis of immunoglobulin and a previously undescribed 17 kDa protein (TEP-2) by the mucosa of the fallopian tube. Hum Reprod 8:1199–1202
Mastroianni L, Jones R (1965) Oxygen tension within the rabbit fallopian tube. J Reprod Fertil 9:99-102
Mastroianni L, Urzua M, Stambaugh R (1970) Protein patterns of monkey oviductal fluid before and after ovulation. Fertil Steril 21:817–820
Mastroianni L, Urzua M, Stambaugh R (1973) The internal environmental fluids of the oviduct. In: Segal SJ, Crozier R, Corfman PA, Condliffe PG (eds) The regulation of mammalian reproduction. Thomas, Springfeld, pp 376–384
Nieder CD, Weitlauf HM, Suda-Hartman M (1987) Studies of stage specific proteins by peri-implantation mouse embryos. Biol Reprod 36:687–699
Oliphant G (1986) Biochemistry and immunology of oviduct fluid. In: Siegler AM (ed) the fallopian tube: Basic studies and clinical contributions. Future, Mount Kisco, New York, pp 129-145
Overstreet JW, Katz DF (1977) Sperm transport and selection in female genital tract. In Johnson MH (ed) Development in mammals, vol 2. Elsevier, Amsterdam, pp 31–65
Patek K, Nilsson L, Johanisson E (1972a) Scanning electron microscopic study of the human fallopian tube. I. The proliferative and secretory stages. Fertil Steril 23:459–465
Patek E, Nilsson L, Johannisson E (1972b) Scanning electron microscopic study of the human fallopian tube. II. Fetal life, reproductive life and menopause. Fertil Steril 23:719–733
Pauerstein CJ (1975) Clincial implications of oviducatal physiology and biochemistry. Gynecol Invest 6:253–264
Pauerstein CJ, Eddy CA (1979a) The role of the oviduct in reproduction: our knowledge and our ignorance. J Reprod Fertil 55:223–229
Pauerstein CJ, Eddy CA (1979b) Morphology of the Fallopian tube. In: Beller FK, Schumacher GFB (eds) The biology of the fluids of the female genital tract. Elsevier, North-Holland, pp 299-317
Pino AM, Devoto L, Soto E, Castro O, Sierralta W (1982) Changes in cytosolic and nuclear estradiol receptors of normal fallopian tube throughout the menstrual cycle. J Steroid Biochem 16:193–197
Pockley AG, Mowles EA, Stocker RJ, Westwood Om, Chapman MG, Bolton AE (1988) Suppression of in vitro lymphocyte reactivity to phytohemagglutinin by placental protein 14. J Reprod Immunol 13:31–39
Pollow K, Intraphuvasak J, Manz B, Grill HJ (1981) A comparison of cytoplasmic and nuclear estradiol and progesterone receptors in human fallopian tube and endometrial tissue. Fertil Steril 36:66–69
Pollow K, Intraphuvasak J, Grill HJ, Manz B (1982) Estradiol and progesterone binding components in the cytosol of normal human fallopian tubes. J Steroid Biochem 16:429–435
Punnonen R, Lukola A (1981) Binding of estrogen and progestin in the human fallopian tube. Fertil Steril 36:610–614
Riddick DH (1975) The composition of rabbit oviductal fluid collected continuously through the gestation. J Reprod Fertil 43:563–566
Robertson DM, Landgren BM 81975) Oestradiol receptor level in the human Fallopian tube during the menstrual cycle and after the menopause. J Steroid Biochem 6:511–513
Seckinger DL, Snyder FF (1926) Cyclic changes in the spontaneous contractions of the human Fallopian tube. Bull Johns Hopkins Hosp 39:371–378
Shams A, Rizk MA, Toppozada HK, Khowessah MM, Abul-Enin M, Said S, Habib YA, Kira LH (1977) Human tubal fluid collection via vagina and its quantitative variations during the menstrual cycle. J Reprod Med 18:61–65

Sjöberg J, Wahlström T, Grudzinskas JG, Sinosich MJ (1986) Demonstration of pregnancy-associated plasma protein-A (PAPP-A)-like material in the fallopian tube. Fertil Steril 45:517–521

Soriero AA (1978) The ageing uterus and fallopian tubes. In: Schneider EL (ed) The geing reproductive system. Raven, New York, pp 85–126

Stegner HE (1961) Das Epithel der Tuba Uterina des Neugeboren. Electronenmikroscopishe Befunde. Z Zellforsch 55:247–262

Talo A, Pulkkinen MO (1982) Electrical activity in the human oviduct during the menstrual cycle. Am J Obstet Gynecol 142:35-147

Talo A, Pulkkinen MO (1984) Electrical activity in the human oviduct after the menopause. Maturitas 5:185–191

Thibault C (1973) Sperm transport and storage in vertebrates. J Reprod Fertil [Suppl] 18:39–53

Tiitinen A, Wahlsrtröm T, Julkunen M, Seppälä M (1986) The content and immunohistochemical localisation of placental protein 10 (PP10) in the fallopian tube. Br J Obstet Gynaecol 93:924–927

Verhage HG, Barehter ML, Jaffe RC, Akbar M (1979) Cyclic changes in ciliation, secretion and cell height of the oviductal epithelium in women. Am J Anat 156:505–521

Voet RL (1983) End organ response to oestrogen deprivation. In: Buchsbaum HJ (ed) The menopause. Springer, Berlin Heidelberg New York, pp 9–22

Voinot JBM (1900) Essai sur l'epithelium de la trompe de la fallope chez la femme. Thesis, Nancy

Waites GT, Bell SC, Walker RA, Wood PL (1990) Immuno-histological distribution of the secretory endometrial protein endometrial α_2-globulin, a glycosylated β-lactoglobulin homologue, in the human fetus and adult employing monoclonal antibodies. Hum Reprod 5:105–111

Tubal Infertility

M. Yildirim

The Normal Fallopian Tube

Anatomy

The fallopian tubes are bilateral organs that originate from the uterine cornua and continue to the right and left with a length of 12–15 cm. Their outer diameter near the ovary is 10–15 mm, and near the uterus, 4–5 mm.

Anatomically, each tube consists of two parts, a fixed part in the uterine muscle and a free part in the peritoneal space. The fixed portion in the uterine muscle is called the interstitial or intramural part. The free portion in the peritoneal space is divided into three parts, beginning from the uterus; these are called the isthmic, ampullar, and infundibular parts. In the infundibulum there are fringes, called fimbriae (Fig. 1).

Interstitial Portion. The length of this rather straight portion, which passes through the uterine muscle, is 0.5–1 cm, and its internal diameter is 0.2–0.5 mm. It is the narrowest part of the fallopian tube. No sphincter has been shown in this portion.

Isthmic Portion. The isthmic portion is situated between the uterus and the ampullar portion of the tube. It has an external diameter of 5–8 mm, an internal diameter of 0.5–1 mm and a length of approximately 4–6 cm. This portion has many more adrenergic receptors, thereby acquiring a sphincter function.

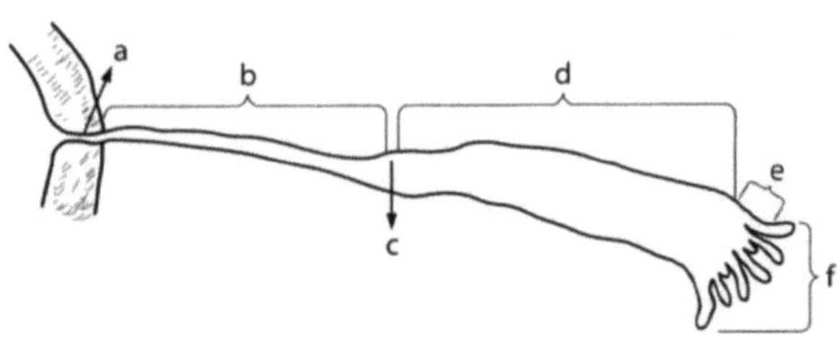

Fig. 1. Segments of the fallopian tube

Ampulla. The widest and the longest part of the fallopian tube is the ampulla. It has a length of 5–8 cm and an internal diameter of 0.5–2 cm. It is the basic portion where fertilization occurs.

Infundibulum. The last part of the tube, the infundibulum, has a length of 1–2 cm. It has 10–12 fimbriae. The longest one, which terminates on the superior pole of the ovary, is called Richard's fimbria. The fimbriae are divided into smaller fimbriatus.

Arteries. Tubal blood is supplied from branches of the uterine artery and only one branch of the ovarian artery. The fallopian tube has three arteries: an internal, a middle, and an external. The internal artery originates from the retrograde artery, which is the terminal artery of the uterine artery, and supplies the isthmic portion. The middle artery originates from the lateral branch of the uterine artery. The external artery comes from the ovarian artery. These three arteries come together and produce an arc in the mesosalpinx. Approximately 30 arterioles originate from this arc and these arterioles form anastomoses between themselves, producing an arterial network. The terminal branches of these arterioles terminate in tubal mucosa.

Veins. Tubal veins drain into the uterine vein and the ovarian vein in a way comparable to the tubal arteries.

Lymphatics. There are three layers of tubal lymphatics: submucosal, intramuscular, and subserosal. The lymphatic network, which is more dense in the ampulla and infundibulum, exerts some physiologic functions within the context of fertilization and migration.

Tubal lymphatics drain into the lumbar, para-aortic, and paracervical ganglia around the uterus.

Nerves. The fallopian tube has sympathetic and parasympathetic innervation. Sympathetic nerves originate from T 10–12 and terminate at the lower mesenteric ganglion. Postganglionic fibers pass through the hypogastric ganglion and terminate at the celiac ganglion. Parasympathetic fibers come from S 2–4.

Histology

The fallopian tube consists of four layers: mucosa, muscle, subserosa, and serosa beginning from the inner surface.

The tubal lumen is completely covered by mucosa. Beneath the mucosa is the lamina propria; together, they form plicae that extend into the lumen. From the tubal ostium to the uterus there are three or four main plicae that in turn produce several small plicae. The mucosal surface in the tubal lumen is thereby increased.

The tubal mucosa contains ciliary, secretory and intercalary cells. Ciliary and secretory cells interact with ovarian hormones. As the estrogen level rises, ciliary movements also increase and the secretory function of secretory cells is increased. In the tubal interstitial portion there are three layers: the inner and outer longitudinal layers and a circular layer between them. However, the free portion of the tube in the peritoneal space consists of only two layers: an inner circular and an outer longitudinal.

The tubal subserosal layer overlying muscle consists of connective tissue and vascular structures. The serosal layer is the peritoneal covering of the tube.

Properties

Peristaltic and antiperistaltic contractions of the fallopian tube reach a maximum at the time of ovulation. Estrogens cause the contractions to increase, as do oxytocin, norepinephrine, ergot derivatives, and $PGF_{2\alpha}$; however, PGE_2 reduces them.

Tubal ciliary activity is directed from the infundibulum to the uterus, and this activity is increased by progesterone.

The tubal lumen contains a liquid produced by transudation, active secretion and peritoneum. This liquid contains glucose, ions, glycogen, enzymes, and amino acids, and is necessary for the food supply and for the transport of the ovum and zygote to the uterine cavity. De Brux and Hafez's (1979) studies showed that tubal liquid movements in the isthmic portion are directed from the uterus to the ampulla whereas in the ampulla portion they are directed bilaterally. There is a tidal motion in the ampulla. We believe that this motion is essential for the fertilization and segmentation of the zygote.

Functions

The fallopian tube forms a passage for transport of spermatozoa. Other functions of the tube are ensuring passage of the ovum into the tube, producing a medium for fertilization, and transportation of the zygote to the uterus. For good function to be achieved, all segments and all layers of the tube must be healthy.

Tubal Investigation

The goal in tubal investigation must be to test the function of the tube rather than to demonstrate its patency. In other words, investigation should be directed towards ensuring that all the layers and segments of the tube are healthy. For this purpose, two basic diagnostic methods, hysterosalpingography (HSG) and laparoscopy, are used. Recently, falloposcopy or salpingoscopy has been added to these methods in some centers.

Hysterosalpingography

In HSG, the uterus and fallopian tubes are visualized radiologically following injection of a radioopaque contrast medium into the uterine cavity. The purpose of this method must be to investigate not only the tubal passage but also the tubal lumen, which is of special interest. This is why the substance used in this technique must be lipid-soluble, not water-soluble. When a lipid-soluble substance is used, the tubal lumen can be investigated in detail.

HSG *must* be performed in sterile conditions whenever colpitis, cervicitis, endometritis, and parametritis coexist; failure to do so can lead to pelvic peritonitis.

It is important that HSG is performed on an appropriate day during the menstrual cycle. It should be avoided during menstruation so as not to cause extravasation, and also should not be performed during the secretion phase. Sometimes infertile patients may have spontaneous pregnancies. During the second phase of the menstrual cycle, when there is a possibility of gestation, HSG may harm the zygote or push it into the abdomen. Additionally, secretory changes occur in the tubal mucosa and in the endometrium. These changes, at the narrowest interstitial and isthmic portions of the tube, may give rise to pseudostrictures that cause the adoption of unnecessary therapeutic measures.

Ideal days for HSG are the 5th–10th days of the menstrual cycle. During the injection into the cavity the doctor must speak with the patient, distracting her attention, and the contrast medium must be given very slowly. If it is given rapidly, the uterus may contract and produce spasm at the cornual level.

HSG evaluation must be done carefully. For this purpose, cervical canal, uterine cavity, tubal lumen, and control films must be evaluated separately.

A long and wide cervical image may represent latent tuberculosis. At the time of ovulation the cervical canal may enlarge, but except for this period, elongation and widening of the cervical canal must force the clinician to consider genital tuberculosis. Nogales and Nogales (1979) studied a large series of 1435 cases of uterine tuberculosis and found elongation of the cervical canal in approximately one-third. In 30% of our genital tuberculosis cases, we have found cervical elongation and widening radiologically.

While evaluating HSG, uterine cavity size, synechiae, and congenital malformations must be investigated separately.

Tubal research in HSG has a distinct importance. Not only the tubal passage, but also the meaning of radiological images that show the type of pathology must be determined. Circular images at the level of the uterus usually show spasm (Fig. 2). However, blockage due to organic pathology produces sharp contours. The tubal lumen must be evaluated carefully. In endometriosis the tubal lumen shows saw-teeth like thin features (Fig. 3). In tuberculosis, tubal plicae show thickening; other images such as the iron-wire, lead-pipe, honeycomb, embryoform, or corn tuft appearances can also occur (Figs. 4–7).

In HSG, evaluation of the control images is also important. Dispersion of radioopaque substance in the peritoneum may give an idea of the peritubal ovarian condition. Additionally, in tuberculosis ovarian and pelvic lymphoid calcifications can be seen (Fig. 8).

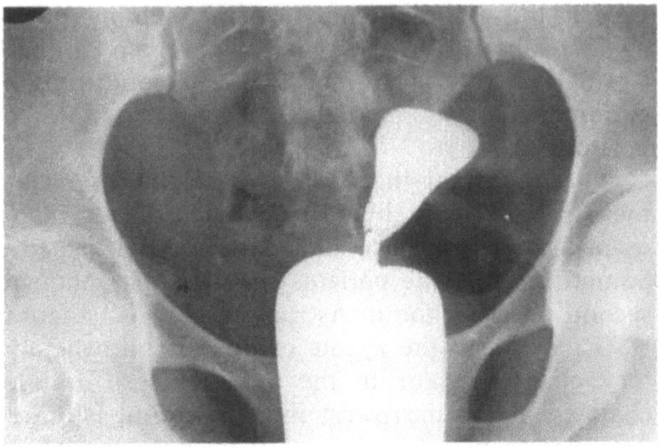

Fig. 2. Cornual spasm

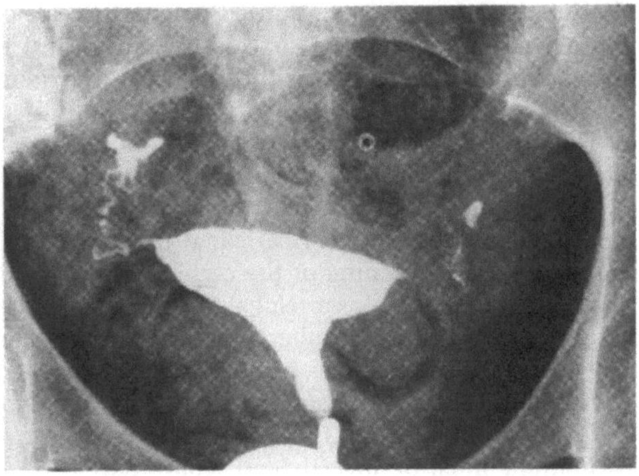

Fig. 3. Endometriotic diverticula in the lumen of the tube and salpingitis isthmica nodosa

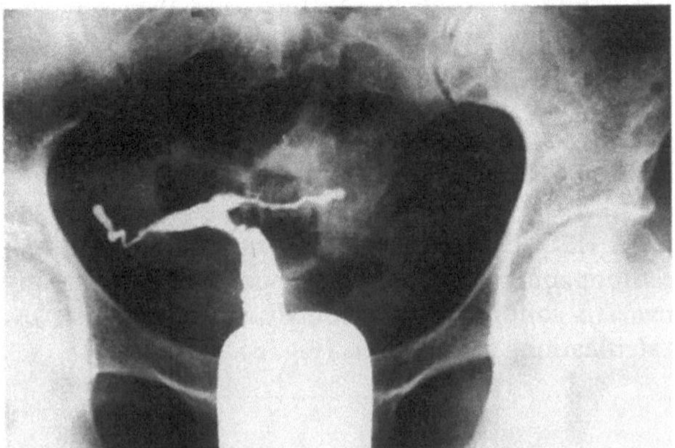

Fig. 4. The "iron-wire" and "lead-pipe" appearances

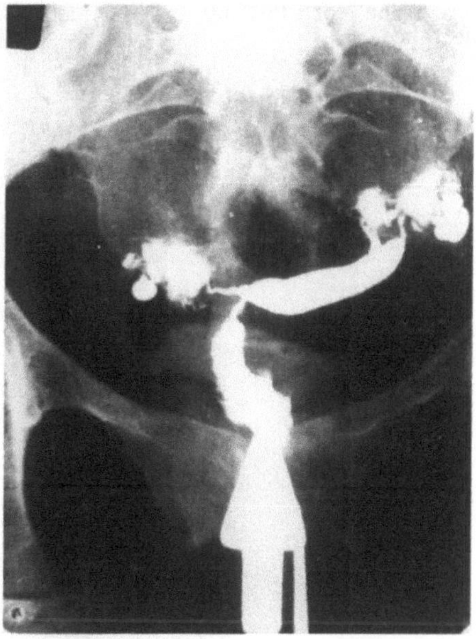

Fig. 5. The "honeycomb" appearance in both tubes

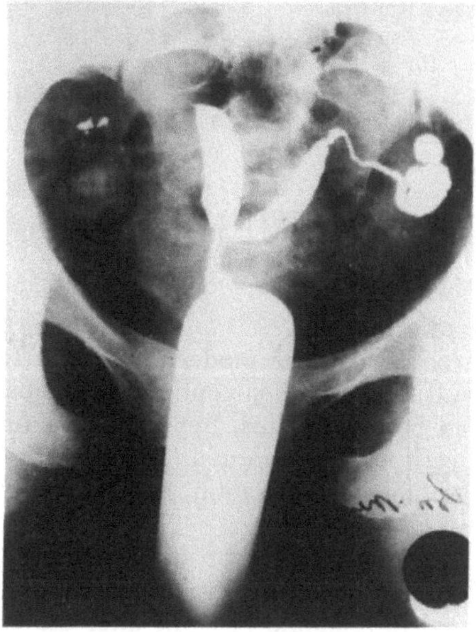

Fig. 6. The "embryoform" appearance

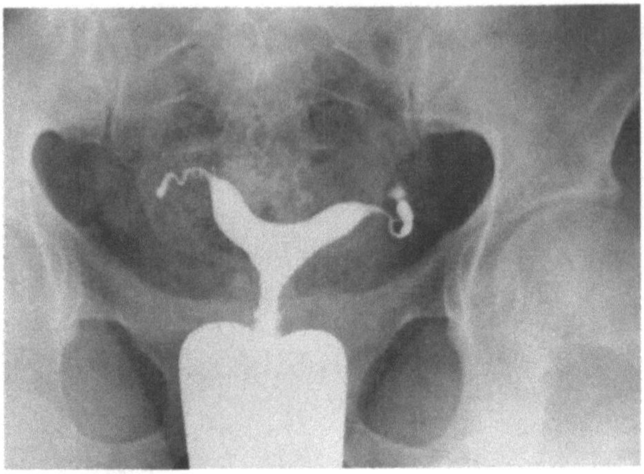
Fig. 7. The "corn tuft" appearance

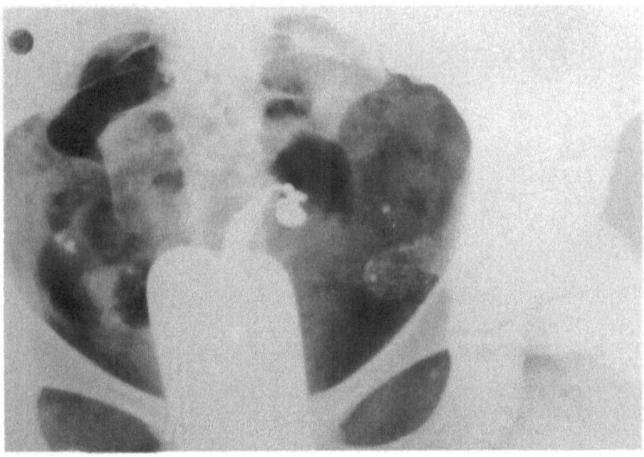
Fig. 8. Calcifications in both ovaries

Laparoscopy

According to the modern approach to infertility, tubal research must begin with HSG and then continue with laparoscopy. By HSG, only the tubal lumen can be investigated, but to have a functional tube all of the segments and layers must be normal. Laparoscopy allows tubal muscle, serosa, fimbriae, the tube-ovary relation, and the pelvic peritoneum to be investigated in detail.

Laparoscopy can be applied at any time except during menstruation. If tubal and ovulatory evaluation is to be done or a premenstrual probe is needed, it should be done after the 21st day of the cycle. If there is a suspicion of the LUF syndrome and if it is intended that it be studied together with the tubal evaluation, this must be done 36–48 h after the increase of basal temperature. If tubal evaluation with possible surgical intervention is planned, this must be done during the first period of the cycle, in particular before the 10th day. The clinician must make a decision as to the appropriate

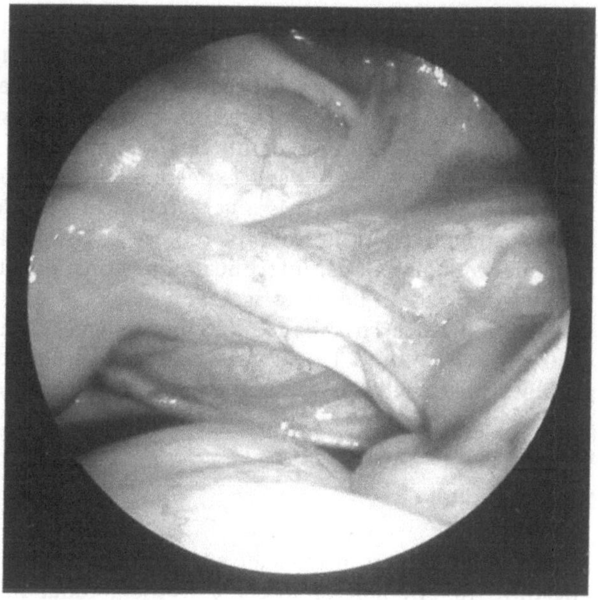

Fig. 9. Lipoid degenerations in the tube

timing of laparoscopy during the cycle, given the purpose of the study; there is no standard time – rather it will vary from one patient to another.

In laparoscopy, all tubal segments and fimbriae must be investigated in detail. A thorough search must be made for tubal serosa, lipoid degeneration (Fig. 9), and fimbrial and interfimbrial adhesions. In the methylene blue test, the patency of the tube is first ascertained; fimbriae must then be washed by saline to remove methylene blue in order to investigate the tubal mucosal condition. If the mucosa is healthy, it will not retain methylene blue. In pathologic conditions and in the presence of mucosal damage, the tubal terminal portion will remain blue despite washing.

In addition to these findings, the ovarian condition, pelvic wall adhesions, ovarian capsule, and follicles under the capsule must be determined when performing laparoscopy.

The important thing is the determination of the exact tubal pathology (e.g., whether it is due to endometriosis or tuberculosis or chlamydia or to a surgical intervention on the pelvic organs). The prognosis will vary according to the reason for the pathology. Some of our colleagues detect only the location of pathology and give no information about its cause; such a failing will render the planned therapy inefficient.

Falloposcopy

At the time of laparotomy or laparoscopy, the use of an optic instrument with entry from the tubal ostium to inspect the tubal lumen is called "salpingoscopy," while entry via the transvaginal route, inspecting all the luminal structures, is called "falloposcopy." These two terms thus have an element of shared meaning, but "falloposcopy" is more correct and will be used here.

The first falloposcopic procedure was performed by Henry-Suchet et al. (1981, 1993); since then, Cornier et al. (1985), Brosens et al. (1987), Kerin et al. (1990), and a number of other clinicians have used this procedure. The technique has, however, been experimental and has not been routinely performed by every center: it is a very refined technique and its use is restricted by the special training that is required. Using falloposcopy, tubal polyps, proximal mucous plugs, interplical adhesions, and tubal mucosal and luminal vascularization can be investigated.

For tubal research, Allahbadia (1992) suggests the use of ultrasound, Stern et al. (1992), colored Doppler ultrasound, and Kadoum et al., hydrogynecography. These methods are still experimental procedures.

Tubal Infertility

Female infertility is often caused by tubal factors (Patton 1984): in fact, in one-third to one-half of infertile women, tubal infertility is present. Consequently, infertility researchers should have sufficient knowledge of tubal infertility and its causes.

Causes of Tubal Infertility

Pelvic Inflammatory Disease Generally the vagina, by virtue of its pH, biologic structure and cervical mucus containing bactericidal and bacteriostatic enzymes, protects internal genital organs against bacteria. However, at the time of menstruation the estrogen level is at its minimum and there is nearly an absence of cervical mucus; consequently this protective system will be very weak. Coitus at this period with a partner with genital tract infection may be the cause of tubal infertility. This possibility must not be forgotten. Additionally, obstetric procedures such as birth, abortion and curettage or PMPC, HSG, and intrauterine procedures done without paying attention to sterility may cause infection of internal genital organs and thus of the fallopian tubes. The damage in such cases will either be located in the tubal lumen or comprise peritubo-ovarian adhesions.

Pelvic Operations Without applying microsurgical rules in pelvic organ surgery, tubal infertility would occur. After myomectomy, cystectomy, wedge resection, metroplasty, surgery for ectopic pregnancy, and, in recent years, the frequently used surgical laparoscopic procedures, peritubo-ovarian adhesions may cause tubal infertility. I believe that in future, the incidence of uterine fibroids will increase. In Turkey the number of married couples is decreasing and marriages tend to occur at the age of 35 or later. In addition, couples frequently have only one child or none at all, and this may give rise to a higher incidence of uterine fibroids.

Infections of Extragenital Origin In this context rupture of the appendix must be borne in mind. Additionally, diverticulitis or urinary tract infections, especially cystitis, can infect internal genital organs and cause perituboovarian adhesions and finally tubal infertility.

Genital Tuberculosis Genital tuberculosis is a secondary organ infection. The primary focus may be in the lungs, intestines, kidneys, or another organ. Definitive diagnosis is made by detection of Koch bacilli; sometimes these cannot be detected, but essentially this is not necessary. The diagnosis of genital tuberculosis can be made by HSG, laparoscopy, histopathologic endometrial study, detection of bacilli in menstrual blood, and inoculation of guinea pigs with Koch bacilli. If tuberculosis is detected by one of these methods, verification by other methods is not necessary.

In order to detect permanent lesions of tuberculosis by HSG, 1–10 years should be allowed to elapse (Siegler 1993). However, after detecting permanent and typical tuberculosis lesions at HSG, the diagnosis does not need to be verified. Classical changes of tuberculosis at HSG are iron-wire, lead-pipe, prayer-bead, saw-like figures in the tubal lumen and a honeycomb appearance. In addition to these features, Yildirim (1989) adds two new typical images of tuberculosis, namely embryoform and corn-tuft appearances at the tubal ends (Figs. 6, 7).

An expert eye may easily detect typical tuberculosis images when performing HSG.

Endometriosis Endometriosis causes infertility by blocking the tubal lumen, damaging the tubal mucosa, or increasing fibroid tissue in tubal muscle and

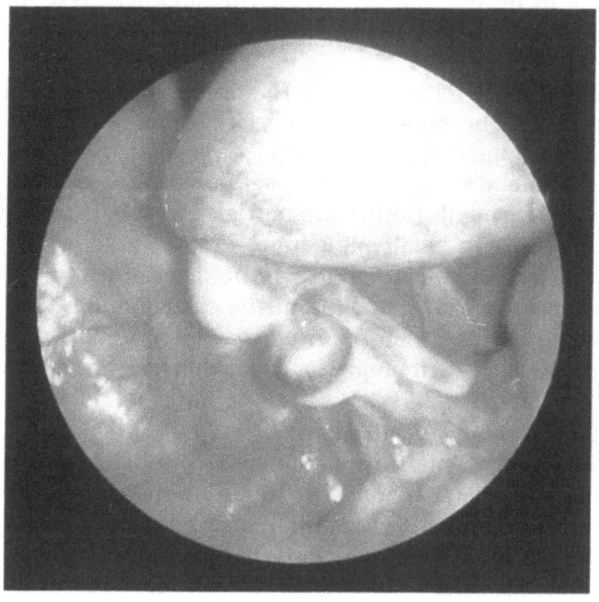

Fig. 10. Endometriosis causing complete blockage in the tube

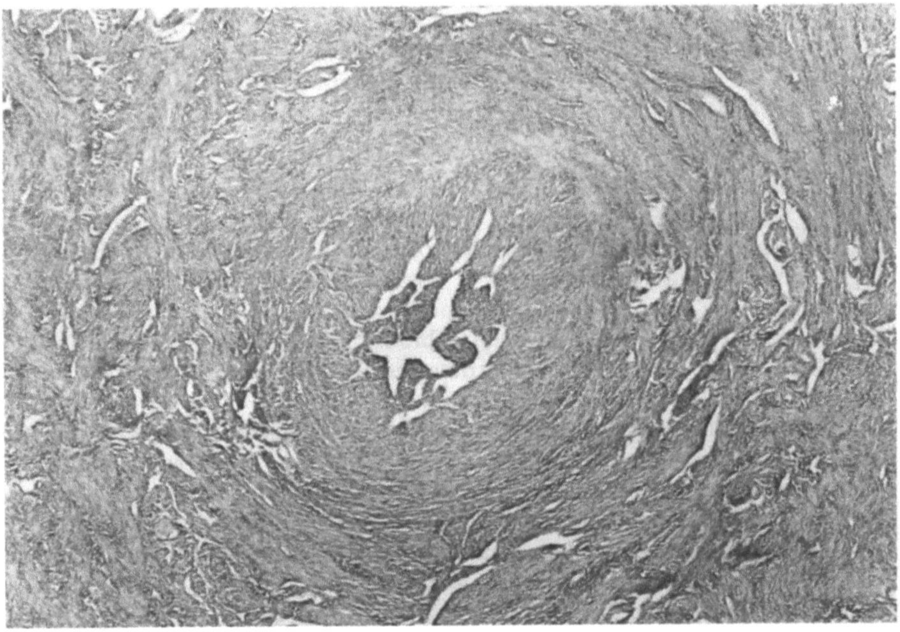

Fig. 11. The obstruction in the tubal lumen. Histopathological appearance

thereby causing constriction of the tubal lumen. The diagnosis of complete tubal occlusion is made by laparoscopy (Fig. 10), but endometriosis-related mucosal damage and constriction of the tubal lumen by increased fibroid tissue in muscle can be detected by a careful HSG investigation. Definitive diagnosis can be made by histopathologic examination of a tubal sample.

Tubal Polyps Philipp and Huber (1939) reported that tubal polypoid structures might produce partial occlusion. Twenty years later, Zenisek (1959) showed such structures by HSG images.

There are two types of tubal polyps, endometrial and fibroid. Endometrial polyps contain both endometrial and tubal epithelium, but in fibroid types there is only tubal epithelium.

Clinically, tubal polyps can be determined at the cornua by HSG (Fig. 11). Laparoscopically, swelling of the cornua and a globular image are typical for polyps. It has been reported that tubal polyps usually coexist with endometriosis, uterine hypoplasia, and abnormal ovulation (Drapier 1979).

Localization of Tubal Lesions

When tubal infertility is the subject, tubal lesions may be divided into proximal and distal lesions. Proximal lesions include obliterative fibrosis, chronic tubal inflammation, salpingitis isthmica nodosa, tubal endometriosis, and tubal polyps (Brosens 1989). Except tubal polyps, all are histopathological signs. Especially obliterative fibrosis, chronic tubal inflammation, and salpingitis isthmica nodosa are accepted as sequelae of other pathologies. The underlying disorder may be infection or endometriosis. In these pathologies, although tubal occlusion is partial, there may be narrow portions in the tubal lumen that will cause infertility. In the proximal portion of the fallopian tube, the nature of pathology that causes infertility can be determined only by histopathologic examination. In all these conditions the only therapy is microsurgery.

Tubal distal lesions include stenosis, phymosis, agglutination, and peritubo-ovarian adhesions that produce malfunction of fimbriae. All of these may be evaluated clinically. Basic reasons for these lesions are infections or operations on pelvic organs.

Treatment of Tubal Infertility

Treatment must be done or planned after a thorough evaluation of the tube. As stated above, after HSG and laparoscopy the data must be carefully evaluated. A forgotten investigation, wrong evaluation, or hurried decision may cause bad results. Additionally the evaluation and decision must be made by an expert on tubal operations. Tubal infertility treatment is divided into two categories, as described below:

Treatment of Proximal Tubal Infertility

Proximal pathologies of the tube can be treated by removing the affected portion microsurgically. The technique was first described by Ehrler (1965); using the microinstruments and operation microscopes available today, the completely or partially occluded damaged portion is removed and then an interstitio-isthmic anastomosis is performed. With this technique, high pregnancy rates are reported (Salut-Baraux 1980). To give more detail: The tube is disconnected from the cornu and healthy tubal lumen is located in muscle. After gradual resection of the disconnected portion, the anastomosis is performed. During the operation it is easy to detect the healthy part by inspecting the tubal lumen and tubal mucosa. Fibrotic and damaged lumen is white or pale, whereas healthy mucosa that will function is bloody and pink.

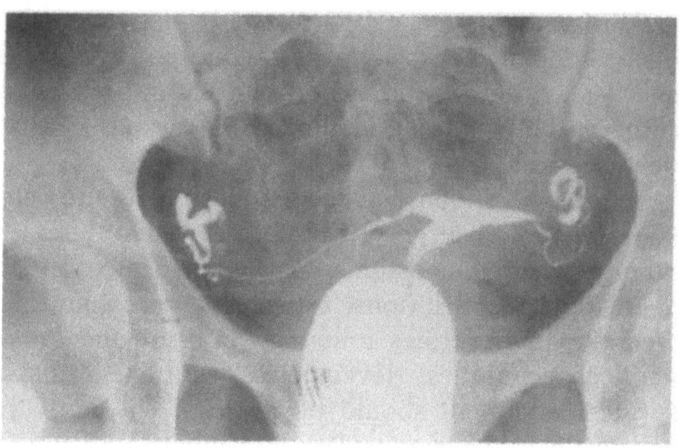

Fig. 12. Cornual polyps in both tubes

Recently, other proximal lesion treatments such as transcervical fluoroscopic recanalization (Platia 1985), transcervical balloon tuboplasty (Confino 1985), transcervical tubal catheterization (Roch 1988), and catheterization with a linear everting catheter (Pearstone 1992) have been reported in the literature, but these have not found wide application and are still experimental procedures.

Treatment of Distal Tubal Lesions

Distal lesions that will cause infertility are as follows: peritubo-ovarian adhesions, stenosis, phymosis, and agglutination.

Peritubo-ovarian adhesions Causes of pelvic adhesions are described above. If tubes are healthy and fimbriae are not damaged by lysis of pelvic adhesions, the pregnancy rate reaches 50%. But following an infection that damages the tube, like tuberculosis, such a result cannot be excepted. Pelvic adhesions can be treated surgically in a straightforward manner.

Stenosis At the final part of tube, just in front of the infundibulum, narrowings and strangulations can sometimes occur. This pathologic state is called stenosis. At HSG "corn tuft" images can be seen. Generally tuberculosis is the cause. If no other pathology is found, this narrow segment can be easily operated on by microsurgery.

Phymosis If the tubal ostium narrows and becomes a small hole in the distal part, this condition is called "phymosis." When it is opened from the external portion, all the fimbrial tufts eviscerate and produce a normal anatomic shape. This can be easily done by laparoscopic surgery.

Agglutination Agglutination involves complete occlusion of the tubal ostium, which has an apple-like configuration. When viewed externally, the terminal portion of the tube shows the appearance of hydrosalpinx. Although the appearance of the tubal terminal portion is invariable, different ampullar aspects can occur.

This pathology can be treated by laparoscopic surgery or microsurgery. The clinician must select the technique in which he has enough experience and is successful. If he has experience in both microsurgery and laparoscopic surgery, the technique is chosen on the basis of general panoramic vision of pelvic organs.

In the case of dense ovarian adhesions to the pelvic wall with intestinal loop adhesions microsurgery is preferred. When there is only agglutination without other adhesions, neostomy can be performed by laparoscopic management.

In tubal distal lesions, especially with agglutination, IVF may be considered. Pregnancy rates following IVF are the same as the rates achieved by surgical techniques. Nevertheless, we believe that in tubal distal pathologies surgical treatment should be the first choice. Although it may be more expensive, it is superior to IVF treatment. Additionally the chance of IVF treatment does not disappear but rather increases. Whether laparoscopic surgery or microsurgery is performed, the advantages of surgical treatment are:

1. When pelvic adhesions are reduced, dysmenorrhea and dyspareunia will disappear.
2. The chance of pregnancies with IVF is present only for one cycle. However, after surgical management, pregnancy is possible every cycle, every month, and every year. For this reason the pregnancy rate is relatively higher than with IVF.
3. Because pelvic adhesions are opened, IVF applications reaching to the ovaries will be easier and without complications.

Recanalization

Nowadays in many countries tubal sterilization is performed for the purpose of birth control. This is done during laparotomies for other reasons or laparoscopically. However, due to a change of partner, the death of a child, the desire for a new baby, or religious reasons, patients sterilized by tubal ligation may want sterilization to be reversed. Today the application of microsurgery enables this to be done successfully. Rates of successful recanalization reported by Gomel (1983) and Dubission (1986) are 78.8% and 78.5% respectively. The pregnancy rate in our series is much higher than in others, but we have not yet published our results. In my opinion, the high success rate in our series is a result of the low rate of pelvic infections in Turkey.

In an alterative new approach, the lysis of pelvic adhesions is first done by means of laparoscopic surgery; then, the tube is removed and anastomosis performed microsurgically with a minilaparotomy, as reported by Silva (1991). In this technique the purpose is to decrease the duration of hospitalization, but other infertility clinicians do not support the technique. In our personal opinion, such an approach will decrease the chance of success: microsurgery is the method of choice!

References

Allahbadia GN (1992) Fallopian tubes and ultrasonography. The Sion experience. Fertil Steril

Brosens IA, Boeckx W, Delattin P, Puttemans P, Basques G (1987) Salpingoscopy: a new preoperative diagnostic tool in tubal infertility. Br J Obstet Gynecol

Brosens I, Gordon A (1989) Tubal infertility. Gower Medical

Confino E, Frieberg J, Gleicher N (1985) Preliminary experience with transcervical balloon tuboplasty. Am J Obstet Gynecol

Cornier E (1985) Per coelioscopic ampullosalpingoscopy. J Gyn Obstet Biol Repr

De Brux J, Hafez ESE Histopathologie de la trompe. In: Brosens I, Cognat M, Constantin A, Thibier M (eds) Oviducte et fertilite. Masson, Paris, p 29

Drapier E, Bremond A, Rochet Y (1979) Les polipes de la portion interstielle de la tromps sont-ils un facteur de la sterilite. Gynecology

Dubisson JP, Aubriot FX, Henrion R (1986) Desterilisations microchirurgicales. Reflexions sur 65 cas. J Gyn Obs Biol Repr

Ehrler P (1965) Anastomose intramurale de la trompe. Une procede nouveau de la plastie tubaire pour supprimer les implantations. Bull Fed Soc Gynec Obstet

Gomel V (1983) Microsurgery in female infertility. Little Brown, Boston

Henry-Suchet J, Tesquier L, Lofredo V (1981) Endoscopies tubaires: premiers resultats. Gynecologie
Henry-Suchet J, Tesquier L, Pez JP et al (1993) Endoscopie tubaire ou tuboscopie. Une exploration complemaintaire utile dans la chirurgie reperatrice des trompes. 31st Meeting of the Gynecological Society of France
Kadoum GS (1992) Hydrogynecography. A new technique establishing vaginal sonography to visualise pelvic adhesions and other pelvic structures. Fertil Steril
Kerin J, Daykhousky L, Segolowitz J et al (1990) Falloposcopy: A new microendoscopic technique for visual exploration of the human fallopian tube from the uterotubal ostium to the fimbria using a transvaginal approach. Fertil Steril
Nogales-Sortis F, Tarancon I, Nogales T (1979) The pathology of female genital tuberculosis. Obstet Gynecol
Patton GW, Kistner RW (1984) Atlas of infertility surgery, 2nd ed. Little Brown, Boston
Pearstone AC, Surrey ES, Kerin SF (1992) The linear everting catheter: a non-hysteroscopic transvaginal technique for access and microendoscopy of the fallopian tube. Fertil Steril
Phillipp E, Huber H (1939) Die Entstehung der Endometriose, gleichzeitig ein Beitrag zur Pathologie des interstitiellen Tubenabschnittes. Zentrabl Gynak
Platia MD, Krudy AG (1985) Transcervical fluoroscopic recanalization of a proximally occluded oviduct. Fertil Steril
Roch J, Thursmond AS, Uchida BT, Sovak M (1988) Selective transcervical fallopian tube catheterization. Technique update. Radiology
Salat-Baroux J, Cutirier JY (1980) Obstruction pathologique de la portion initiale de la istme tubaire. J Gyn Obstet Biol Repr
Siegler AM (1993) Hysterosalpingography. Fertil Steril
Silva PD, Schaper AM, Meisch JK, Schauberger CW (1991) Outpatient microsurgical reversal of tubal sterilization by a combined approach of laparoscopy and minilaparotomy. Fertil Steril
Stern J, Peters AJ, Coulam CB (1992) Colour doppler ultrasonography assessment of tubal patency: a comparison study with traditional technique. Fertil Steril
Yildirim M (1989) ARTA. Assisted reproduction technology/andrology. International Congress, Casablanca, Sept 27–29, 1989
Zenisek L (1959) Die Salpingogramme bei der Endometrium Hyperplasie. Fortschr Röntgenstr

Endocrinology and Immunology

Endocrine Testing for In Vitro Fertilization

U. P. Merten and I. Turanli

Introduction

During recent years in vitro fertilization (IVF) and embryo transfer has been successfully introduced in hospital and private practice. The success of IVF depends on the number of embryos transferred into the uterus. Ovarian hyperstimulation results in multiple follicular maturation. Oocytes are extracted by laparoscopy and fertilized in vitro. To estimate the hyperstimulation of the ovaries and to avoid overstimulation, frequent sonographic examination of the ovaries and regular control of endocrine parameters are necessary (Runnebaum and Rabe 1987), even if the most important factor determining the pregnancy rate during IVF or gamete intrafallopian transfer (GIFT) is the number of embryos or oocytes transferred (Edwards and Steptoe 1983; Interim Licensing Authority 1991).

Endocrine testing in the diagnosis of fertility in monitoring the cycle and pregnancy and in IVF adds valuable information as the sensitivity and specificity of these tests have increased greatly and a high level of accuracy and precision has been achieved when they are used by specialists. Up to 50% of cases of reduced female fertility can be related to endocrine dysfunction (Freundl et al. 1990), and the choice of hormones to be tested depends on the specific question and the clinical picture investigated.

Specimens

Hormones can be measured in serum and urine specimens. The advantage of using 24-h urine is that it is the simplest way of obtaining a sample. The disadvantages of using urine are the time-consuming nature of the procedure, the late availability of a sample and the influence of oral fluid intake on the concentration of hormones in the urine (Trotnow 1987). The advantage of using serum as a sample relates primarily to the avoidance of the disadvantages and errors when collecting urine samples. Further, the analytical accuracy of serum tests is higher. An LH elevation is seen 12 h earlier in serum than in urine, which is of considerable importance in IVF programs. The disadvantage of using serum samples relates to the necessity of frequent venal puncture.

Table 1 Endocrine testing in gynecology

Diagnosis of fertility:	
Prolactin	Thyroid hormones
Luteinizing hormone (LH)	Corticotropin (ACTH)
Follicle-stimulating hormone (FSH)	Cortisol
Estradiol	Testosterone
Progesterone	Dehydroepiandrosterone
(including stimulation and suppression tests)	
Cycle monitoring:	
LH	
Estradiol	
Progesterone	
Pregnancy monitoring:	
Choriogonadotropin (β-chain) (hCG)	
Estradiol	
Progesterone	
Choriomammotropin (hPL)	
Estriol	
Progesterone	
α_1-Fetoprotein (AFP)	

In Vitro Fertilization

In the diagnosis of fertility the speed of hormone testing and availability of results are of less relevance than when the female cycle or a pregnancy has to be monitored or when cycle optimization with timed insemination or IVF techniques is used. With both of the latter methods, time necessary for the analytical procedures is of major importance as the results of relevant hormone tests (Table 1) have to be reported within a very short time.

Estradiol

Estradiol is produced by the growing follicle at the time of ovulation. Estradiol levels and sonography of the ovaries are needed in order to choose the dose and time of injection of hCG in order to stimulate the necessary number of follicles. As this is a multiple follicular maturation process, estradiol is elevated above physiological levels to more than 500 ng/l, but should not exceed 2000 ng/l. Next to the hormone concentration, the speed of increase in levels is important for ovulation. Therefore to identify the correct moment for hCG therapy, multiple tests during stimulation with clomiphene and/or HMG are necessary to ascertain the current concentrations, rising levels or even a down-regulation with diminishing levels of estradiol. Fast and highly precise estradiol testing can be performed within 2 h (Table 2).

Table 2 Estradiol

Test name:	Estradiol (17-β-estradiol)
Diagnostic value:	Monitoring of cycle
Specimen:	1.0 ml serum (or heparin-plasma) Store at +4 °C for several days Can be mailed without refrigeration within 24 h
Reference range:	Pubertal 5–15 ng/l Follicular 20–200 ng/l Midcycle 120–375 ng/l Luteal 60–260 ng/l Postmenopausal 6–22 ng/l
Diagnostic information:	Increased: feminization in children, estrogen-secreting tumor, gynecomastia, hepatic cirrhosis Decreased: primary and secondary ovarian insufficiency, anovalution, corpus luteum insufficiency, Turner's syndrome
Interference by:	Clomiphene (increase) Oral contraceptives (decrease)

Table 3 Luteinizing hormone

Test name:	Luteinizing hormone (LH), Lutropin
Diagnostic value:	Diagnosis of primary and secondary ovarian failure
Specimen:	1.0 ml serum (or heparin-plasma) Store at +4 °C for several days Can be mailed without refrigeration within 24 h
Stimulating test:	GnRH test (LH/FSH-RH test) Clomiphene test
Reference range:	Prepubertal <6 U/l Follicular 3–10 U/l Midcycle 20–100 U/l Luteal 3–17 U/l Postmenopausal 20–100 U/l
Diagnostic information:	Primary ovarian dysfunction (repeated increase of LH and/or FSH, and normal or increased GnRH test): - Gonadal dysgenesis 45,Xo (Turner's syndrome) 46,XY (Swyer's syndrome) - Resistant ovary syndrome - Cytostatic and/or radiotherapy - Stein-Leventhal syndrome Secondary ovarian dysfunction (decreased LH and FSH, no GnRH stimulation): - Pituitary or hypothalamic impairment - Isolated gonadotropic deficiency - Anosmia or hyposmia (Kallmann's syndrome) - Gestagen-negative amenorrhea - Isolated gonadotropic deficiency FSH/LH quotient <1 indicates polycystic ovarian syndrome (hyperandrogenemic dysfunction of ovaries)
Interference by:	Clomiphene, spironolactone (increase) Digoxin, megestrol, oral contraceptives, estrogens (decrease)

Luteinizing Hormone (LH)/Lutropin

Oocytes are removed 36 h after LH elevation or, in the case of low endocrine LH production, after hCG therapy. Therefore accurate LH test results have to be obtained with the greatest possible speed (Table 3). This can be done within 2 h. Multiple samples can be collected during the day and night before hCG injections are planned. By testing these in parallel, an LH elevation can be recognized early and the time estimated in which the LH concentration doubles.

Progesterone

Progesterone tests should be performed together with LH tests for additional safety as progesterone starts to rise approximately at the same time as LH. If declining estradiol levels are accompanied by a rapid increase in progesterone, this indicates luteinization of follicles. The progesterone test also can be performed within 2 h (Table 4).

Table 4 Progesterone

Test name:	Progesterone
Diagnostic value:	Detection of ovulation and evaluation of corpus luteum function
Specimen:	1.0 ml serum Store at +4 °C for several days Can be mailed without refrigeration within 24 h
Reference range:	Pubertal <0.3 ng/l Follicular 0.26–1.24 ng/l Midcycle 0.44–4.67 ng/l Luteal 3.29–17.4 ng/l Luteal peak 6.09–17.9 ng/l Postmenopausal <0.3 ng/l
Diagnostic information:	(highest level 6–8 days after ovulation, declining 3 days before menstruation) 1) Ovulation probably positive if progesterone value is >7.0 ng/l on the 7th day after expected time of ovulation 2) Corpus luteum insufficiency possible if progesterone level is <15 ng/l on the 7th day and <10 ng/l on the 10th day after expected time of ovulation 3) Increase: Congenital adrenal hyperplasia due to 21β-hydroxylase, 17β-hydroxylase, and 11β-hydroxylase deficiency, chorion epithelioma of ovary, molar pregnancy 4) Decreased: threatened abortion, galactorrhea-amenorrhea syndromes 5) Diagnosis of progesterone is useful to monitor patients having ovulation during induction with hCG, hMG, FSH/LH-RH or clomiphene
Interference by:	Clomiphene (increase) Ampicillin, PGF2α, ethinylestradiol, oral contraceptives (decrease)

Other Hormones

Besides the three hormones discussed above, various other tests can be performed: FSH (Table 5), GnRH stimulation test (Table 6), prolactin (Table 7), prolactin stimulation test (Table 8), and hCG (Table 9).

Table 5 Follicle-stimulating hormone

Test name:	Follicle-stimulating hormone (FSH), Follitropin
Diagnostic value:	Diagnosis of primary and secondary ovarian failure
Specimen:	1.0 ml serum (or heparin-plasma) Store at +4 °C for several days Can be mailed without refrigeration within 48 h
Stimulating test:	GnRH test (LH/FSH-RH test) Clomiphene test
Reference range:	Prepubertal <12 U/l Follicular 3–10 U/l Midcycle 7–20 U/l Postmenopausal 40–100 U/l
Diagnostic information:	Primary ovarian dysfunction (repeated increase of LH and/or FSH, and normal or increased GnRH test): - Gonadal dysgenesis 45,Xo (Turner's syndrome) 46,XY (Swyer's syndrome) - Resistant ovary syndrome - Cytostatic and/or radiotherapy - Stein-Leventhal syndrome Secondary ovarian dysfunction (decreased LH and FSH, no GnRH stimulation): - Pituitary or hypothalamic impairment - Isolated gonadotropic deficiency - Anosmia or hyposmia (Kallmann's syndrome) - Gestagen-negative amenorrhea - Isolated gonadotropic deficiency FSH/LH quotient <1 indicates polycystic ovarian syndrome (hyperandrogenemic dysfunction of ovaries)
Interference by:	Clomiphene, spironolactone (increase) Digoxin, megestrol, oral contraceptives, estrogens (decrease)

Table 6 GnRH (LH/FSH-RH) stimulating test

Test name:	Gonadotropin-releasing hormone (GnRH)/LH/FSH-releasing hormone stimulating test
Diagnostic value:	Gestagen, negative amenorrhea
Specimen:	1.0 ml serum (or heparin-plasma) Store at +4 °C freeze if stored for over 48 h Can be mailed without refrigeration for 24 h
Stimulating test:	Draw 5.0 ml blood for basal LH and FSH testing, GnRH-stimulating with 100 mg i.v. 30 min after injection draw 5.0 ml blood for LH test 45 min after injection draw 5.0 ml blood for FSH test
Diagnostic information:	Pituitary disease (no or little response) Hypothalamic disease (normal or prepubertal response) Primary gonadal failure (exaggerated and prolonged response)

Table 7 Prolactin

Test name:	Prolactin (PRL)
Diagnostic value:	Diagnosis of hyperprolactinemia
Specimen:	1.0 ml serum Blood should be drawn between 8.00 and 10.00 a.m. (circadian rhythm) Stable at +4 °C over 4–8 days Can be mailed without refrigeration within 24 h
Stimulating test:	Prolactin-stimulating test (metoclopramide HCl) (Paspertin) 5.0 mg i.v.
Reference range:	f 1–16 (25) ng/l [20–320 (500) mU/l] m 1–11 (20) ng/l [20–220 (400) mU/l]
Diagnostic information:	Value >250 ng/l (500 mU/l) in pituitary tumors (macro-adenomas) Value <250 ng/l (500 mU/l) Prolactinomas (microadenomas) Amenorrhea and/or galactorrhea, polycystic ovarian syndrome, hypothalamic-pituitary disease, renal failure, ectopic PRL production Infection: HVH encephalitis, basal gran. meningitis Primary hypothyroidism: hypothalamic stimulation Decrease possible in lesions of hypothalamus and/or pituitary
Interference by:	- Butyrophenone (Haloperidol) - Cimetidine, domperidone, methyldopa - Metoclopramide, estrogens, pimozide - Perphenazine, promazine, reserpine, Sulpivid, - Stress (breast palpation prior to blood drawing)

Table 8 Prolactin-stimulating test

Test name:	Prolactin-stimulating test with metoclopramide (Paspertin)
Diagnostic value:	Diagnosis of hyperprolactinemia
Specimen:	1.0 ml serum Blood should be drawn between 8.00 and 10.00 a.m. (circadian rhythm) Stable at +4 °C over 4–8 days Can be mailed without refrigeration within 24 h
Stimulating test:	Draw 5.0 ml blood for the prolactin Metoclopramide HCl (Paspertin) 5 mg i.v., after 30 min draw 5.0 ml blood for stimulated prolactin
Reference range:	w 1–16 (25) ng/l 20–320 (500) mU/l m 1–11 (20) ng/l 20–220 (400) mU/l
Diagnostic information:	Interpretation of results: 1) Basal <16 stimulated <250 ng/l = normal 2) Basal >16 stimulated >250 ng/l = hyperprolactinemia 3) Basal <16 stimulated >250 ng/l = latent hyperprolactinemia 4) Basal >16 stimulated <250 ng/l = hyperprolactinemia with decreased pituitary storage ability
Interference by:	- Butyrophenone (Haloperidol) - Cimetidine, domperidone, methyldopa - Metoclopramide, estrogens, pimozide - Perphenazine, promazine, reserpine, Sulpivid - Stress (breast palpation prior to blood drawing)

Table 9 Human chorionic gonadotropin

Test name:	Choriogonadotropin, human chorionic gonadotropin (hCG)
Diagnostic value:	Pregnancy (testing for and monitoring) Trophoblastic disease
Specimen:	1.0 ml serum (or EDTA-plasma) Store at $+4\,^{\circ}$C (freeze if stored for over 48 h) Can be mailed without refrigeration within 24 h
Reference range:	Nonpregnant females <10 U/l during pregnancy: 7–10 days (post conception) >10 U/l 1st week: 10–30 U/l 3rd week: 560–22600 U/l 5th week: 20400–81200 U/l 7th week: 6400–71300 U/l 2nd trimester: 530–43100 U/l 3rd trimester: 140–23900 U/l
Diagnostic information:	Increased: multiple pregnancy hydatidiform mole, choriocarcinoma, ovarian teratoma, ectopic hCG production (tumor of lung, stomach, liver, pancreas, colon) Decreased: ectopic pregnancy, threatened abortion

Methods and Quality Assurance

Radioimmunoassays (RIAs) are widely used for hormone tests and are constantly being improved in quality. This results in faster and more reliable analysis. During the last decade, different enzyme immunoassays, fluorescence immunoassays, and luminescence immunoassays (LIAs) have been introduced. Evaluation of these methods has indicated sufficient comparability, but deviations in borderline areas (i.e., lower and upper limits of decision) create problems if a laboratory plans to change from one method to another. If such a change is necessary both methods have to be run in parallel and both results should be reported for a certain period.

Internal and external quality control procedures are necessary for all immunoassays. Rules and regulations regarding quality control procedures in the medical laboratory are tending to become more similar in different countries.

Internal quality control represents a form of self-control on the part of the laboratory to ensure accurate and precise results. This can be done with control charts which list every result of control sera. Shewart's control chart (Büttner et al. 1974) is a simple method to indicate precision of an analytical test. More details on quality control of RIAs can be found in Wood (1987).

Each test has to be checked for its *accuracy* by using certain accuracy control samples. Using immunoassays the specificity of antibodies is of major importance as different antibodies can recognize different epitopes of the same antigen, leading to different specificity. Further antibodies can bind to the epitopes with different avidity which results in a different sensitivity for the test and produces different results of different tests. Control samples for accuracy and precision as well as samples from patients have to be tested in duplicate, even if for certain tests, such as LIAs, a high precision of results is obtained (Kayser et al. 1986).

Internal quality control requires regular use of control samples for tests of accuracy and *precision*. Test precision from day to day has to be checked by precision control samples.

Today hormone testing is nearly exclusively performed with kits supplied by manufacturers; only a very few laboratories prepare their own reagent sets. Therefore quality control rules for self-production of test kits will not be discussed in this context.

Analysers are being introduced into the market, offering a variety of (black box) methods including calibration curves to be stored and used over a longer period. This has to be viewed with the utmost caution. The stability of a calibration curve has to be checked daily with control samples. It is not sufficient to test only one control sample and to use mathematical corrections of a calibration curve.

External quality control serves as an independent means of judging accuracy and overall quality of laboratory performance, in addition to internal quality control. Participation in at least two to four surveys during one year is advised, especially if no standard methods are applied and the use of a multitude of antisera results in a different specificity of applied test kits. Models for optimized external quality control programs have been described (Merten 1982, Röhle and Breuer 1982) and surveys are offered regularly by different institutions (INSTAND, DGKC, CAP) in different countries (Germany, USA, UK, France) by manufacturers (Wellcome) and even by the World Health Organization (Human Reproduction Unit) in Geneva.

In Germany the rules and regulations of the Bundesärztekammer indicate which measures should be used in internal and external quality control (Bundesärztekammer 1987). These include as a necessity complete internal quality control and external quality control by regular participation in surveys.

In a *survey* an organization sends to the laboratory unknown samples to be analyzed for certain constituents. Results are returned to the organization within a certain time and are compared with results obtained by other laboratories and reference laboratories. Results of the laboratory have to meet certain requirements (limits) to receive a certificate of excellence. Therefore external control of a laboratory's results leads to reliable reports of endocrine parameters necessary for IVF patients.

Summary

Hormone analysis in fertility diagnosis, IVF, and pregnancy monitoring must be of high quality for the safety of the patient. The future of the patient and her child depends on the accuracy, precision, and reproducibility of these tests. To achieve the desired quality, each laboratory should perform with each test an internal quality control for accuracy and precision and should participate regularly in surveys for each constituent analyzed in the laboratory. In addition to this, each result of a laboratory must have a direct medical importance; it should not only be a result of a chemical test. To ensure that the needs of patients and gynecologists and also the laboratory requirements are met adequately, constant dialogue between clinical pathologists and gynecologists is necessary; this should result in more profound knowledge of the problems involved in endocrinology.

References

Büttner H, Hausert E, Stamm D (1974) Auswertung, Kontrolle und Beurteilung von Meßergebnissen. In: Bergmeyer (ed) Methoden der enzymatischen Analyse. VCH, Weinheim, vol 1, 2nd edn. p 283

Edwards RC, Steptoe PC (1983) Current status of in-vitro fertilisation and implantation of human embryos. Lancet ii:1265–1269

Interim Licensing Authority for Human In-Vitro-Fertilisation and Embryology. Sixth report (1991) ILA Secretariat, London

Freundl G, Heywinkel E, Hofmann N (1990) Gynäkologisch-andrologische Interaktion. Gynäkologe 23:209–213 Kinderlosigkeit als Dauerproblem

Kayser C, Schmitt Y, Kruse-Jarres JJ (1986) Gegenüberstellung von Lumineszenz- und Radio-Immuno-Assay am Beispiel von vier Hormon- bzw. Tumormarker-Tests. Ärztl Lab 32:267–270

Merten R (1981) Die Effektivität von Ringversuchen als externe Qualitätssicherung im medizinischen Laboratorium - Bewertungsmaßstäbe und ihre Auswirkung. Lab Med 5(A+B):6, 68, 197, 257; (1982) 6(A+B):17

Richtlinien der Bundesärztekammer (1988) Qualitätssicherung der quantitativen Bestimmungen im Laboratorium. Deutsches Ärzteblatt I:697–712

Röhle G, Breur G (1982) Über die Notwendigkeit und die Problematik von Ringversuchen in der Endokrinologie. Acta Endocrinol (Kbh) 3:33–38

Runnebaum B, Rabe T (eds) (1987) Gynäkologische Endokrinologie. Springer, Berlin Heidelberg New York

Trotznow S (1987) In: Runnebaum B, Rabe T (eds) Gynäkologische Endokrinologie. Springer, Berlin Heidelberg New York

Wood WG (1987) Qualitätssicherung bei radioimmunologischen in-vitro-Analysen. In: v Boroviczeny KG, Merten R, Merten UP (eds) Qualitätssicherung im Medizinischen Laboratorium. Springer, Berlin Heidelberg New York, pp 405–444

The Ovary

A. Helvacioglu

Introduction

In the words of Albert Schweitzer, the most precious thing about man, however creative he may be, is man himself. "Man" endures through the intricate reproductive process in which the ovary plays a lead role. The ovary is a multicompartmental structure with different and variable biologic properties. Responding to cyclic pituitary gonadotropin secretion, it secretes sex steroids and glycoproteins and produces the ovum. Current information suggests that the ovary is very instrumental in the activities of the hypothalamo-pituitary-ovarian axis.

Steroidogenesis

Analysis of ovarian venous effluents revealed that the ovaries secrete pregnenolone, progesterone, 17α-hydroxyprogesterone (17OHP), dehydroepiandrosterone, adrostenedione, testosterone, estrone, and 17β-estradiol. When microdissected follicles were studied, estrone and estradiol were found to be the major products of the follicle, while progesterone and 17OHP were mainly secreted by the corpus luteum. Studies employing C_{21} and C_{19} precursors revealed the isolated granulosa cell capable of producing mostly progesterone, estrogens, and 17OHP. Isolated theca cells produced progesterone and androstenedione.

Estrogen biosynthesis

Follicle stimulating hormone (FSH) and luteinizing hormone (LH) stimulate membrane-associated adenylate cyclase enzyme, which in turn converts intracellular ATP to cAMP. The latter binds to the regulatory subunit of a protein kinase whereupon the catalytic subunit of the enzyme is activated and dissociated (Fig. 1). The catalytic subunit phosphorylates key intracellular proteins central to the signal transduction sequence. LH also activates the phospholipase C-protein kinase C system in granulosa cells. This system is usually antagonistic to gonadal steroidogenesis. Existence of these who different pathways may further regulate steroidogenesis in the cells. According to two cell/two gonadotropin theory, follicular estrogen biosynthesis requires

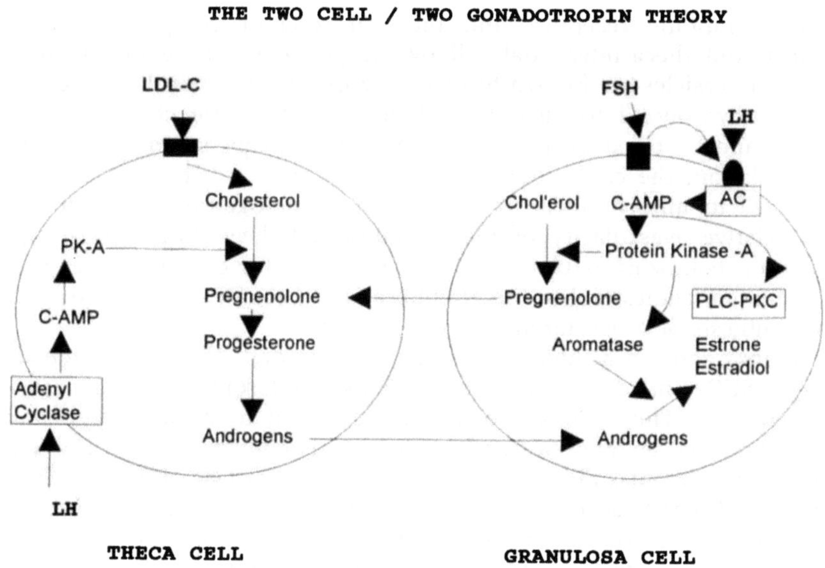

Fig. 1. Steroidogenesis in the ovary. *PK-A*, protein kinase A; *AC*, adenylate cyclase; *PLC*, phospholipase C; *PKC*, phosphokinase C; *cAMP*, cyclic AMP. See text for further details

theca-interstitial cells to produce C_{19} precursors which are then aromatized in the granulosa cells to estrogens (Fig. 1). Aromatase activity of granulosa cells was estimated to be at least 700 times greater than that of theca cells from large preovulatory follicles. So, granulosa cells are the principal site of estrogen synthesis in the dominant preovulatory follicle. Androgens, mainly adrostenedione, produced by LH-stimulated theca cells, are the main substrate for estrogen biosynthesis by FSH-stimulated granulosa cells. Estrone is readily converted to estradiol by the steroidogenic enzyme 17β-hydroxysteroid dehydrogenase, which is located in the granulosa cell. The aromatization process involves the loss of angular C_{19} precursors' methyl group and the stereospecific elimination of the 1β and 2β hydrogens of the A ring of the androgen precursor. Thus, for each mole of estrogen formed, a total of three hydroxylation reactions are required.

Aromatase gene exceeds 70 kb and is the largest of cytochrome P450 family of steroidogenic genes. Aromatase transcription is highly regulated with four major promoter sites that respond to cytokines, cyclic nucleotides, gonadotropins, phorbol esters, glucocorticoids and growth factors [1]. Therefore all of these agents may be instrumental in estradiol production through their effects on the aromatase gene expression.

Progestin biosynthesis

Steroidogenesis begins with cholesterol, which is derived primarily from circulating lipoproteins (Fig. 1). Low-density lipoproteins (LDL) are bound to specific membrane receptors and the LDL-receptor complexes enter the granulosa and theca-interstitial cell by receptor-mediated endocytosis. The endocytotic vesicles are known to fuse to lysosomes wherein LDL-cholesterol esters are hydrolyzed to yield free cholesterol. The free cholesterol is re-esterified and is stored in the cytoplasm in lipid droplets. Under gonadotropin stimulation, the cholesterol ester is hydrolyzed and the free cholesterol transported to mitochondria to be used in steroidogensis. In the follicular phase, relative avascularity of the granulosa cell layer limits progesterone production. Following ovulation, vascularization of the corpus luteum supplies abundant cholesterol to the granulosa and theca interna cells to be used in the synthesis of progesterone.

Granulosa and theca interna cells contain abundant cholesterol side chain cleavage (SCC) and delta 5-4 isomerase/β-hyroxysteroid dehydrogenase (3β-HSD) enzymes. Thus LDL-cholesterol is converted to delta-5 pregnenolone by mitochondrial enzyme SCC, which in turn is converted into delta-4 progesterone via cytoplasmic enzyme delta-5-4 isomerase/3β-HSD. The human granulosa cell has been reported to have low levels of 17α-hydroxylase activity, and thus converts a very small amount of progesterone into 17OHP. Functional roles of the steroidogenic enzymes 20α-hydroxysteroid dehydrogenase and 5α-reductase at the level of the human granulosa cell are not completely known.

Androgen biosynthesis

The biosynthesis of the C_{19} androgens takes place in the theca-interstitial cells. This cell type contains enzymes necessary to generate C_{21} precursors, as well as 17α-hydroxylase/17–20 desmolase activity capable of converting C_{21} products (pregnenolone, progesterone) to C_{19} (dehydroepiandrosterone and androstenedione), which could be viewed as an exclusive feature of the theca-interstitial cell.

Protein Biosynthesis

The granulosa and theca-interstitial cells are capable of producing a large number of proteins as shown by gel fractionation studies. Functions of only a few of these – inhibin, activin, follistatin, and gonadotropin surge-inhibiting factor – are known at present.

Inhibin

Inhibin is an FSH-inducible 32-kDa heterodimer glycoprotein, with a covalently linked common 18-kDa α-subunit and two distinct 14 kDa β-subunits (β_A and β_B) which show approximately 85% identity. The α/β_A heterodimer is called inhibin A and the α/β_B heterodimer is called inhibin B; they possess similar physiological properties. All three subunits are encoded by separate mRNAs [2]. Peripherally inhibin has potent bioactivity for inhibiting FSH secretion. However, in two distinct clinical conditions in which FSH modulation differs from that of LH, i.e., polycystic ovarian disease (PCOD) and luteofollicular transition phase of the normal menstrual cycle, inhibin was not responsible for the distinct FSH changes [3]. Autocrine and paracrine functions of inhibin are studied in experimental animals and suggest a significant role in the modulation of gonadotropin-mediated folliculogenesis, follicle maturation, and corpus luteum (CL) formation. Functional studies in the rate suggest that inhibin attenuates granulosa cell production of estrogen and stimulates androgen biosynthesis in the thecal cell [4].

In human ovaries mRNA expression studies suggest that both thecal and granulosa cells are able to synthesize inhibin/activin subuntis and follistatin with differential expression in small and dominant follicles and CL, and that this system has a role in the growth and development of oocytes [5]. Inhibin is produced by the granulosa and theca cell in normal women, in women with PCOD, thecal and stromal cells exhibit distinct positive staining for α, β_A, and β_B subunits, suggesting that thecal and stromal cells might be the main cellular site of inhibin production in PCOD [6]. Nevertheless, these in vitro functions may not reflect the in vivo situation, since the bioavailability of inhibin is dependent upon the presence of a high-affinity binding protein, follistatin, which binds to both inhibin and activin through the common β-subunit [7].

Activin

Activin is a homodimer of the β subunits of the inhibin (β_A/β_B, β_B/β_B, or β_A/β_A) and has bioactivity opposite to that of inhibin. Functional studies in the rat suggest that activin potentiates granulosa cell production of estrogen, and inhibits androgen biosynthesis in the thecal cell [4]. The bioavailability of activin is also dependent upon the presence of a high-affinity binding protein, follistatin [7]. In human ovaries activin is also synthesized by both thecal and granulosa cells, with differential expression in small and dominant follicles and CL, and has a role in the growth and development of oocytes [5].

Follistatin

Follistatin is an FSH-inducible granulosa cell-derived, 315 amino acid single chain polypeptide and appears to suppress the release of pituitary FSH but not LH. It is a high-affinity binding protein, and binds to both inhibin and activin through the common β-subunit [7]. In human ovaries mRNA expression studies suggest that both thecal and granulosa cells are able to synthesize follistatin with differential expression in small and dominant follicles and CL [5].

Gonadotropin surge-inhibiting factor (GnSIF)

GnSIF refers to a nonsteroidal substance with an unknown exact biochemical nature. It is short lived and inhibits the FSH and LH surges. GnSIF may be the substance preventing endogenous gonadotropin surge during controlled ovarian hyperstimulation.

Follicular Growth and Development and Ovulation

Although optimal follicular development depends largely on gonadotropic and steroidogenic action at the level of ovarian granulosa cells, classical concepts of ovarian regulation have been extended in recent years to include a complex system of endocrine, paracrine, and autocrine factors. Among the many factors involved in the regulation of ovarian function, insulin growth factors (IGFs) and growth hormone (GH) have been studied to a greater extent. A list of growth factors and their roles in ovarian function is summarized in Table 1. Clinical and experimental observations suggest a potential role of GH in ovarian function. GH receptors are found to be widely distributed in the female reproductive system of the rat [8], including the granulosa cell, and GH-binding protein is found to be present in human periovulatory follicular fluid [9]. Levels of GH-binding protein in the follicular fluid were found to be positively related to young age, high serum estradiol level, and high follicular fluid estradiol concentration [9]. Moreover, GH has been shown to increase the in vitro effects of both IGF-I and IGF-II [10]. Consequently, it is possible ot assume that both GH and IGFs play important roles in the control of follicular growth and development through reciprocal potentiation. Furthermore, epidermal growth factor and IGF-1 have been shown to augment spontaneous maturation in immature human oocytes [11]. GH also augments progesterone production by human luteal cells in a dose-dependent manner and synergizes with human chorionic gonadotropin [12].

Progressively increasing insulin levels and IGF-1 activity during puberty have been suggested to cause PCOD in susceptible women [13]. In lean PCOD patients low serum IGFBP-1 levels were associated with poor clomiphene citrate reponse [14]. Furthermore, PCOD patients demonstrated relative deficiency in GH reserve [15], suggesting direct or indirect involvement of GH and growth factors in the development of PCDO.

The pioneering studies of McNatty et al. [16] on the microenvironment of human antral follicles were the first to indicate a correlation between high intrafollicular androgen/estradiol ratios and the inability of the oocyte to complete meiotic maturation. Presence of androgen receptors in the granulosa and thecal cells of primate follicles [17] supports a direct paracrine/autocrine role for androgen during folliculogenesis and luteinization. Alteration of endogenous androgen/estradiol ratio by inhibiting aromatase activity led to abrogated oocyte nuclear maturity without any change in follicular growth, suggesting that either decreased estradiol or increased androgen adversely affects oocyte maturation in rhesus monkeys [18]. Labelled C_{19} steroid infusion studies in normal women strongly suggested that the follicular testosterone functions as a follicular regulator, enhancing follicular aromatase activity when adequate amounts of FSH are available [19]. Nevertheless, high follicular concentrations of reduced androgens (e.g., DHT) may act as a competitive inhibitors of granulosa cell aromatase activity.

Table 1 Role of growth factors in ovarian function (from [22])

Factor	Granulosa	Theca	Corpus luteum	Other
Insulin	Receptors present Augments basal and hCG-induced P Enhances E_2-stimulated P	Enhances LH/hCG-induced Adione, E_2, P, T Increases basal secretion of E_2, P, T, Adione	Enhance secretion of oxytocin and P	Receptors present in stroma
IGF-I (somatomedin C)	Has type I receptors that are increased by FSH Made here Enhances cAMP-induced P Enhances FSH-induced P, E_2, cAMP, adenylyl cyclase, luteinization, LH receptors, proteoglycans Enhances PMSG-induced aromatase and P Stimulated by LH, FSH, cAMP, GH, EGF Enhances HDL-induced P Enhances P and inhibin production	Has type I receptors Increases hCG-induced E_2, P, T, Adione Increases basal secretion of P	Increases secretion of oxytocin and P	Stimulated by GH in whole ovary Enhances aromatase in luteinized granulosa Enhances androsterone from theca-interstitial cells Stimulated in ovary by hCG
IGF-II (MSA)	Made here Enhances steroidogenesis Has type II receptors Stimulated by LH and FSH Increases ornithine decarboxylase	Enhances hCG-induced P, T, E_2		Stimulated by GH, hCG, hPL, PRL, and FSH in luteinized granulosa
TGF*β*	Inhibits EGF-induced growth Enhances FSH-induced LH receptors, aromatase, EGF receptors, and inhibin Inhibits EGF-induced IGF-I Inhibits basal and FSH-stimulated P Increases production of E_2, cAMP, inhibin Increases growth	Produced here Increases basal and hCG-induced E_2 production Inhibits hCG-induced P, T, Adione Inhibits basal P, Adione		
EGF/TGF*α*	Inhibits FSH-induced aromatas, E_2 Stimulates growth/mitosis Has receptors Receptors are stimulated by FSH and inhibited by LH Stimulates P and E_2 Enhances FSH receptor binding Inhibits LH receptor binding, inhibin secretion	TGF*α* made here (not EGF) Decreases basal and hCG-stimulated E_2 Stimulates growth		Augments basal and hCG-induced P in luteinized granulosa Present in theca-interstitial cells
FGFa	Produced here Inhibits FSH-induced LH receptors Inhibits FSH-induced cAMP, E_2		Produced here	

P, progesterone; T, testosterone; PMSG, pregnant mare serum gonadotropin; HDL, high-density lipoprotein; hPL, human placental lactogen; Adione, androstenedione; TGF, transforming growth factor; MSA, multiplication-stimulating activity; hCG, human chorionic gonadotropin; GH, growth hormone; EGF, epidermal growth factor; FGFa, acidic fibroblast growth factor

Putative Intraovarian Regulators

An increasing body of evidence suggests that transforming growth factor $\beta 1$, basic fibroblast growth factor, interleukin-1, tumor necrosis factor α, catecholamines, luteinization inhibitor, gonadotropin binding inhibitors, oocyte maturation inhibitor, renin, angiotensin, and oxytocin are some of the paracrine factors that modify the actions of the pituitary gonadotropins, resulting in the selectivity of the ovarian follicular maturation process. Recently it has been shown that atretic follicles in normal human ovaries stained for renin and angiotensin in both theca and granulosa cells and there was constant expression of renin and angiotensin in the typical follicles of PCOD, suggesting an association between the ovarian renin-angiotensin system and PCOD [20].

Fertility Drugs and Ovarian Cancer

It is now well established that the risk of ovarian cancer is altered by a number of identifiable factors relevant to fertility and reproductive health. Factors such as parity and pill use have protective effects, whereas the effect of infertility and related treatment is far less certain. The possibility of an increased risk of developing ovarian cancer related to fertility-related drug treatment has been raised. In 1993, The International Federation of Fertility Societies (IFFS) concluded that women who choose to use drug treatment for infertility probably will be exposed to an annual additional risk of <1 in 5000 [21].

References

1. Simpson ER, Mahendroo MS, Means GD, Kilgore MW, Corbin CJ, Mendelson CR (1993) Tissue-specific promoters regulate aromatase cytochrome P450 expression. Clin Chem 39:317–324
2. Mason AJ, Niahll HD, Seeburgh PH (1986) Structure of two human ovarian inhibins. Biochem Biophys Res Commun 35:957–964
3. Le Nestour E, Marraoui J, Lahlou M, Roger M Ziegler DE, Bouchard PH (1993) Role of estradiol in the rise in FSH levels during the luteal-follicular transition. J Clin Endocrinol Metab 77:439–442
4. Hsueh AJW, Dahl KD, Vaughan J et al. (1987) Heterodimers and homodimers of inhibin subunits have different paracrine action in the modulation of luteinizing hormone-stimulated androgen biosynthesis. Proc Natl Acad Sci USA 84:5082–5086
5. Roberts VJ, Barth S, El-Roeiy A, Yen SSC (1993) Expression of inhibin/activin subunits and follistatin messenger ribonucleic acids and proteins in ovarian follicles and the corpus luteum during the human menstrual cycle. J Clin Endocrinol Metab 77:1402–1410
6. Yamoto M, Minami S, Nakano R (1993) Immunohistochemical localization of inhibin subunits in polycystic ovary. J Clin Endocrinol Metab 77:859–862
7. Shimonaka M, Inouye S, Shimasaki S, Ling N (1991) Follistatin binds to both activin and inhibin through the common beta-subunit. Endocrinology 128:3313–3315
8. Lobie PE, Breipohl W, Aragon JG, Waters MJ (1990) Cellular localization of the growth hormone receptor/binding protein in the male and female reproductive systems. Endocrinology 126:2214–2221

9. Amit T, Dirnfeld M, Barkey RJ, Peleg I, Hacham H, Abramovici H, Blumenfeld Z (1993) Growth hormone-binding protein (GH-BP) levels in follicular fluid from human periovulatory follicles: correlation with serum GH-BP levels. J Clin Endocrinol Metab 77:33–39
10. Barreca A, Artini PG, Del Monte P, Ponzani P, Pasquini P, Cariola G, Volpe A, Genazzani AR, Giordano G, Minuto F (1993) In vivo and in vitro effect of growth hormone on estradiol secretion by human granulosa cells. J Clin Endocrinol Metab 77:61–67
11. Gomez E, Tarin JJ, Pellicer (1993) Oocyte maturation in humans: the role of gonadotropins and growth factors. Fertil Steril 60:40–46
12. Di Simone N, Castellani R, Lanzone A, Caruso A, Mancuso S (1993) Human GH enhances P production by human luteal cells in vitro. II. Evidence of a distinct effect of two luteal cell types. Fertil Steril 60:47–52
13. Nobels F, Dewailly D (1992) Puberty and polycystic ovarian syndrome: the insulin/insulin-like growth factor I hypothesis. Fertil Steril 58:655
14. Tiitinen AE, Laatikainen TJ, Seppala MT (1993) Serum levels of insulin-like growth factor binding protein-1 and ovulatory responses to clomiphen citrate in women with polycystic ovarian disease. Fertil Steril 60:58–62
15. Acar B, Kadanali S (1993) Diminished growth hormone response to L-dopa in polycystic ovarian disease. Fertil Steril 60:984–987
16. McNatty KP, Smith DM, Makris A, Osathanondh R, Ryan KJ (1979) The microenvironment of the human antral follicle: interrelationships among the steroid levels in antral fluid, the population of granulosa cells, and the status of the oocyte in vivo and in vitro. J Clin Endocrinol Metab 49.851–860
17. Horie K, Takakura K, Fujiwara H, Suginami H, Liao S, Mori T (1992) Immunohistochemical localization of androgen receptor in the human ovary throughout the menstrual cycle in relation to estrogen and progesterone receptor expression. Hum Reprod 7:184–190
18. Zelinski-Wooten MB, Hess DL, Baughman WL, Molskness TA, Wolf DP, Stouffer RL (1993) Administration of an aromatase inhibitor during the late follicular phase of gonadotropin treated cycles in rhesus monkeys: effects on follicle development, oocyte maturation, and subsequent luteal function. J Clin Endocrinol Metab 76:988
19. Haning RV, Hackett Jr RJ, Flood CA, Loughlin JS, Zhao QY, Longcope C (1973) Testosterone, a follicular regulator: key to anovulation. J Clin Endocrinol Metab 77:710–715
20. Palumbo A, Pourmotabbed G, Carcangiu ML, Andrade-Gordon P, Roa L, DeCherney A, Naftolin F (1993) Immunohistochemical localization of renin and angiotensin in the ovary: comparison between normal women and patients with histologically proven PCOD. Fertil Steril 60:280-284
21. International Federation of Fertility Societies (IFFS) (1993) Fertility drugs and ovarian cancer. Fertil Steril 60:406–408
22. Hylka VW, Dizerega GS (1991) Reproductive hormones and their mechansim of action. In: Mishell DR, Davajan V, Lobo RA (eds) Infertility, contraception and reproductive endocrinology. 3rd edn. Blackwell Scientific, Boston, p 47

Thyroid Gland, Gravidity and Puerperium

H. G. Bohnet

This chapter aims at elucidating some special aspects of thyroidal disturbances and diseases. Hormonal and metabolic alterations during pregnancy exert complex influences on thyroidal function. The primary cause is an estrogen-induced surplus synthesis of thyroxine-binding globulin (TBG) in the liver, producing significantly higher serum levels of total T3 and T4. As a consequence, it is far more difficult to diagnose disturbances of thyroidal function during pregnancy and childbed when TBG decline occurs. Treatment is extremely difficult due to permeability of the placenta by certain medications or substances (e.g., thyreostatics, iodine) as opposed to others (thyroxine).

From the first few weeks of pregnancy, increased renal iodine clearance has been reported, leading to a decline in serum level of anorganic iodine. Increased glomerular filtration rates cause higher iodine loss by micturation. By (physiologic) enlargement of the organ and supported by the thyroid-stimulating hormone (TSH)-stimulating characteristic of gonadotropic human chorionic (hCG), the thyroid gland aims at binding more iodine to maintain euthyroidism. The thyroid gland, however, must not exceed the upper normal volume of 18 ml.

From the beginning of the second trimenon, thyroidal function is controlled by fetal hypothalamus and hypophysis initiating their own production of T3 and T4, i.e., increasing additional iodine requirements that can hardly be met by nutrition, despite the use of iodine salt in private households or by nationwide introduction, as is done in Switzerland. These are the reasons why all pregnant women, regardless of any struma, should receive additional iodine, either 200 µg/day or 1500 µg/week.

Hormonal Levels of Thyroid Gland and In Vitro Diagnosis

Presently it is almost unanimously agreed that the reference interval for TSH and the free thyroidal hormones does not differ in the presence or absence of pregnancy. Basal TSH serum levels reach their lowest rates during the first trimenon [18, 55], coinciding with the highest serum concentrations of hCG. This is considered to have a partially thyroid gland-stimulating effect corresponding to an activity of 0.2 micro units TSH per unit hCG in the bioassay, from which an equivalent range of between 3 and 10 micro units/ml TSH is calculated depending on the hCG concentration.

Around the second trimenon, TSH levels show slight increases within the normal range. A significant but not linear negative correlation with free T4 is observed, leading to the conclusion that free hormone concentrations of T3 and T4 decline in the course of pregnancy, reaching lower normal limits towards delivery date. There is now increasing doubt about whether these alterations can (still) be considered physiologic. They are rather interpreted as being the result of relative iodine shortages. In the course of the lactation period, lasting several weeks and presumably depending on the maternal iodine supply level, increases in thyroidal hormone concentrations become manifest while TSH levels decline.

From what has been described so far, it may be concluded that the determination of TSH and fT4 furnish very precise data (except for TRH tests) on the thyroidal function during pregnancy, puerperium, and the lactation period as well as at other times. During the first trimenon, TSH response to TRH is weaker than during the second. It has not been clearly established whether this fact is solely attributable to higher estrogen secretion or whether relative iodine insufficiency with consecutive decline of T4 is involved as well. If determination of TSH and fT4 is replaced by a TRH test during pregnancy, approximately a third more thyroidopenia cases become evident. The determination of total T3 and T4 is not suitable for diagnosing disturbances of thyroidal function during pregnancy.

Struma

Almost 30 years ago a decline in serum iodine level during pregnancy was described, apparently normalizing within a few weeks after delivery. Examinations proved a doubling of struma diseases originating from iodine shortage during pregnancy as compared to women that were not pregnant. Results from studies recently conducted in Northern Germany prove that struma prevalence affects approximately one quarter of gynecological patients, a rate rising to almost two thirds of patients affected in the third trimenon of pregnancy. Comparably high rates have been described in earlier studies conducted in various areas of Germany. If iodine supply is optimum, as, e.g., in Iceland, struma prevalence does not increase during pregnancy. Any struma, mainly prevalent during pregnancy, requires consultation considering hormonal aspects (TSH, fT4, antithyreoperoxidase), since simultaneous hypothyreosis necessitates immediate treatment. Primary occurrence of thyroidal nodes during pregnancy or childbed requires examination for malignity (thyroidal carcinoma).

Hypothyreosis and Lymphocytic Thyroiditis (Hashimoto' Syndrome)

National studies have shown that nearly every fourth pregnant woman or woman in childbed develops latent hypothyreosis. In one eighth of women, thyroidal dysfunction becomes manifest. Insufficient iodine supply provokes an isolatedly reduced fT4 in another one eighth of women. In fetuses unable to produce sufficient thyroidal hormones, iodine shortage may cause neurocerebral development disturbances, among which cretinism, a very serious disease, has now disappeared in Europe. A working team guided by Man et al. has examined the progress in development in children of hypothyroid mothers 8 months after their birth and at the age of 7 years. Normal development was only observed in one half of the children in cases where no optimum regulation of hypothyreosis was achieved during pregnancy. Even at the age of 7 years, scores in psychological tests were still inferior. Other research teams reported similarly high rates of development disturbances in children. The earlier a hypothyroid newborn child receives levothyroxine treatment, the more favorable the prognosis: the first 3 months of life are decisive. In less severe maternal hypothyreosis, the impact on fetal development is less harmful as a result of two mechanisms. First, the fetus in its early intrauterine life has access to maternal thyroidal hormones, i.e., the placental barrier is not yet fully developed. Second, the entire second trimenon is marked by a severe increase in fetal TSH, resulting in serum concentrations of 5–10 micro units/ml provoking a maximum stimulation of self-produced thyroidal hormones by the fetus, documented by an increase in thyroidal hormone volume in the amniotic fluid. Furthermore, it has the function of a reservoir, shown by the fact that the intra-amniotic administration of thyroxine is absorbed or utilized by the fetus.

Pregnancies of hypothyroid women are complicated or endangered under various conditions. Results from examinations carried out at a very early stage show reduced thyroidal hormone concentrations in two thirds of those women that had abortions. One third of hypothyroid pregnant women have an abortion if levothyroxine is inadequately substituted, whereas abortion rates of adequately substituted patients only reach about 10%. In the case of autoimmunothyreopathy, spontaneous abortion rates double. Data collected retrospectively by Davis et al. indicate a frequency of anemia (ferritin inadequacy) of approximately 30% with refractory response to chalybeate drug therapy. Preeclampsia frequency was reduced in latent hypothyreosis (17%) as compared to manifest disturbances (44%). Still births double in hypothyroid pregnant women. One third of the newborn children of hypothyroid mothers are relatively small.

In addition to iodine insufficiency, chronic lymphocytic thyroiditis may provoke hypothyreosis with occasional struma development during pregnancy. Apart from the incidences described, another type of thyroiditis – atropic Hashimoto thyroiditis – may, however seldom, occur, usually in older pregnant women. In total, its frequency during pregnancy and puerperium reaches 5%–10%. Postnatal Hashimoto thyroiditis promotes (childbed) depressions.

Hypothyreosis during pregnancy is always treated using L-thyroxine. Additional iodine administration is indicated in cases where immunothyreopathy is excluded. Field reports confirm that daily administration of 100 µg L-thyroxine plus 100 µg iodine in minor hypothyreosis easily produces euthyreote metabolic situations preventing struma growth. A normalization of thyroid volume cannot be achieved during pregnancy and childbed. It is recommended that at least 200 µg iodine/day is administered (recommendations have already been submitted). In severe hypothyreosis, L-thyroxine doses vary depending on the results of TSH and fT4 determination. We know from experience that doses of L-thyroxine administered to achieve euthyreosis before pregnancy must be increased by one third to one half of the dose during pregnancy, requiring further maintenance of a level of 25% of the original dose during puerperium. Daily doses of 150 µg are, however, rarely exceeded.

(Minor) euthyreote struma diagnosed at the beginning of pregnancy should be treated by iodine. Since daily iodine doses of 200 µg are required in struma, prophylaxis therapeutic administration should be increased (250–500 µg/day).

Hyperthyreosis and Basedow's Disease

Immunohyperthyreosis mainly becomes manifest in women in the third decade of life, while struma autonomies tend to affect older people. This would explain a relatively high number of pregnant women suffering from Basedow's disease. However, this is not actually the case. A rate of 1–10 per 1000 has been reported. Various examinations have occasionally shown lower (0.3%) or higher (1%) rates of TSH receptor antibodies during pregnancy and childbed.

The very rare coincidence of Basedow's disease and pregnancy might be explained by an extreme subfertility of the women concerned, becoming manifest in a significantly increased abortion rate (20%–40%). Similar conclusions were drawn from the fact that 90% of all cases of Basedow's disease were found prior to a pregnancy, with defined therapeutic strategies (thyroidectomy) being applied before the woman becomes pregnant again.

Minor or latent functional hyperthyreosis has less harmful effects on female fertility than immunopathy. Thus may explain the higher frequency of hyperthyreote metabolic occurrence during pregnancy than anticipated: both latent and manifest hyperthyreosis amount to 5% during pregnancy and reach up to 3% postnatally. Other reports indicate a considerably lower number (up to 2%). A distinction is necessary between functional hyperthyreosis existing prior to pregnancy and hyperthyreosis induced by pregnancy itself.

In mole pregnancies and trophoblast tumors, hyperthyreosis may become manifest. It is not yet known whether elevated hCG levels or increased secretion of chorial TSH-like factors induce the phenomenon. Depending on the intensity of hyperemesis, it is possible to diagnose hyperthyreosis, which obviously requires treatment.

Clinical diagnosis of hyperthyreosis developing during pregnancy is difficult in most cases. It is often neglected since even in healthy pregnant women a tendency towards tachycardy, warm skin, or temperature intolerance may exist. Weight loss is rare, although weight gain may fail to occur. Frequent watery stool and any vomiting during pregnancy requires laboratory diagnosis. Determination of TSH furnishes very precise results with additional determination of fT3 values in the serum. Results that are not clear require a TRH test, whereas the determination of total T3 and T4 is not necessary.

From experience we know that any form of hyperthyreosis existing prior to pregnancy will improve in the course of gravidity, which is, however, not reflected in the risk of abortion. In patients with Basedow's disease, it is presumed that a change in the immunologic balance may have a positive influence, since TSH receptor antibody titer may decline (amino 6), whereas a postnatal exacerbation frequently occurs. Other mechanisms, e.g., elevation of TBG-6 with ensuing cutoff of thyroid hormones combined with increased iodine demand during gravidity, provoking relative iodine shortage usually in the mother, might favorably influence metabolism, notably in hyperthyreosis that is not immunologically induced. Therapy must be adapted accordingly.

In severe forms of hyperthyreosis that become manifest during pregnancy, thyreostasis is imperative, while minor forms may be treated later. Thyroidization should principally be a monotherapy. Combined use of thyreostatics and levothyroxine are contraindicated, since thyreostatic requirements are elevated, exposing the fetus to high doses of the substance and provoking thyreose insufficiency, while they are met in the mother by thyroxine administration. Lowest doses of a.m. thyreostatics should be administered to achieve borderline euthyreosis, i.e., minor hyperthyreosis is tolerated, allowing basal TSH suppression, while fT3 may reach the upper margin. With these therapeutic proceedings the possibility cannot be excluded that thyreostasis may cause an enlargement of the thyroid gland or struma. An operation during gravidity should be avoided if possible. If serious mechanical complications occur, however, it may become imperative.

In cases of preexisting hyperthyreosis, the doses of thyreostatics must be reduced during pregnancy. We know from experience that doses administered prior to gravidity must be reduced by half towards the delivery date and increased again during puerperium, reaching 75% of the original dose. In women treated as described, the fetal malformation rate is lower than in those receiving no treatment. Consequently, there is no proof of hypothyreosis in newborns. In the case of maternal Basedow's disease, attention must be paid in the event of thyroidal hyperfunction, since TSH receptor antibodies may have entered the fetus in utero, resulting in stimulation of the thyroid gland of the newborn due to a long medicinal half-life.

Although thyreostatics enter maternal milk, a mother may nourish her newborn once optimum adaptation of maternal metabolism is ensured. This highlights the necessity of thyroidal parameter controls at regular intervals of 2 weeks to start with and 4 weeks thereafter. An adequate iodine supply to the newborn must be ensured by doses of, e.g., 50 μg iodine, as contained in instant milk and pap.

References

1. Aboul-Khair SA, Crooks J, Turnbull AC, Hytten FE (1964) The physiological changes in thyroid function during pregnancy. Clin Sci 27:195
2. Amino N, Tanizawa O, Miyai K (1978) Changes of serum immunoglobulins IgG, IgA, IgM, and IgE during pregnancy. Obstet Gynecol 52:415
3. Bauch K, Meng W, Ulrich FE, Grosse E, Kempe R, Schönemann F, Sterzel G, Seitz W, Möckel G, Weber A, Tiller R, Rockel A, Dempe A, Seige K (1986) Thyroid status during pregnancy and post partum in regions of iodine deficiency and endemic goiter. Endocrinol Exp 20:67–77
4. Bohnet HG, Kato K, Trapp M, Weise HC, Leidenberger FA (1986) Different hormonal patterns in human menopausal gonadotropin-treated, clomiphene-treated and untreated conception cycles. Fertil Steril 45:469
5. Bohnet HG, Fiedler K, Leidenberger FA (1981) Subclinical hypothyreoidism and infertility. Lancet II:1278
6. Bohnet HG, Seeler M (1992) Häufigkeit von Schilddrüsenfunktionsstörungen post partum. Gynäkol Praxis 16:265–268
7. Bohnet HG, Knuth UA, Seeler MJ, Stranzinger JM (1992) Schilddrüsenkrankheiten in der Schwangerschaft und Stillperiode. In: Pfannenstiel P (ed) Schilddrüse und Zeiten hormoneller Umstellung: Pubertät, Schwangerschaft und Klimakterium. pp 54–58
8. Bohnet HG (1991) Strumaprophylaxe und -therapie. Der informierte Arzt. IMP 12 (16a):1563–1566
9. Bohnet HG (1985) Prolaktin und weibliche Sterilität. Leitfaden für die Praxis. Grosse, Berlin
10. Bouillon R, Nalsens M, Vanassehe FA (1982) Hyperthyroxinemia: a cause for hyperemesis gravidarum. Am J Obstet Gynecol 143:922
11. Burrow GN (1985) The management of thyrotoxicosis in pregnancy. N Engl J Med 313:562–565
12. Crooks J, Tulloch MI, Turnbull AC et al. Comparative incidence of goitre in pregnancy in Iceland and Scotland. Lancet 2:625
13. Davis LE, Lucas MJ, Hankins GDV, Roark ML, Cunningham FG (1989) Thyrotoxicosis complicating pregnancy. Am J Obstet 160:63–70
14. Ekins R (1985) Roles of serum thyroxine-binding proteins and maternal thyroid hormones in fetal development. Lancet: 1129–1132
15. Fehr P, Bohnet HG Postpartale Hypothyreosehäufigkeit in der Schweiz (manuscript in preparation)
16. Frilling A, Goretzki PE, Horster FA, Grußendorf M, Röher HD (1990) Subtotale Schilddrüsenresektion als Therapiekonzept bei thyreotoxischer Krise. Dtsch Med Wochenschr 115:735–739
17. Gärtner R (1990) Struma – Pathophysiologie und Definition des Krankheitsbildes. In: Köbberling J, Pickardt CR (eds) Struma. Springer, Berlin Heidelberg New York, pp 7–13
18. Glinoer D, De Nayer P, Bourdoux P, Lemone M, Robyn C, Van Steirteghem A, Kinthaert J, Lejeune B (1990) Regulation of maternal thyroid during pregnancy. J Clin Endocrinol 71:276–287
19. Goodwin TM, Montoro M, Mestman JH (1992) Transient hyperthyroidism and hyperemesis gravidarum: clinical aspects. Am J Obstet Gynecol 167:648–652
20. Goretzki PE (1988) Wachstumsregulation der menschlichen Schilddrüse – TSH gesteuert? Thieme, Stuttgart
21. Graves RJ (1925) Clinical Lectures. Med Surg J 7(2):516–517
22. Greenman GW, Gabrielson MO, Howard-Flanders J, Wessel MA (1962) Thyroid dysfunction in pregnancy. N Engl J Med 267:426
23. Gutekunst R, Smolarek H, Wächter W, Scriba PC (1985) Strumaepidemiologie. Schilddrüsenvolumina bei deutschen und schwedischen Schulkindern. Dtsch Med Wochenschr 110:50–54
24. Gutekunst R (1990) Jodmangel bei Kindern und Erwachsenen. In: Köbberling J, Pickardt CR (eds) Struma. Springer, Berlin Heidelberg New York
25. Harada A, Hersman JM, Reed AW et al. (1979) Comparison of thyroid stimulators and thyroid hormone concentrations in the sera of pregnant women. J Clin Endocrinol Metab 48:793

26. Harris B, Fung H, Johns S et al. (1989) Transient post-partum thyroid dysfunction and postnatal depression. J Affect Disord 17:243–249
27. Hashimoto H (1912) Zur Kenntnis der Lymphomatösen Veränderung der Schilddrüse (Struma Lymphomatosa). Arch Klin Chir 97:219–248
28. Hayslip CC, Fein HG, O'Donnell VM, Friedman DS, Klein TA, Smallridge RC (1988) The value of serum antimicrosomal antibody testing in screening for symptomatic postpartum thyroid dysfunction. Am J Obstet Gynecol 159:203–209
29. Hehrmann R (1980) Klinik und Therapie der Hypothyreose des Erwachsenen. Intern Welt 3:423–433
30. Hehrmann R (1990) Medikamentöse Therapie der Jodmangelstruma bei Kindern, Jugendlichen, jungen Erwachsenen und Schwangeren. Sozialpädiatrie 12:92–101
31. Heldin NE, Westermark B (1988) Epidermal growth factor but not thyrotropin stimulates the expression of c-fos and c-myc messenger ribonucleic acid in porcine thyroid follicle cells in primary culture. Endocrinology 122:1042–1046
32. Hoff HG, Windeck R, Reinwein D (1982) Die Behandlung von Schilddrüsenerkrankungen während der Schwangerschaft. Therapiewoche 32:1028–1039
33. Horster FA, Wildmeister W, Beysel D (1990) Zur Diagnostik und Therapie von Schilddrüsenkrankheiten. Scripta Medica Merck 2
34. Jonckheer MH, Michotte Y, van Steirteghem AC, Deconinck F (1983) The adaptation of the human thyroid gland to a physiological regimen of iodide intake: evidence for a transitory inhibition of thyroid hormone secretion modulated by the intrathyroidal iodine stores. J Endocrinol Invest 6:267–271
35. Kalle E (1989) Letters to the Editors. NucCompact 20:181–183
36. Klein AH, Hobel CJ, Sack J, Fisher DA (1978) Effect of intra-amniotic fluid thyroxine injection on fetal serum and amniotic fluid iodothyronine concentrations. J Clin Endocrinol Metab 47:1034
37. Klein AH, Meltzer S, Kenny FM (1972) Improved prognosis in congenital hypothyroidism treated before age three months. J Pediatr 81:912
38. Kodama K, Sikorska H, Bayly R et al. (1984) Use of monoclonal antibodies to investigate a possible role of thyroglobulin in the pathogenesis of Graves ophthalmopathy. J Clin Endocrinol 59:67–73
39. Kriss JP, Pleshokov V, Chien JR (1964) Isolation and identification of the long acting thyreoid stimulator and its relation to hyperthyroidism and circumscribed pretibial myxedema. J Clin Endocrinol Metab 24:1005–1028
40. Krüskemper HL et al. (1985) Intern. Welt 8:47–49
41. Löbig H, Schatz H (1991) Schilddrüsenfunktion und Schilddrüsenantikörper in der Schwangerschaft und in der Postpartalperiode. Med Welt 42:45–52
42. Man EB, Heinemann M, Johnson CE et al. (1951) The precipitable iodine of serum in normal pregnancy and its relation to abortions. J Clin Invest 30:137
43. Mandel SJ, Larsen PR, Seely EW, Brent GA (1990) Increased need for thyroxine during pregnancy in women with primary hypothyroidism. N Engl J Med 323:91–96
44. Mann K (1992) Schilddrüse und Klimakterium. In: Pfannenstiel P (ed) Schilddrüse und Zeiten hormoneller Umstellung: Pubertät, Schwangerschaft und Klimakterium. pp 70–78
45. Mertz DP, Sanwald R, Müller I (1959) Über den diagnostischen Wert der effektiven Halbwertszeit von J131 als Parameter für den Jodumsatz in der Schilddrüse. Dtsch Med Wochenschr 84:1901–1906
46. Momotani N, Ito K, Hamada N, Ban Y, Nishikawa Y, Mimura T (1984) Maternal hyperthyroidism and congenital malformation in the offspring. J Clin Endocrinol 20:695–700
47. Niswander KR, Gordon M, Berendes HW (1972) The women and their pregnancies. Saunders, Philadelphia
48. Pekonen F, Teramo K, Ikonen E, Österlund K (1984) Women on thyroid hormone therapy: pregnancy course, fetal outcome, and amniotic fluid thyroid hormone level. Obstet Gynecol 63:635
49. Pfannenstiel P, Saller B (1991) Schilddrüsenkrankheiten: Diagnose und Therapie, 2nd edn. BMV, pp 72–79
50. Pfannenstiel P, Colbow B (1990) Schilddrüsenkrankheiten in der Schwangerschaft. Gynäkologe 23:47–52
51. Plummer HS (1913) Clinical and pathological relationships of simple and exophthalmic goiter. Trans Assoc Am Phys 43:159–167

52. Pop VJM et al. (1991) Postpartum thyroid dysfunction and depression in an unselected population. N Engl J Med 324/25:1815–1816
53. Potter JD (1980) Hypothyroidism and reproductive failure. J Surg Gynecol Obstet 150:251
54. Raue F, Kohlwagen R, Ziegler R (1991) Morbus Basedow und Schwangerschaft. Med Welt 42:31–32
55. Reiners C (1991) Schilddrüsenfunktion und -funktionsparameter in der Schwangerschaft. Med Welt 42:18–24
56. Roitt IM (1993) Autoimmunerkrankungen – Begriffsumfang und Ätiologie. In: Leitfaden der Immunologie. Blackwell, Berlin, p 325
57. Rothenbuchner G, Schmidt K-J (1989) Thyroxin – ein „Geriatricum"? BMV, pp 38–39
58. Schmidt K-J, Rothenbuchner G, Reiser HH, Diehl K, Schuster H, Lagemann K, Herzberg U (1980) Die blande Struma. Therapiewoche 30:4201
59. Schmidt K-J, Rothenbuchner G, Reiser HH, Diehl K, Schuster H, Herzberg U (1980) Die kausale Therapie der primär-blanden Struma mit L-Thyroxin. Dtsch Med Wochenschr 105:1015
60. Scriba PC, Börner W, Emrich D et al. (1985) Schilddrüsenfunktionsdiagnostik und die Diagnose von Schilddrüsenkrankheiten der Deutschen Gesellschaft für Endokrinologie, Sektion Schilddrüse. Intern Welt 8:50–57, 78–86
61. Stagnaro-Green A, Roman SH, Cobin RH, El-Harazy E, Alvarez-Marfany M, Davies TF (1990) Detection of at risk pregnancy by means of highly sensitive assays for thyroid autoantibodies. JAMA 1422
62. Struve C, Ohlen S (1990) Einfluß früherer Schwangerschaften auf Struma- und Knotenhäufigkeit bei schilddrüsengesunden Frauen. Dtsch Med Wochenschr 115:1050–1053
63. Stübner D, Gärtner R, Greil W, Gropper K, Brabant G, Permanetter W, Horn K, Pickardt CR (1987) Hypertrophy and hyperplasia during goiter growth and involution in rats – separate bioeffects of TSH and iodine. Acta Endocrinol (Copenh) 116:537–548
64. Volpe R, Row VV (1985) Evidence of antigen specific suppressor T lymphocytes in the pathogenesis of autoimmune thyroid disease. In: Walfish P, Wall JR, Volpe R (eds) Autoimmunity in the thyroid. Academic, Orlando, pp 79–94
65. Volpe R (1985) Autoimmune thyroid disease – a perspective. Mol Biol Med 3:25–51
66. Volpe R (1989) Autoimmune Thyreoiditis. In: Burrow GN, Oppenheimer JH, Volpe R (eds) Thyroid function and disease. Saunders, Philadelphia, pp 191–207
67. Volpe R (1989) Subacute thyreoiditis. In: Burrow GN, Oppenheimer JH, Volpe R (eds) Thyroid function and disease. Saunders, Philadelphia, pp 179–190
68. Volpe R (1987) Immunoregulation in autoimmune thyroid disease. N Engl J Med 316:44–46

Infertility Treatment and Genetic Disorders

M.S. Beksaç and A.N. Cakar

Introduction

One of the main interests of fetal medicine is to investigate the teratogenic potential of ovulation induction agents and assisted reproductive technologies. In this context, the higher incidence of genetic problems due to the causal factors of infertility and intrinsic ovulation disorders must also be considered.

Genetic Problems in Stimulated Cycles

Between 40% and 60% of spontaneous abortions are considered to be due to genetic problems (Wramsby et al. 1987; Edmons et al. 1982). Chromosomal abnormalities are reported to be associated with fetal wastage in ovulation induction pregnancies (Boué and Boué 1973). The reported abortion rate for pregnancies achieved during gonadotropin-induced cycles is 17%–34% compared with 10%–15% in natural cycles (Ransom et al. 1993; Bohrer and Kemmann 1987). Some authors have also suggested a causal relationship between clomiphene citrate and multigenic multifactorial disorders such as neural tube defects (James 1977; Kurachi et al. 1983). However, we should always consider the possibility that the genetic disorders may be associated with subfertility rather than the drug itself.

The chromosome status of embryos and congenital malformations in in vitro fertilization (IVF) babies are of great interest from an ethical/legal point of view (Zenzes et al. 1992; Rizk et al. 1991; Medical Research International and SART 1992). The variety of ovulation induction protocols and assisted reproductive technology (ART) procedures makes it difficult to determine whether there is an increase in the incidence of congenital structural or chromosomal abnormalities in ART babies due to cycle stimulation of in vitro procedures.

Oocyte

It has been reported that in infertile women undergoing clomiphene citrate (CC) stimulation, nearly 50% of oocytes have an abnormal karyotype (Wramsby et al. 1987). This may explain the high frequency of chromosome abnormalities (aberrations) occurring in early abortions and the low pregnancy rate after IVF. However, it is difficult to define the exact mechanism responsible for these unwanted changes. Both stimulated folliculogenesis and the teratogenic effect of the ovulation induction drugs may be responsible for impaired oocytes.

When chromosomes of the first polar body are examined, they are indistinct and clearly different from the chromosomes of the oocyte. The formation of micronuclei can be observed in unfertilized oocytes (also in early cleavage stages after IVF) and this can reasonably be regarded as derived from small groups of chromosomes (Wramsby et al. 1987). Five to ten percent of eggs fertilized in vitro may have three pronuclei, indicating anomalous fertilization in addition to gamete abnormalities (Rudak et al. 1984; Angell et al. 1983). The likelihood that an oocyte fertilized in vitro will develop to full term after embryo replacement is about 10% (Biggers 1981; Lopata 1983). Higher pregnancy rates have been achieved by multiple embryo replacement (Edwards and Steptoe 1983). In vivo, however, fecundity during unstimulated cycles is about 25% (Edmons et al. 1982). This difference is probably due to genetic problems resulting from the teratogenic effect of ovulation induction drugs or ART procedures. Abnormal fetuses are most likely eliminated, since no increase in genetic disorders has been reported among children born after ART procedures (Seppälä 1985). Several studies on chromosomal abnormalities in oocytes from mammals have found an excess of hypohaploidy and attributed it to artificial loss due to the preparation procedure (Röhrborn 1972; Hansmann and Probeck 1979). It is also proposed that aberration in the number of chromosomes in an oocyte is caused not only by non-disjunction but also by anaphase lag (Wramsby et al. 1987).

It has been reported that 80% of all cases of trisomy D and G are due to non-disjunction in the female meiosis (Ishikiriyama and Niikawa 1984). Stimulated cycle oocytes may well be more likely to be chromosomally abnormal compared to spontaneously ovulating oocytes and this may be one of the important reasons for increased abortion rate after induction of ovulation (Wramsby et al. 1987; Boué and Boué 1973).

Preimplantation Embryo

The reported rates of chromosomal abnormality in preimplantation embryos range between 12- and 50% (Zenzes and Casper 1992). Preimplantation embryos have specific chromosomal errors not found in embryos from spontaneous abortions (Zenzes et al. 1992).

As mentioned above, the frequency of chromosomal abnormality before week 8 of gestation is about 50% (Wramsby et al. 1987; Edmons et al. 1982; Eiben et al. 1990). Estimates of overall rates of chromosome abnormalities in spontaneous abortions and fetal deaths, adjusted for gestational age, are around 32% (Hook 1992).

The most common chromosome abnormalities found in preimplantation embryos are aneuploidy, mosaicism and triploidy (Zenzes and Casper 1992). Aneuploidy, which results from non-disjunction or anaphase lag during meiosis, is an important cause of spontaneous abortions and birth defects

(Zenzes et al. 1992). Such segregational errors are also demonstrated in cytological preparations of oocytes and spermatozoa (Zenzes et al. 1990). On the other hand, mosaicism and triploidy mainly arise after fertilization. Mosaicism occurs as a result of postzygotic nondisjunction and is the most frequent abnormality (Zenzes et al. 1992). Haploid and polyploid (mainly triploid) embryos are also frequent in the preimplantion period. Subclinical (chemical) pregnancy is observed in 3%–8% of apparently normal cycles, and this rate seems to be increased in stimulated cycles and IVF programs.

In Vitro Fertilization Babies

The results of IVF pregnancies are not directly comparable with population data on naturally conceived pregnancies because of differences in risk factors such as maternal age, parity, preceding history of infertility, and poor reproductive performance (Rizk et al. 1991; Medical Research International and SART 1992). Multiple births are frequent, constituting 20%–24% of all deliveries, and 25% of all deliveries are preterm (Rizk et al. 1991; Medical Research International and SART 1992). In comparison, about 1% of natural conceptions result in multiple births. The high proportion of preterm and low birth weight babies is largely a result of multiplicity. However, there is still a relatively high proportion of preterm singleton deliveries: about 14% (Rizk et al. 1991). The comparative figure for natural conceptions is 7% (Rizk et al. 1991).

The overall stillbirth, perinatal and infant mortality rates in IVF babies are double those of babies born after natural conception (Rizk et al. 1991; Medical Research International and SART 1992). However, once standardization is made for multiplicity, the increased mortality becomes non-significant (Rizk et al. 1991).

Factors which could raise the risk of congenital malformations after ART procedures include the relatively advanced age of infertile couples, the underlying causes of infertility, the drugs used to induce ovulation and the ART procedures themselves. It is of particular interest to determine whether there is an increase in the incidence of genetic disorders in IVF or other ART babies. Overall, 2.5%–3% of the babies have major congenital malformations, which is comparable with the expected values from naturally conceived babies. No specific malformations are significantly increased, but higher than expected number of central nervous system, chromosomal, urogenital, and limb malformations are observed.

The rate of chromosomal abnormalities in spontaneous abortions following superovulation was found to be 83%, compared to 61% for abortions following natural conceptions (Bove and Bove 1973). Chromosomal abnormalities at birth are found to be 0.5% in IVF programs, which is within the expected range when standardized for maternal age (Rizk et al. 1991). However, slight increases in the number of malformations within the central nervous system, the urogenital system, and limbs and in chromosomal disorders emphasize the need for careful fetal neonatal surveillance.

Future of Human Genome and Preimplantation Genetics

Advances in methods used to detect specific genes or gene products have contributed to the development of methods to identify genetic disorders early in life. In situ hybridization (FISH) allows one to directly visualize DNA sequences of interest and is ideal for numerical chromosome analysis. Recent developments also enable the use of this technique for specific gene problems (Critser 1992; Grifo et al. 1992; Cakar et al. 1993; Ataç et al. 1994). In addition, it is not fraught with the hazards of contamination that plaques polymerase chain reaction technology. The potential to use this technology in conjunction with IVF techniques to genetically analyze an embryo before transfer could offer patients at genetic risk an alternative. However, genetic diagnoses are currently limited to the postimplantation period and are performed by classical techniques such as chronic villus sampling, amniocentesis and fetal blood sampling.

Conclusion

Reproductive failure is closely associated with genetic disorders. Infertility treatment itself may also affect different stages of reproductive life and fetal development. We believe that more epidemiological studies are necessary to make possible better prenatal diagnosis programs and to reduce perinatal morbidity and mortality especially in high-priority pregnancies of infertility clinics.

References

Angell RR, Aitken RJ, van Look PFA, Lumsden MA, Templeton AA (1983) Chromosome abnormalities in human embryos after in vitro fertilization. Nature 303:336–338

Ataç FB, Cakar AN, Dağdeviren A (1994) Fluorescent in situ hybridization (FISH). Gynecol Obstet Reprod Med (in press)

Biggers JD (1981) In vitro fertilization and embryo transfer in human beings. N Engl J Med 304:336–342

Bohrer M, Kemmann E (1987) Risk factors for spontaneous abortion in menotropin-treated women. Fertil Steril 48:571–575

Boué JG, Boué A (1973) Increased frequency of chromosomal anomalies in abortions after induced ovulation. Lancet 1:679–680

Critser ES (1992) Preimplantation genetics. Arch Pathol Lab Med 116:383–387

Cakar AN, Dağdeviren A, Ataç FB, Beksaç MS, Beksaç M (1993) A rapid method for sex determination in prenatal diagnosis. Turk J Med Res 11:5:228–230

Edmons DK, Lindsay KS, Miller JF, Williamson E, Wood PJ (1982) Early embryonic mortality in women. Fertil Steril 38:447–453

Edwards RG, Steptoe PC (1983) Current status of in-vitro fertilisation and implantation of human embryos. Lancet 2:1265–1270

Eiben B, Bartels I, Bähr-Porsch S et al (1990) Cytogenetic analysis of 750 spontaneous abortions with the direct-preparation method of chorionic villi and its implications for studying genetic causes of pregnancy wastage. Am J Hum Genet 47:656–663

Grifo JA, Boyle A, Tang Ya-Xu, Ward DC (1992) Preimplantation genetic diagnosis. Arch Pathol Lab Med 116:393–397

Hansman I, Probeck HD (1979) Detection of nondisjunction in mammals. Environ Health Perspect 31:161–165
Hook EB (1992) Chromosome abnormalities: Prevalence , risks, and recurrence. In: Brock DJH, Rodeck CH, Feguson Smith MA (eds) Prenatal diagnosis and screening. Churchill Livingstone, Edinburgh, pp 351–392
Ishikiriyama S, Nukawa N (1984) Origin of extra chromosome in Patau syndrome. Hum Genet 68:266–268
James WH (1977) Clomiphene, anencephaly, and spina bifida. Lancet 1:603
Kurachi A, Aono T, Mingawa J, Miyake A (1983) Congenital malformations of newborn infants after clomiphene-induced ovulation. Fertil Steril 40:187–189
Lopata A (1983) Concepts in human in vitro fertilization and embryo transfer. Fertil Steril 40:289–301
Medical Research International and SART (1992) In vitro fertilization-embryo transfer (IVF-ET) in the United States: 1990 results from the IVF-ET Registry. Fertil Steril 57:15–24
Ransom MX, Bohrer M, Blotner MB, Kemman E (1993) The difference in miscarriage rates between menotropin-induced and natural cycle pregnancies is not surveillance related. Fertil Steril 59:567–570
Rizk B, Doyle P, Tan SL, Rainsburg P, Betts J, Brinsden P, Edwards R (1991) Perinatal outcome and congenital malformations in in-vitro fertilization babies from the Bounr-Hallam group. Hum Repro 6:1259–1264
Röhrborn G (1972) Frequencies of spontaneous non-disjunction in metaphase II oocytes of mice. Humangenetic 16:123–125
Rudak E, Dor J, Mashiack S, Nebel L et al (1994) Chromosome analysis of multinuclear human oocytes fertilized in vitro. Fertil Steril 38–45
Seppälä M (1985) The World Collaborative Report on in vitro fertilization and embryo replacement: current state of the art in January 1984: Ann NY Acad Sci 442:558–563
van Blerkom J, Henry G, Porreco R (1984) Preimplantation human embryonic development from polypronuclear eggs after in vitro fertilization. Fertil Steril 41:686–696
Wramsby H, Fredga K, Liedholm P (1987) Chromosome analysis of human oocytes recovered from preovulatory follicles in stimulated cycles. N Engl J Med 316:121–124
Zenzes MT, Casper RF (1992) Cytogenetics of oocytes, zygotes and embryos after in vitro fertilization. Hum Genet 88:367–375
Zenzes MT, de Geyter CH, Bordt J et al (1990) Abnormalities of sperm chromosome condensation in the cytoplasm of immature human oocytes. Human Reprod 7:842–846
Zenzes MT, Wang P, Casper RF (1992) Chromosome status of untransferred (spare) embryos and probability of pregnancy after in-vitro fertilization. Lancet 340:391–394

Recurrent Pregnancy Loss

A. Arici and O. Bukulmez

Introduction

Spontaneous miscarriage itself is an extremely common disorder during pregnancy. About 15%–20% of clinically detected pregnancies result in spontaneous abortion prior to 20 weeks' gestation (Warburton and Frazer 1964; Poland et al. 1977; Stray-Pedersen and Stray-Pedersen (1984). By using daily sensitive plasma and urine assays for human chorionic gonadotropin (hCG), 39% of the postimplantation pregnancies were reported to be lost (Wilcox et al. (1988). Also, it was concluded that 30% of embryos fail to implant and another 30% of early pregnancies could only be recognized by sensitive β-hCG assays (Chard 1991).

Recurrent pregnancy loss is usually defined as three or more spontaneous consecutive pregnancy losses. Compared to sporadic abortion, it is relatively uncommon, affecting 1%–3% of couples during pregnancy (Hill 1992). The same term has, however, also been used in a number of studies including those with two consecutive spontaneous abortions. Observations have shown that the greatest change in risk of losing a subsequent pregnancy occurs after two consecutive abortions, and there are no differences in the prevalence of etiologic factors among couples with three or more abortions (Roman 1984; Coulam 1991).

For decades gynecologists believed that after three but not fewer fetal losses, the risk of subsequent losses rises sharply to 80%–90%. This conclusion was reached in 1938 by the theoretical calculations of Malpas (Malpas 1938). Until proven incorrect by Warburton and Frazer (1964), the clinical trials evaluating various treatment plans were mostly based on this information. These investigators showed the likelihood of recurrent abortion to be only 25%–35%, irrespective of whether a woman has had one, two, three or more abortions previously. Later studies regarding the recurrence risks after first, second and third abortions revealed different figures due to the differences in population samples and the methods of analysis. In a recent study, pregnancy loss rates following one to four consecutive abortions were reported to increase from 16%–54% (Knudsen et al. 1991). The frequency of miscarriage also increase with advancing maternal and paternal age (Warburton and Frazer 1964); Knudsen et al. 1991). However, after repeated abortions in younger and older women, similar pregnancy loss rates were observed. This leads one to think that additional age-independent factors are involved in women with recurrent pregnancy loss.

The past obstetric history is also of much importance in estimating the recurrence risk for spontaneous abortion. The likelihood of fetal loss was reported to be 46% if a woman had had at least one fetal loss at any time of pregnancy and no liveborn infants (Poland et al. 1977). Primigravid women and those with a history of live births have a low incidence of abortion. Women with only pregnancy loss histories have an increased risk for recurrence of miscarriage (Regan et al. 1989). Some authors suggest a recurrence risk of 25%–35% in couples having at least one liveborn infant and up to 40% if they have none (Simpson and Golbus 1992). Overall, the outcome is not so unfavorable. There are a number of reports with a successful pregnancy role of 60%–70% without intervention, making the management decisions more difficult (Poland et al. 1977, Goldzieher and Benigno 1958; Vlaanderen and Treffers 1987). Usually any evaluation of a couple with recurrent pregnancy loss should take into account both the high inherent pregnancy wastage rate in human reproduction and also the possible etiologies common to this particular patient population. At present, conventionally identifiable etiologic factors can be shown in about 60% of the couples who suffer from recurrent spontaneous abortion. It is also extremely difficult to assign percentages to the different causes of recurrent pregnancy wastage. Differences in definitions and in the basic workup of each investigator make direct comparisons between studies difficult if not impossible. Since developing embryos and trophoblasts are immunologic targets due to their paternally inherited genetic products, numerous immunologic theories have been suggested for the unexplained recurrent pregnancy losses. This article will cover the common etiologies of recurrent early pregnancy failure with special emphasis on the current immunologic implications.

Genetic Causes

Chromosomal abnormalities have been detected in 50%–60% of first trimester spontaneous abortions compared with 5%–10% of second trimester losses and less than 1% of liveborn infants; thus the earlier the abortion, the greater the likelihood of chromosomal abnormality (Carr 1972). About half of these are autosomal trisomies (Dewald and Michels 1986; Warburton 1987). Monosomy X is the single most common chromosomal abnormality in spontaneous abortions, accounting for up to 24%; then come triploidy and tetraploidy with proportions of 15% and 7% respectively (Hassold et al. 1980). In the study of Guerneri and co-workers, tissues for cytogenetic analysis were obtained by chorionic villus sampling as soon as possible after ultrasound diagnosis of abortion (Guerneri et al. 1987). With this technique, a higher proportion of specimens could be cultured than in earlier reports, and 77% of the specimens exhibited chromosomal abnormalities. This rate was also higher than in studies based on spontaneously expelled conceptional material. So the true proportion of chromosomal abnormalities in the first trimester may be more than 50%.

In contrast to the sporadic spontaneous abortion, repeated aneuploidy was not found to be so common in recurrent aborters, who were more likely to have losses of chromosomally normal conceptions (Daya and Clark 1992). Also the risk of a second abortion was reported to be higher following abortion of a fetus with karyotypic abnormalities than following karyotypically normal miscarriages (Boue et al. 1975; Geisler and Kleinebrecht 1978). In one study, the highest incidence of cytogenetic abnormalities was found in couples with abortion and a normal child (Portnoi et al. 1988). These data suggest that chromosomally normal abortions are less random than the defective ones. Studies by Simpson and co-workers revealed the translocation rate among repeated aborters to be between 0.3% and 0.9%, which in fact is lower than once believed (Simpson et al. 1981, 1989). The data question the value of routine chromosomal analysis in recurrent aborters. In two relatively recent reports it has been shown that the rate of aneuploid conceptions is significantly higher in couples experiencing recurrent pregnancy loss than in controls (Braekeleer and Dao 1990; Drugan et al. 1990). So prenatal diagnosis in any subsequent pregnancy was recommended to couples with a history of two or more abortions. Nonetheless, balanced parental translocations are the most important chromosomal abnormality detectable among couples with recurrent early pregnancy losses, especially in those with a positive family history and a history of congenitally malformed infant.

The recurrent euploid pregnancy loss may also be caused by so-called molecular mutations including lethal genes, oncogenes, or mutations in homeobox genes which appear to control the expression of ensembles of genes through transcriptional regulation (McDonough 1988). Human leukocyte antigen (HLA) haplotyping of both parents is controversial. Beyond the immunologic considerations, increased pregnancy losses seen in couples that share HLA types may be due to sharing a recessive lethal developmental gene linked to HLA. Especially in cases with "empty sac" blighted ovum, karyotyped cells are mostly euploid 46, XY (McDonough 1988). So there might be a possibility of X-linked dominant diseases with embryonic lethality in hemizygous males. A single point mutation in paternal X-chromosome related to paternal age could also occur. It has also been found that male gametes from couples with recurrent abortion carry a significantly greater number of chromosome breaks and eccentric fragments compared to normal controls, but the total rates of aneuploidy and structural anomalies do not differ (Rosenbusch and Sterzik 1991).

Genetic causes, if detected, have no treatment. But couples may need genetic counselling, prenatal diagnosis, artificial donor insemination, or adoption.

Anatomic Defects

Failure of müllerian duct fusion or canalization, either total or partial, reportedly occurs in one of every 700 women (Glass and Golbus 1994). The incidence usually varies from 0.1% to 10% of patients investigated. This is an area that attracts most attention in the evaluation of pregnancy loss. Fetal wastage is believed to be increased in all trimesters. The classical associations with müllerian anomalies are midtrimester abortion, premature labor and fetal presentation abnormalities (McWilliams and Gibbons 1991). Patients with unicornate, bicornate and septate uterus have the highest abortion rates. Although anomalies of the müllerian system have been found in 10%–15% of women with recurrent abortion, only a minority of women with uterine anomalies experience reproductive failures (Tho et al. 1979; Stray-Pedersen and Stray-Pedersen 1984). Often, the majority of the anomalies remain unrecognized. Most of these women have successful pregnancies and those with a history of pregnancy loss usually achieve successful pregnancies without any treatment. Indeed, the sole indication for septal incision or unification operation is poor reproductive performance in which pregnancy loss is thought to occur as a result of the anomaly. So the decision depends primarily on the previous reproductive performance modified by the ease with which pregnancy is achieved, the woman's age, and the waiting period after the diagnosis of the condition (Corson 1992). Also it should be considered that open abdominal surgery carries the risk of both pelvic and intrauterine adhesion formation, which may increase the later incidence of infertility by up to 30% (Bennet 1987). The results of hysteroscopic excision of uterine septum are promising and devoid of the complications of the abdominal approach.

Other anatomic defects implicated in the etiology of recurrent pregnancy loss are intrauterine synechia, uterine leiomyoma, endometrial polyps and incompetent cervix. Intrauterine synechiae are present in about 5% of patients with recurrent abortion, although they are frequently secondary to the interventions and complications that are relevant to pregnancy itself, such as postabortal or postpartum currettage and related endomyometritis. At present, hysteroscopic scissor dissection of synechiae with concomitant laparoscopy to minimize the uterine perforation is the treatment of choice. Postoperative use of antibiotics, insertion of an intrauterine device, and estrogen/progesterone therapy to stimulate the proliferation of endometrium are recommended (Corson 1992). Leiomyomas are also approached by either hysteroscopy and/or laparoscopy, especially after pretreatment with gonadotropin-releasing hormone agonists. For patients with a classic history of cervical incompetence, uncontrolled trials suggest cerclage to be effective (Ayers et al. 1982).

As a whole, diagnosis of anatomic disorders can be made in 38%–55% of patients with repeated pregnancy wastage (Kutteh and Carr 1993). Although such disorders may not be the direct cause of abortion, hysterosalpingography or hysteroscopy is an essential part of the evaluation for recurrent pregnancy loss.

Endocrinologic Causes

Metabolic and endocrinologic causes account for more than 15% of cases of recurrent pregnancy loss (Ninia 1994). The most frequently implicated ones are luteal phase defects and poorly controlled diabetes mellitus. There is no evidence that mild thyroid dysfunction can cause recurrent abortion (Harger et al. 1983). Although the glucose tolerance test is one of the first orders for most physicians, there is no conclusive evidence that unsuspected diabetes or overt diabetes that is adequately controlled is a cause of recurrent abortion (Kalter 1987). So there is no value in the routine ordering of a glucose tolerance test.

Although the incidence of luteal phase defect is difficult to determine due to lack of uniform diagnostic criteria, it has been reported to occur in 23%–60% of patients with recurrent pregnancy loss, which is a higher incidence compared to infertility patients (3%–4%) (Fritz 1988). Diagnosis is mostly based on basal body temperature measurements, luteal phase progesterone levels, and timed endometrial biopsies. Although a biphasic basal body temperature chart strongly suggests an ovulatory cycle, a monophasic chart does not indicate an ovulatory dysfunction. Hormonal evidence of ovulation can be shown in up to 75% of monophasic cycles (Bauman 1981). However, it is helpful in determination of the length of the luteal phase. A luteal phase of less than 11 days may be associated with luteal phase defect (Downs and Gibson 1983; Lenton et al. 1984). There is significant overlap among single midluteal serum progesterone levels obtained from controls and patients with luteal phase defect. Also, a poor correlation exists between a single progesterone level and the endometrial biopsy (Shangold et al. 1983). All of these observations are related to the pulsatile nature of progesterone secretion (Filicori et al. 1984). Because of this, multiple serum samples during the luteal phase are necessary, with added inconvenience and expense. Endometrial biopsy with histologic dating is considered the standard diagnostic test for inadequate luteal phase by identifying both the deficient progesterone production and the abnormal endometrial responsiveness. Classically, it is performed 2–3 days prior to the time of the expected menses. False-negative results are increased in biopsies performed before the 25th day. Sampling is made from high in the fundus to avoid a dyssynchronous lower uterine segment (Rein 1991). Endometrium that is 2 days or more out of phase with the menstrual cycle in two successive cycles in considered diagnostic. It is now agreed that correct timing of endometrial sampling should be made by LH assays which can be performed easily using commercial urine LH kits. So, interpretation of the endometrial biopsy should be based on days after ovulation, which is the time between the 8th and the 11th postovulatory day (Li et al. 1987). Treatment options for luteal phase inadequacy include clomiphene citrate, vaginal progesterone suppositories, bromocriptine if serum prolactin level is also elevated, and luteal support with hCG.

Recent studies have focused on the quality of the luteal phase, which is dependent on preovulatory endocrine events. Adverse effects of high levels of LH on follicular development have been shown in ovulation induction therapy (Jacobs and Hombourg 1990). In some patients both infertility and repeated miscarriage might be related to abnormalities in the follicular development. In a study of ovulation induction in polycystic ovarian syndrome patients using low-dose hMG, poor response to treatment with successful ovulation but no conception or early pregnancy loss correlated with raised baseline or midfollicular LH levels (Hamilton-Fairley et al. 1991). There were no successful pregnancies in women whose LH levels were persistently elevated. The same conclusion was reached in another study evaluating the relationship between pregnancy follicular phase serum LH levels and outcome of prepregnancy (Regan et al. 1990). In women with regular and spontaneous menstruation with elevated 8th day LH levels, the incidence of abortion was 65% in contrast to 12% in women with normal LH levels. The authors suggested that follicular phase LH testing is a useful test in predicting abortion. Detrimental effects of inappropriately high LH were related to the premature activation of occyte maturation and perhaps to its direct regulatory function on the endometrium (Regan 1992). Treatment of this condition might comprise suppression of endogenous LH secretion by gonado-tropin-releasing hormone agonists followed by hMG ovulation induction therapy.

Immunologic Causes

As stated earlier, the cause of recurrent pregnancy loss is unexplained by basic workup in up to 60% of couples (Stray-Pedersen and Stray-Pedersen 1984). The concept that some unexplained pregnancy losses might have an immunologic basis has attracted attention especially during the last decade. One of the proposed mechanisms is alloimmune-mediated, i.e., the conceptus, acting as a semiallogenic graft, is rejected similar to transplantation rejection. Allogenicity refers to genetic dissimilarities between individuals of the same species. Another mechanism is autoimmunity even in women with no clinical autoimmune disease.

Alloimmunity

Chromosome 6 contains genes of the major histocompatibility complex (MHC) that regulate immune responses. These genes code for class I MHC antigens, i.e., human leukocyte antigens (HLA) A, B, and C, and class II MHC antigens that include HLA-DR, -DP, and -DQ. Class I molecules are present on almost every cell in the body and are crucial for defining the self. They are recognized by CD8+ T cells. Exogenous antigens like proteins and bacteria are presented by antigen-presenting cells to the immune system via class II molecules which are recognized by CD4+ T cells (Lanzavecchia 1990). There are no HLA antigens on the spermatozoa (Billington 1992), oocyte, and embryo at the early cleavage and blastocyst stages (Desoye et al. 1988; Roberts et al. 1992).

Trophoblasts are the only fetal cells exposed directly to the maternal blood. Although they do not carry classical HLA antigens, it has been shown that villous and nonvillous cytotrophoblasts of the placenta and cytotrophoblasts of the amniochorion express a recently discovered HLA-G which is a class I antigen (Kovats et al. 1990). The lack of expression of HLA antigens and the presence of nonclassical HLA-G antigen on the trophoblasts have been thought to prevent the occurrence of immune attack by hindering the co-recognition of any other form of surface antigen that the trophoblasts express. Trophoblasts also carry so-called trophoblast-lymphocyte cross-reactive (TLX) antigens which are presumably near HLA (McIntyre et al. 1983). They have been proposed to be important in some kinds of maternal recognition and protection of blastocyst by the production of blocking factors. According to one hypothesis, their lack of recognition via antigen sharing leads to absence of blocking antibodies, resulting in abortion. It was noted by Beer (1986) that the problem of recurrent abortion resolved in some women after they had changed sexual partners. However, in a series of patients who had been pregnant by two different spouses it was concluded that recurrent abortion is not partner specific, although there may be a strong familial disposition in families where recurrent miscarriage occurs (Christiansen et al. 1990). Another study in an ethnically homogeneous Chinese population showed that there was an excess HLA sharing between husband and wife in couples experiencing primary and secondary recurrent spontaneous abortions (Ho et al. 1990). Recurrent aborters have been reported to develop less antipaternal lymphocytotoxic antibody than controls (Carp et al. 1990). This knowledge has been used to identify patients for whom immunotherapy might be beneficial. However, in a prospective study, the development of this antibody was found to be dependent on gestational age of pregnancy (Regan et al. 1991). Since antipaternal lymphocytotoxic antibodies are rare prior to 28 weeks' of gestation, it could not be used as a diagnostic test for recurrent aborters. Also antibody levels have been shown to diminish between pregnancies.

The hypothesis that blocking factor deficiency may be a cause of recurrent abortion is based on pathophysiologic assumptions. According to these assumptions, there is an antifetal cell-mediated immune response that must be blocked during the pregnancy. The blocking antibodies that develop in successful pregnancies are thought to prevent immune attack by blocking antigenic sites.

Immunotherapeutic procedures have been invented in order to induce the production of blocking factors, complement-dependent antipaternal lymphocytotoxic antibodies, or suppressor cells of prevent maternal rejection of the fetus. Three types of antigen used for this purpose have been paternal or third-party leukocytes, placental syncytiotrophoblast plasma membrane, and immunoglobulin. Nevertheless, the efficacy and safety of this treatment remain obscure. The first randomized controlled trial of immunotherapy was the only one to show a statistically significant benefit. In that study, recurrent aborters were randomized to treatment with either paternal leukocytes or their own lymphocytes once before conception. Women immunized with paternal leukocytes were more likely to have a successful pregnancy than the latter group (Mowbray et al. 1985; Fraser et al. 1993). In the trial by Cauchi et al., the group given the placebo had a nonsignificant higher rate of successful pregnancy (Cauchi et al. 1991). Two other trials of immunotherapy also failed to show statistically significant effects on pregnancy outcome (Ho et al. 1991; Johnson et al. 1991). Meta-analyses of these studies revealed that immunotherapy did not significantly improve pregnancy rates (Fraser et al. 1993).

The role of blocking factors and complement-dependent antipaternal lymphocytotoxic antibodies in determing the outcome of pregnancy in unexplained recurrent pregnancy aborters was evaluated in another immunotherapy trial (Hwang et al. 1992). Blocking factors were measured by mixed lymphocyte reaction. After immunization with the husband's or a third party donor's lymphocytes, a substantial rise in the titer of blocking factors could be produced in all patients regardless of whether they had a successful pregnancy or a repeated abortion. The blocking factor levels before and after immunization did not correlate with the outcome of the subsequent pregnancy. The authors concluded that neither mixed lymphocyte reaction blocking factors nor antipaternal lymphocytotoxic antibodies were essential for successful pregnancy.

Immunotherapy with leukocytes also carries risks of virus transmission, erythrocyte sensitization, autoimmune disease, increased abortion and infertility rates, fetal growth retardation, and graft-versus-host disease (Hill 1991; Clark and Daya 1991; Kats et al. 1992). In short, there is currently no strong evidence supporting the beneficial effect of immunotherapy in recurrent pregnancy loss.

It has been proposed that aberrant cellular immunity in response to trophoblast antigen stimulation may be involved in the pathogenesis of recurrent abortion through embryotoxic factor production by leukocytes (Hill et al. 1992; Ecker et al. 1993). Recently, it was shown that women with recurrent abortion of unknown cause exhibited in vitro evidence of T-cell immunity to trophoblast antigen stimulation which was undetected in controls (Yamada et al. 1994). So, T-cell immunity to trophoblast antigens may aslo play a role in alloimmune pregnancy loss.

Autoimmunity

Autoimmune diseases occur with an overwhelming preponderance in women (Talal 1979). In studies of pregnancy in women with systemic lupus erythematosus, the pregnancy loss rates were higher (Dudley and Branch 1991). Lubbe et al. were the first to suggest that abnormal autoimmunity in clinically asymptomatic women may be associated with reproductive failure (Lubbe et al. 1984). Long before then, an association of a unique circulating anticoagulant and a false-positive Wasserman serology test with recurrent pregnancy wastage had been reported (Laurell and Nilsson 1957). The so-called lupus anticoagulant was found to be an autoantibody usually of IgG and rarely of IgM type (Lubbe and Liggins 1985). It is one of the recognized antiphospholipid antibodies in recurrent pregnancy loss.

Antiphospholipid antibodies are directed to the negatively charged phospholipids which are constituents of all cell membranes. Their presence has been linked to adverse maternal and fetal outcome including spontaneous abortion, stillbirth, intrauterine growth retardation, preeclampsia, thromboembolism, and thrombocytopenia, i.e., antiphospholipid syndrome.

Lupus anticoagulant was first described in patients with systemic lupus erythematosus who displayed false-positive serological tests for syphilis and a plasma inhibitor of in vitro clotting assays (Conley and Hartman 1952). The term is a misnomer since many patients with these antibodies do not have lupus and it is mostly associated with thrombotic events (Lubbe and

Liggins 1985). It interferes with the binding between the platelet wall phospholipid and activated factors V and X to form prothrombin activator complex (Thiagarajan et al. 1980). The definitive diagnosis of lupus anticoagulant activity requires three criteria to be met: (1) prolongation of a phospholipid-dependent clotting assay; (2) documentation that prolongation is not due to a clotting factor deficiency, and (3) confirmation that the prolongation is phospholipid specific (Lockwood and Rand 1994). The initial test should contain a low phospholipid concentration for which an activated partial thromboplastin time (aPTT) with platelet-poor plasma is appropriate. In order to rule out a factor deficiency in the presence of a prolonged aPTT, test material is mixed with plasma, observing the normalization of the test. If there is no correction with plasma, the test is repeated by adding an excess amount of platelet phospholipid for final confirmation. False-negative screening tests can be ruled out with the dilute Russell viper venom test (dRVVT) and confirmed by adding platelet phospholipids. Kaolin clotting time and plasma clot time are other sensitive screening tests but since they do not use added phospholipid they cannot be used for confirmation (Kutteh and Carr 1993). The use of aPTT appears to be the most sensitive screening procedure (Triplett 1989). Changes in the coagulation system during pregnancy make the diagnosis difficult. In strongly suspected cases with normal aPTT, a second screening test should be employed (Triplett 1992). To rule out the possibility that heparin may be responsible for a prolonged screening test, thrombin time should be used. Thrombin time is prolonged in the presence of heparin or in the absence of fibrinogen, but it is normal if the prolongation of aPTT or dRVVT is due to the presence of lupus anticoagulant or factor deficiency.

Other antiphospholipid antibodies of clinical interest are anticardiolipin antibodies. They are quantified by either radioimmunoassay or enzyme-linked immunosorbent assay. It was first suggested that anticardiolipin antibody detection is a more sensitive test than lupus anticoagulant in identifying women with increased risk of pregnancy loss (Lockshin and Druzin 1985). Later it was proposed that it is more sensitive but that lupus anticoagulant has greater specifity in identifying patients at risk (Derksen et al. 1988); also, the results of lupus anticoagulant tests are more reproducible (Peaceman et al. 1992).

Previous pregnancy history is important in determining the significance of a positive laboratory test for antiphospholipid antibody. The reported incidence of antiphospholipid antibodies among recurrent aborters varies from 5%–50% (Regan 1992). A significantly higher rate of positive tests is noted in women with recurrent losses and a history of thrombosis or in women who have documented systemic lupus erythematosus. The precise pathophysiologic mechanisms of these antibodies are not so clear. Inhibition of prostacycline generation (Wolf et al. 1982), diminished protein C activity (Cariou et al. 1988) inhibition of antithrombin III (Cosgriff and Martin 1981) alteration of platelet-endothelium interactions (Harris et al. 1985), and interference with postreceptor signal transduction processes (Gleicher et al. 1992) have been suggested by in vitro experiments.

The availability of treatment for patients with recurrent pregnancy loss and antiphospholipid antibodies necessitated the screening and identification of at-risk patients early in pregnancy. Treatment is clearly indicated for pregnant patients with a history of previous thrombosis, recurrent fetal loss, or thrombocytopenia if they have correctly diagnosed lupus anticoagulant activity or medium to high concentrations of anticardioplipin G or M antibodies confirmed in two laboratories and on two occasions more than 6 weeks apart (Harris 1987; Lockwood and Rand 1994). The need for treatment of patients without previous pregnancy losses or thrombosis but incidentally found lupus anticoagulant and anticardiolipin antibodies is controversial. Also, it has been shown in a case-control study that presence of lupus anticoagulant or anticardiolipin antibodies is not a risk factor for women who present with spontaneous abortion or fetal death but have had no previous spontaneous fetal loss (Infante-Rivard et al. 1991).

Treatment options for antiphospholipid syndrome are based on two approaches. The first is to reduce the antibody burden, and the second, to reduce the procoagulant effects of antiphospholipid antibodies. The former approach includes treatment with prednisone or, in refractory cases, azathioprine or plasmapheresis with or without immunoglobulin therapy. To counteract the procoagulant effects, low-dose aspirin (50–81 mg/day) and heparin (10 000–20 000 U/day s.c.) are used. In a comparative trial of prednisone (10–40 mg/day) plus low-dose aspirin (81 mg/day) versus low-dose aspirin alone in the treatment of anticadiolipin antibody-positive patients, the co-administration of prednisone with low-dose aspirin did not improve the outcome and even provoked obstetric complications like preterm delivery (Silver et al. 1993). A similar study comparing aspirin (80 mg/day) plus prednisone (40 mg/day) and aspirin plus heparin (10 000 U twice a day) revealed similar live birth rates (around 75%); however, preterm deliveries were again more common in the prednisone-treated group (Cowchock et al. 1992).

Recently, it was documented in experimental antiphospholipid syndrome in mice that in vivo administration of recombinant interleukin-3 was beneficial (Fishman et al. 1993). The pregnancy loss rates dropped from 32% to 4% following administration of interleukin-3, which also corrected the antiphospholipid syndrome-associated thrombocytopenia.

A high prevalence of elevated titers of antinuclear antibodies in recurrent aborters has been reported but it is not clear whether the elevated titers preceded or followed the pregnancy losses (Xu et al. 1990). Routine screening for antinuclear antibodies in patients with recurrent pregnancy loss is not recommended.

Miscellaneous Causes

Although there are numerous studies regarding the infectious etiologies of recurrent pregnancy loss, these data remain inconclusive since there are no well-designed and placebo-controlled treatment studies. Recently, no association was found betwen the immunoglobulin G antibodies to *Chlamydia trachomatis* and recurrent spontaneous abortion (Rae et al. 1994).

A family history of recurrent abortion and earlier age at menarche have also been revealed to be more common in women with recurrent pregnancy loss (Parazzini et al. 1991).

Conclusion

Any investigation of a patient with recurrent pregnancy loss should include a detailed history and physical examination paying attention to previous pregnancy outcomes, medications, menstrual pattern, family history of pregnancy loss and congenital anomalies, galactorrhea, evidence of systemic disease and cervical or uterine anomalies. Laboratory investigation covers complete blood count, aPTT, anticardiolipin antibodies, LH, prolactin, and, if indicated, a search for autoimmune diseases. Parental karyotyping is also indicated. Pelvic ultrasound may help in the diagnosis of polycystic ovaries and uterine anomalies. Selected cases should definitely undergo hysterosalpingography and, if indicated, laparascopy for final diagnosis.

Treatment should be directed at correcting any identifiable causes of early pregnancy losses. In these cases, therapy can significantly increase the probability of carrying a subsequent pregnancy to term. In those couples where no cause can be identified, it is essential for the physician to provide continuing emotional support, since 70% of couples in this group will eventually carry a pregnancy to term whether or not they receive treatment. Physicians should resist the temptation to use treatment modalities that have not been scientifically validated. Ideally, any treatment modality should be proven to be more effective than chance by entry into a randomized, double-blind trial and should be shown to be more effective than the 70% spontaneous remission rate.

References

Ayers J, Peterson E et al (1982) Early therapy for the incompetent cervix in patients with habitual abortion. Fertil Steril 38:177–181

Bauman J (1981) Basal body temperature: unreliable method of ovulation detection. Fertil Steril 36:729–733

Beer A (1986) New horizons in the diagnosis, evaluation and therapy of recurrent spontaneous abortion. Clin Obstet Gynecol 13:115–124

Bennett M (1987) Congenital abnormalities of the fundus. In: Bennett, Edmonds (eds) Spontaneous and recurrent abortion. Blackwell, London, pp 109–129

Billington W (1992) The normal fetomaternal immune relationship. Baillieres Clin Obstet Gynaecol 6:417–438

Boue J, Boue A et al (1975) Retrospective and prospective epidemiological studies of 1500 karyotyped spontaneous human abortions. Teratology 12:11–26

Braekeleer M, Dao T (1990) Cytogenetic studies in couples experiencing repeated pregnancy losses. Hum Reprod 5:519–528

Cariou R, Tobelem G et al (1988) Effect of lupus anticoagulant of antithrombogenic properties of endothelial cells – inhibition of thrombomodulin dependent protein C activation. Thromb Haemost 60:54–58

Carp H, Toder V et al (1990) Recurrent miscarriage: a review of current concepts, immune mechanisms, and results of treatment. Obstet Gynecol Surv 45:657–669
Carr D (1972) Cytogenetic aspects of induced and spontaneous abortions. Clin Obstet Gynecol 15:203–219
Cauchi M, Lim D et al (1991) Treatment of recurrent aborters by immunization with paternal cells-controlled trial. Am J Reprod Immunol 25:16–17
Chard T (1991) Frequency of implantation and early pregnancy loss in natural cycles. Baillieres Clin Obstet Gynaecol 5:179–189
Christiansen O, Mathieson O et al (1990) Idiopathic recurrent spontaneous abortion. Acta Obstet Gynecol Scand 69:597-601
Clark D, Daya S (1991) Trials and tribulations in the treatment of recurrent spontaneous abortion. Am J reprod Immunol 25:18–24
Conley C, Hartman R (1952) Hemorrhagic disorder caused by circulating anticoagulant in patients with disseminated lupus erythematosus. J Clin Invest 31:621–622
Corson S (1992) Operative hysteroscopy for infertility. Clin Obstet Gynecol 35:229–241
Cosgriff T, Martin B (1981) Low functional and high antigenic antithrombin III level in a patient with the lupus anticoagulant and recurrent thrombosis. Arthritis Rheum 24:94–96
Coulam C (1991) Epidemology for recurrent spontaneous abortion. Am J Reprod Immunol 26:23–27
Cowchock F, Reece A et al (1992) Repeated fetal losses associated with antiphospholipid antibodies: a collaborative randomized trial comparing prednisone with low-dose heparin treatment. Am J Obstet Gynecol 166:1318–1323
Daya S, Clark D (1992) Alloimmunity. Principles and practice of medical therapy in pregnancy. Appleton, Norwalk, pp 407-413
Derksen R, Hasselaar P et al (1988) Coagulation screen is more specific than the anticardiolipin antibody ELISA in defining a thrombotic subset of lupus patients. Ann Rheum Dis 47:364–371
Desoye G, Dohr G et al (1988) Lack of HLA class I and class II antigens on the human preimplantation embryos. J Immunol 140:4157–4159
Dewald G, Michels V (1986) Recurrent miscarriages: cytogenetic causes and genetic counseling of affected families. Clin Obstet Gynecol 29:865–885
Downs K, Gibson M (1983) Basal body temperature graph and the luteal phase defect. Fertil Steril 40:466–468
Drugan AFK III et al (1990) Prenatal genetic diagnosis following recurrent early pregnancy loss. Obstet Gynecol 75:381–384
Dudley D, Branch D (1991) Antiphospholipid syndrome. A model for autoimmune pregnancy loss. Infertil Reprod Med Clin North Am 2:149–164
Ecker J, Laufer M et al (1993) Measurement of embryotoxic factors is predictive of pregnancy outcome in women with a history of recurrent abortion. Obstet Gynecol 81:84-87
Filicori M, Butler J et al (1984) Neuroendocrine regulation of the corpus luteum in the human. Evidence for pulsatile progesterone secretion. J Clin Invest 73:1638–1647
Fishman P, Falach-Vaknine E et al (1993) Prevention of fetal loss in experimental antiphospholipid syndrome by in vivo administration of recombinant interleukin-3. J Clin Invest 91:1834–1837
Fraser E, Grimes D et al (1993) Immunization as therapy for recurrent spontaneous abortion: a review and meta-analysis. Obstet Gynecol 82:854–859
Fritz M (1988) Inadequate luteal function and recurrent abortion: diagnosis and treatment of luteal phase deficiency. Semin Reprod Endocrinol 6:129–143
Geisler M, Kleinebrecht J (1978) Cytogenetic and histologic analyses of spontaneous abortions. Hum Genet 45:239–251
Glass R, Golbus M (1994) Recurrent abortion. Maternal-fetal medicien, principles and practice. Saunders, Philadelphia, 3rd edn., pp 445–451
Gleicher N, Harlow L et al (1992) Regulatory effect of antiphospholipid antibodies on signal transduction: a possible model for autoantibody-induced reproductive failure. Am J Obstet Gynecol 167:637–642
Goldzieher J, Benigno B (1958) The treatment of threatened and recurrent abortion: a critical review. Am J Obstet Gynecol 75:1202–1214
Guerneri S, Bettio D et al (1987) Prevalence and distribution of chromosome abnormalities in a sample of first trimester internal abortions. Hum Reprod 2:735–739

Hamilton-Fairley D, Kiddy D et al (1991) Low-dose gonadotropin therapy for induction of ovulation in 100 women with polycystic ovary syndrome. Hum Reprod 6:1095–1099
Harger J, Archer D et al (1983) Etiology of recurrent pregnancy losses and outcome of subsequent pregnancies. Obstet Gynecol 62:574–581
Harris E (1987) Syndrome of the black swan. Br J Rheumatol 26:324–326
Harris E, Ghavari A et al (1985) Anticardiolipin antibodies in autoimmune thrombocytopenic purpura. Br J Haematol 59:231–234
Hassold T, Chen N et al (1980) A cytogenetic study of 1000 spontaneous abortions. Ann Hum Genet 44:151–178
Hill J (1991) The rationale for leukocyte immunization in women with recurrent spontaneous abortion: fact or fiction? Colloque INSERM Libbey Eurotext, Paris, pp 263–269 Cellular and molecular biology of the maternofetal relationship
Hill J (1992) Immunological contributions to recurrent pregnancy loss. Baillieres Clin Obstet Gynecol 6:489–505
Hill J, Polgar K et al (1992) Evidence of embryo- and trophoblast-toxic cellular immune response(s) in women with recurrent spontaneous abortion. Am J Obstet Gynecol 166:1044–1052
Ho H, Gill TI et al (1990) Sharing of human leukocyte antigens in primary and secondary recurrent spontaneous abortions. Am J Obste Gynecol 163:178–188
Ho H, Gill TI et al (1991) Immunotherapy for recurrent spontaneous abortions in a Chinese population. Am J Reprod Immunol 25:10–15
Hwang J, Ho H et al (1992) The role of blocking factors and antipaternal lymphocytotoxic antibodies in the success of pregnancy in patients with recurrent spontaneous abortion. Fertil Steril 58:691-696
Infante-Rivard C, David M et al (1991) Lupus anticoagulants, anticardiolipin antibodies and fetal loss. A case-control study. N Engl J Med 325:1063-1066
Jacobs H, Hombourg R (1990) The endocrinology of conception. Baillieres Clin Endocrinol Metab 4:195–205
Johnson P, Ramsden G et al (1991) A combined randomised double-blind and open study of trophoblast membrane infusion (TMI) in unexplained recurrent miscarriage. In: Cellular and molecular biology of the materno-fetal relationship. Colloque INSERM/Libbey Eurotext, Paris, pp 277–284
Kalter H (1987) Diabetes and spontaneous abortion: a historical review. Am J Obstet Gynecol 156:1243–1253
Kats I, Fisch B et al (1992) Cutaneous graft-versus-host-like reaction after paternal lymphocyte immunization for prevention of recurrent abortion. Fertil Steril 57:927–929
Knudsen U, Hansen V et al (1991) Prognosis of a new pregnancy following previous spontaneous abortions. Eur J Obstet Gynecol Reprod Biol 39:31–36
Kovats S, Main E et al (1990) A class I antigen, HLA-G, expressed in human trophoblast. Science 248:220-223
Kutteh W, Carr B (1993) Recurrent pregnancy loss. Textbook of reproductive medicine. Appleton and Lange, Norwalk, pp 559-570
Lanzavecchia A (1990) Receptor mediated antigen uptake and its effect on antigen presentation to class II-restricted T lymphocytes. Annu Rev Immunol 8:773–793
Laurell A, Nilsson I (1957) Hypergammaglobulinemia, circulating anticoagulant and biologic false-positive Wasserman reaction. J Lab Clin Med 49:694
Lenton E, Landgreen B et al (1984) Normal variation in the length of the luteal phase of the menstrual cycle: identification of the short luteal phase. Br J Obstet Gynaecol 91:685–689
Li T, Rogers A et al (1987) A comparison between two methods of chronological dating of human endometrial biopsies during the luteal phase, and their correlation with histological dating. Fertil Steril 48:928–932
Lockshin M, Druzin M (1985) Antibody to cardiolipin as a predictor of fetal distress or death in pregnant patients with systemic lupus erythematosus. N Engl J Med 313:152–156
Lockwood C, Rand J (1994) The immunobiology and obstetrical consequences of antiphospholipid antibodies. Obstet Gynecol Surv 49:432–441
Lubbe W, Liggins G (1985) Lupus anticoagulant and pregnancy. Am J Obstet Gynecol 153:322–327
Lubbe W, Butler W et al (1984) Lupus anticoagulant in pregnancy. Br J Obstet Gynaecol 91:357–363

Malpas P (1938) Study of abortion sequences. J Obstet Gynaecol Br Emb 45:932–949
McDonough P (1988) The role of molecular mutation in recurrent euploidic abortion. Semin Reprod Endocrinol 6:155–164
McIntyre J, Faulk W et al (1983) Human trophoblast-lymphocyte cross-reactive (TLX) antigens define a new alloantigen system. Science 222:1135–1137
McWilliams R, Gibbons W (1991) Müllerian anomalies and recurrent pregnancy loss. Infertil Reprod Med Clin North Am 2:55–74
Mowbray J, Gibbings C et al (1985) Controlled trial of treatment of recurrent spontaneous abortion by immunisation with paternal cells. Lancet i:941-943
Ninia J (1994) Recurrent pregnancy loss. The Female Patient 19:26–32
Parazzini F, Bocciolone L et al (1991) Risk factors for spontaneous abortion. Int J Epidemiol 20:157-161
Peaceman A, Silver R et al (1992) Interlaboratory variation in antiphospholipid antibody testing. Am J Obstet Gynecol 166:1780-1787
Poland B, Miller J et al (1977) Reproductive counselling in patients who have had a spontaneous abortion. Am J Obstet Gynecol 127:685-691
Portnoi M-F, Joye N et al (1988) Karyotypes of 1142 couples with recurrent abortion. Obstet Gynecol 72:31–34
Rae R, Smith I et al (1994) Chlamydial serologic studies and recurrent spontaneous abortion. Am J Obstet Gynecol 170:782–785
Regan L (1992) Recurrent early pregnancy failure. Curr Opin Obstet Gynecol 4:220–228
Regan L, Braude P et al (1989) Influence of past reproductive performance on risk of spontanenous abortion. Br Med J 299:541–546
Regan L, Owen E et al (1990) Hypersecretion of luteinising hormone, infertility and miscarriage. Lancet 336:1141-1144
Regan L, Braude P et al (1991) A prospective study of the incidence, time of appearance and significance of anti-paternal lymphocytotoxic antibodies in human pregnancy. Hum Reprod 6:294–298
Rein M (1991) Luteal phase defect and recurrent pregnancy loss. Reprod Med Clin North Am 2:121–136
Roberts J, Taylor C et al (1992) Expression of the CD46 antigen and the absence of class I MHC antigen on the human oocyte and preimplantation blastocyst. Immunology 75:202-205
Roman E (1984) Fetal loss rates and their relation to pregnancy order. J Epidemiol Commun Health 38:29–35
Rosenbusch B, Sterzik K (1991) Sperm chromosomes and habitual abortion. Fertil Steril 56:370–372
Shangold M, Berkeley A, et al (1983) Both midluteal serum progesterone levels and late endometrial histology should be assessed in all in infertile women. Fertil Steril 40:627–630
Silver RK, MacGregor S et al (1993) Comparative trial of prednisone plus aspirin versus aspirin alone in the treatment of anticardiolipin antibody-positive obstetric patients. Am J Obstet Gynecol 169:1411-1417
Simpson J, Golbus M (1992) Genetics of pregnancy losses. In: Genetics in obstetrics and gynecology, 2nd edn. Saunders, Philadelphia, pp 181-200
Simpson J, Elias S et al (1981) Parental chromosomal rearrangements associated with repetitive spontaneous abortions. Fertil Steril 36:584–590
Simpson J, Meyers C et al (1989) Translocations are infrequent among couples having repeated spontaneous abortions but no other abnormal pregnancies. Fertil Steril 51:811–814
Stray-Pedersen B, Stray-Pedersen S (1984) Etiological factors and subsequent reproductive performance in 195 couples with a prior history of habitual abortion. Am J Obstet Gynecol 148:140–146
Talal N (1979) Sex factors, steroid hormones and the host response. Proceedings of the Kroc Foundation Conference. Arthritis Rheum 22:1153
Thiagarajan P, Shapiro S et al (1980) Monoclonal immunoglobulin M coagulation inhibitor with phospholipid specifity. J Clin Invest 66:397–405
Tho P, Byrd J et al (1979) Etiologies and subsequent reproductive performance of 100 couples with recurrent abortion. Fertil Steril 32:389–395
Triplett D (1989) Screening for the lupus anticoagulant. Res Clin Lab 19:379–389
Triplett D (1992) Obstetrical implications of antiphospholipid antibodies. Baillieres Clin Obstet Gynaecol 6:507-518

Vlaanderen W, Treffers P (1987) Prognosis of subsequent pregnancies after recurrent spontaneous abortion in first trimester. Br Med J 295:92–93

Warburton D (1987) Chromosomal causes of fetal death. Clin Obstet Gynecol 30:268–277

Warburton D, Frazer F (1964) Spontaneous abortion risk in man: data from reproductive histories collected in a medical genetics unit. Am J Hum Genet 16:1–25

Wilcox A, Weinberg C et al (1988) Incidence of early loss of pregnancy. N Engl J Med 319:189–194

Wolf FD, Carreras L et al (1982) Decidual vasculopathy and extensive placental infarction in a patient with repeated thromboembolic accidents, recurrent fetal loss, and a lupus anticoagulant. Am J Obstet Gynecol 142:829–834

Xu L, Chang V et al (1990) Antinuclear antibodies in sera of patients with recurrent pregnancy wastage. Am J Obstet Gynecol 163:1493–1497

Yamada H, Polgar K et al (1994) Cell-mediated immunity to trophoblast antigens in women with recurrent spontaneous abortion. Am J Obstet Gynecol 170:1339–1344

Immunology

A. Helvacioglu

Introduction

Data have been accumulating in the literature to suggest that significant interactions occur between the immune system and the reproductive system. It has been proposed that the major histocompatibility complex (MHC) can influence hormonally mediated functions in addition to its crucial role in immunological functions and disease resistance [1, 2]. Graft rejection is a specific immunological reaction. Grafts are rejected either by sensitized T cells or antibody-inducing platelet aggregation or type II hypersensitivity reactions (e.g., antibody-dependent cell-mediated cytotoxicity). MHC is responsible for provoking the most intense graft reactions. Differences between the MHC of the father, mother, and fetus may render the sperm, embryo, and fetus to be potential grafts to the maternal immune system, resulting in reproductive failure. Recent information related to the immunological factors that may influence recurrent pregnancy loss, endometriosis, ovarian failure, infertility, and immunologic conditions affecting the male, such as sperm antigens and formation of sperm antibodies, will be summarized below. The reader may find an excellent basic review of this topic in Aksel's article [3]: thus only recent research is summarized here.

Immunological Factors in Conception and Implantation

In the last three decades, the problem of immunological infertility has been extensively investigated, but there is still no absolute aggreement in the literature on the real clinical significance of antisperm antibodies in male infertility. In vitro fertilization (IVF) has been recommended as a method for achieving fertilization in couples with male autoimmune infertility. In men with congenital absence of the vas deferens, the presence of high titers of antisperm antibodies did not compromise their ability to father children via successful IVF, suggesting that autoimmunity to sperm should not be considered a reason for failure of IVF [4]. Contrasting data exist to show a positive correlation between male autoimmunity and IVF failure; fertilization failure in these IVF cycles was related to the localization of antibodies to the sperm head. Spermatozoa with head-bound antibodies had a lower amplitude of lateral head displacement and did not bind to the zona pellucida (ZP) [5]. Immune responses against the human sperm-specific antigen FA-1 have been implicated in the etiology of involuntary human infertility. The mode of action of anti-FA-1 antibodies in inhibiting fertility may be by way of interference with the egg-sperm receptor-binding mechanism. Existing data suggest that FA-1 has a lectin-binding property that binds and neutralizes the sperm ligand activity of purified ZP3 from the zona pellucida of oocytes [6]. Furthermore, anti-FA-1 antibodies prevent sperm from interacting with and penetrating the zona pellucida of oocytes, possibly by blocking capacitation and the acrosome reaction [7]. The ELISA method using the sperm-specific antigen FA-1 should help in elucidating the role of discrete sperm antibodies in human infertility, since cervical mucus and sera of antisperm-antibody positive women have been found to contain IgA and IgG antibodies against sperm-specific antigen FA-1 [8].

The diagnostic tests commonly used to detect antisperm antibodies pose several diagnostic and technical problems related to sensitivity and specificity. Mixed antiglobulin reaction (MAR) and immunobead tests (IBT) can only be performed on highly motile spermatozoa. In addition, detection of antisperm immunoglobulins in cervical mucus is difficult. Furthermore, antisperm antibodies detected by ELISA within seminal fluid may not be representative of the Ig detected on the surface of sperm from the same ejaculate. Consequently, the search for new tests to detect antisperm antibodies continues. One of the proposed novel techniques is flow cytometry analysis of living spermatozoa subjected to indirect immunofluorescence staining with mouse anti-human immunoglobulin monoclonal antibodies. This method has 100% specificity and 90% sensitivity in verifying that IgG antisperm antibodies are on the surface of living spermatozoa [9]. Sperm antibody can be independently synthesized in the reproductive tract [10], and the occurrence of sperm antibodies in cervical mucus cannot be explained merely on the basis that they are transudated from the blood. The dichotomy between local and systemic humoral responses, reflected by the differences in the specificities of systemic and local antisperm antibodies, is exhibited not only in infertile females but also in infertile males [11].

If sperm are coated with antisperm antibody, they are rapidly phagocytized. At present we have little understanding of the factors that influence the antisperm antibodies in secretions of the female reproductive tract, nor do we understand why serum and reproductive tract secretions should express antisperm antibodies differently.

Immunological Factors in Recurrent Pregnancy Loss

Predisposing factors for recurrent pregnancy loss include uterine abnormalities, endometrial infections, cervical incompetence, hormonal imbalance, and parental balanced chromosomal abnormalities. The etiology in approximately half of these abortions is still unknown. Therefore immunological factors as a cause of recurrent abortion have regained popularity as a subject of research. Antiphospholipid antibodies causing fetal demise, and abnormal maternal immune responses to paternal or trophoblast alloantigens with insufficient production of blocking antibodies or suppressor cells, causing a maternal rejection response, are the two frequently proposed immunological causes for recurrent pregnancy loss.

Recurrent Pregnancy Loss Associated with the Presence of Antiphospholipid Antibodies

Systemic lupus erythematosus (SLE) is considered to be the prototype of autoimmune diseases and is known to be associated with an increased incidence of spontaneous abortions, fetal death, and preterm deliveries (Fig. 1). Recurrent pregnancy losses in women with SLE may be closely associated with the presence of IgG and IgM antiphospholipid antibodies and the level of antibody titers correlates well with the incidence of pregnancy failures (Fig. 2). IgG anticardiolipin antibody (ACA) isotype was found to be more

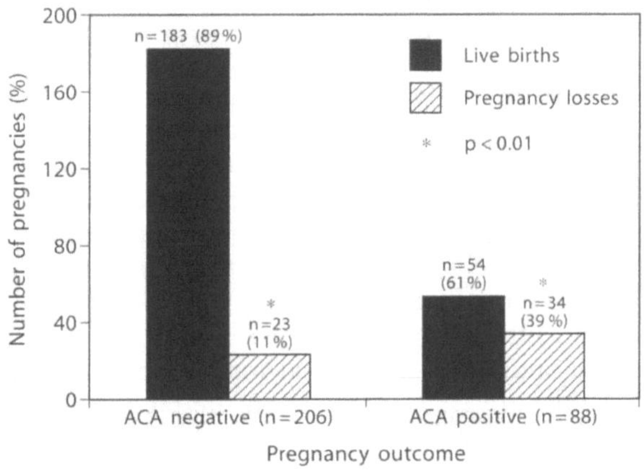

Fig. 1. Pregnancy losses in women of childbearing age with SLE. Women of reproductive age were grouped based on the presence or absence of anticardiolipin antibodies (*ACA*), and pregnancy outcomes are shown. *Solid columns*, number of successful pregnancies; *hatched columns*, number of pregnancy losses. (From [38])

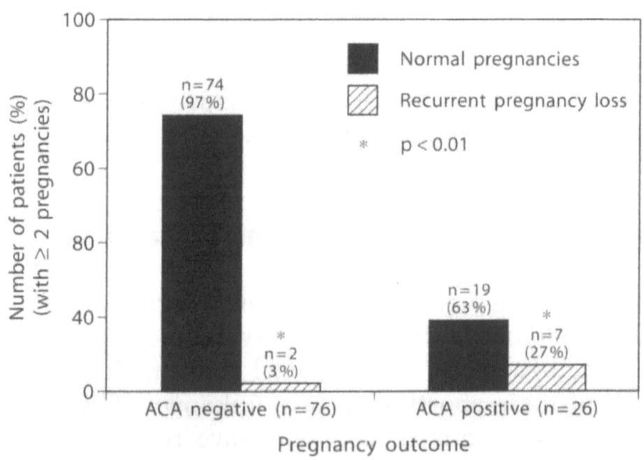

Fig. 2. Recurrent pregnancy losses in women of reproductive age with SLE. Women with two or more pregnancy losses were grouped basend on the presence or absence of anticardiolipin antibodies (*ACA*) and pregnancy outcomes are shown. *Solid columns*, number of women with successful pregnancy outcomes; *hatched columns*, number of women with recurrent pregnancy loss. (From [38])

closely linked to pregnancy loss than IgM and IgA isotypes [12]. Despite the presence of antiphospholipid antibodies, a number of patients may have uncomplicated pregnancies; however, an increase in ACA titers may result in pregnancy wastage (Figs. 1, 2) [13]. The prevalence of positive ACA among women without SLE but with recurrent abortions that were otherwise unexplained varies between 8% and 42% [14].

The mechanism of pregnancy loss is associated with a thrombotic tendency resulting in decidual and placental insufficiency. Probably via the mechanisms of prostacyclin production inhibition [15], inhibition of prekallikrein factor production [16], antiendothelial cell thrombomodulin activity, acquired deficiency of protein C and S and antithrombin III activity, and inhibition of the release of venous plasminogen activator. Nevertheless, the finding of increased baseline serum prostacyclin metabolite in women with positive antiphospholipid antibodies may suggest a condition of long-term stimulation or altered metabolism of prostacyclin [17].

An association between recurrent spontaneous abortions and circulating IgG antibodies to sperm tails in women was suggested in one study, but not confirmed by others [18]. As treatment, steroids, low-dose heparin, low-dose acetyl salicylic acid, or a combination of these have been suggested. However, no controlled study exists to justify their use. Recently, intravenous preparations of Ig have become available for clinical use in women with recurrent pregnancy loss and high levels of antiphospholipid antibodies. The mechanism of action of Ig treatment may be through the blockade of antibody binding to receptors on macrophages, increase in T suppressor cells, or decrease in antibody synthesis. Dose of Ig, treatment duration and treatment interval are all empirical at this time.

Problems in Maternal Recognition of the Fetal Allograft

Abnormal maternal immune responses to paternal or trophoblast alloantigens with insufficient production of blocking antibodies or suppressor cells, causing a maternal rejection response, may lead to fetal death pregnancy loss (Fig. 3). Differences between MHC of the mother and fetus may be beneficial to the fetus [19] but as a potential graft it must be protected against transplantation attack by the mother; suggested defense mechanisms are lack of class I and II MHC antigens on syncytiotrophoblast, a mucopolysaccharide coat around trophoblast, and local production of immunosuppressant.

There are scattered data in the literature implying the possible role of MHC in recurrent pregnancy loss and other reproductive diseases. Lack of HLA allosensitization may increase the risk of pregnancy-induced hypertension [20]. Furthermore, it has been theorized that MHC-linked recessive genes affect both fetal viability and susceptibility to cancer. In a large ethnically homogeneous Chinese population, HLA sharing occurred in significant excess in normal couples with primary or secondary recurrent spontaneous abortions and in couples in whom a gestational trophoblastic tumor developed in the woman [21].

Leukocyte immunotherapy of aborters with paternal or third party leukocytes is suggested to improve pregnancy outcome in women with a previous

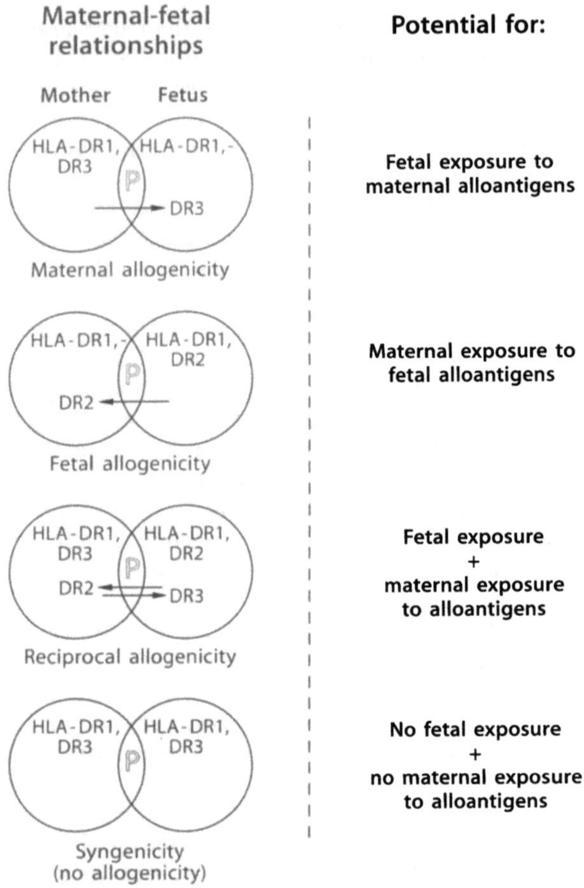

Fig. 3. The four different types of maternal-fetal HLA relationship and potential for maternal and/or fetal exposure to alloantigens (using an HLA-DR example). (From [20])

history of idiopathic recurrent abortion. The efficacy of this treatment is still controversial and its mechanism of action is obscure [22]. Furthermore, potential life-threatening complications such as graft-versus-host-like reaction is a possibility following such therapy [23]. Such treatment should be conducted in research centers equipped to handle these patients.

Immunological Factors in Infertility and Endometriosis

Although the etiology of endometriosis is still unknown, accumulating data suggest that immunological mechanisms may be involved in the pathophysiology of endometriosis and associated infertility. Some of these proposed mechanisms are autoimmune etiology [24], nonspecific activation of the peritoneal factors [25], and a defect in cell-mediated immunity [26]. Natural killer (NK) cell activity was decreased in women with endometriosis [27], as was the lymphocyte proliferation response to autologous endometrium [28], suggesting that impaired clearance of ectopic endometrium by NK cells may contribute to the development of the disease.

Normally the peritoneal fluid contains macrophages and lymphocytes along with several other types of blood cells and desquamated endometrial and mesothelial cells [29]. This cellular composition is modified in patients with endometriosis [30]. Macrophages are the predominant cell type observed in the peritoneal fluid and in the cavity of patients with endometriosis. Presence of a 20-kDa chemotactic factor has been shown in the peritoneal fluid of women with endometriosis, attracting isolated peripheral neutrophils, HL60-differentiated neutrophils, and U937 cells [31]. This chemotactic factor may also trigger macrophage activation, leading to the release of cytokines, cytotoxic factors, and cell growth effectors such as epidermal growth factor (EGF), transforming growth factor-α (TGF-α), TGF-β, and fibroblast growth factor (FGF). Cytokines and cytotoxic factors may be responsible for the observed aseptic inflammation in the peritoneal fluid of endometriosis patients, leading to endometriosis-associated infertility. On the other hand, cell growth effectors may contribute to proliferation of endometrial implants in vivo [32]. Patients with medical suppression as treatment for endometriosis have been found to have the lowest chemotactic activity [33]. Endometriotic implants per se, and or aberrant ovarian function, may be the reason for the macrophage transformation seen in endometriosis patients. The ovarian product inhibin induced a significant dose-related increase in monocyte chemotaxis while activin increased the migrational activity of monocytes [33]. It is important to determine whether alterations in NK activity associated with endometriosis are a cause or effect of the disease. It is possible that a genetically controlled NK cell aberrancy could contribute to the pathophysiology of the endometriosis [27, 34, 35]. So far, no one has reported immunological suppression of a patient with endometriosis to effect a better conception rate. Before definitive conclusions can be drawn regarding potential immunopathophysiological mechanisms in endometriosis, adequately controlled large clinical trials are needed.

Ovarian Failure

The finding of immune complexes around the follicles suggested an immune etiology in some patients with premature ovarian failure. During controlled ovarian hyperstimulation treatment of infertility in oligo-anovulatory women and in poor responders to human menopausal gonadotropin (hMG), circulating antibodies to ovarian tissue and to gonadotropin receptors were [36]. These autoantibodies were also detected in a large population of women with polyendocrinopathies [37]. Although sporadic pregnancies are reported following oral contraceptive pill suppression followed by high-dose hMG stimulation, there is no permanent cure for the disease at present. Women in premature menopause need to be watched carefully for their thyroid and pancreas functions, since detection of antiorgan antibodies, leading to multiple endocrine organ failure, is common in these women.

Conclusions

The current status of knowledge concerning the interaction between the immune and reproductive systems has been reviewed. It may be hypothesized that the human reproductive system may secrete cytokines that, in turn, may have an effect on cell growth and differentiation, similar to their pleiotropic effects on the immune system and other tissue. Furthermore, cytokines originating from the oocytes and the developing embryo may also signal the maternal immune or endocrine systems and thereby influence recognition of pregnancy. Further understanding of these interactions may lead to new concepts in fertility regulation.

References

1. Klein J (1986) The natural history of the major histocompatibility complex. Wiley, New York
2. Pende A, Ioverno A, Setti M, Bosco O, Musso NR, Vergassola C, Lanza L, Indiveri F, Lotti G (1993) Evidence for interactions between HLA systems class I and β-adrenergic receptors in human mononuclear leukocytes. J Clin Endocrinol Metab 77:1329–1333
3. Aksel S (1992) Immunologic aspects of reproductive diseases. JAMA 268:2930–2934
4. Patrizio P, Silber SJ, Ord T, Moretti-Rojas I, Asch RH (1982) Relationship of epididymal sperm antibodies to their in vitro fertilization capacity in men with congenital absence of the vas deferens. Fertil Steril 58:1006–1010
5. Zouarie R, DeAlmeida M, Rodrigues D, Jouannet P (1993) Localization of antibodies on spermatozoa and sperm movement characteristics are good predictors of in vitro fertilization success in cases of male autoimmune infertility. Fertil Steril 59:606–612
6. Naz RK, Sacco AG, Yurewicz EC (1989) Human spermatozoal FA-1 binds with ZP3 of porcine zona pellucida. J Reprod Immun 57:1072–1077
7. Kaplan P, Naz RK (1992) The fertilization antigen-1 does not have proteolytic/acrosin activity, but its monoclonal antibody inhibits human sperm capacitation and acrosome reaction. Fertil Steril 58:396–402
8. Menge AC, Naz RK (1993) IgG, IgA, and IgA subclass antibodies against fertilization antigen-1 in cervical secretions and sera of infertile couples. Fertil Steril 60:658–663
9. Nikolaeva MA, Kulakov VI, Ter-Avanesov GV, Terekhina LN, Pshenichnikova TJ, Sukhikh GT (1993) Detection of antisperm antibodies on the surface of living spermatozoa using flow cytometry: preliminary study. Fertil Steril 59:639–644
10. Shulman S, Hu C (1992) A study of the detection of sperm antibody in cervical mucus with a modified immunobead method. Fertil Steril 58:387–391
11. Shai S, Naot Y (1992) Identification of human sperm antigens reacting with antisperm antibodies from sera and genital tract secretions. Fertil Steril 58:593–598
12. Kutteh W, Lyda EC, Abraham SM, Wacholtz MC (1993) Association of anticardiolipin antibodies and pregnancy loss in women with systemic lupus erythematosus. Fertil Steril 60:449–455
13. Lockwood CJ, Roberto R, Feinberg RF, Clyne LP, Coster B, Hobbins JC (1989) The prevalance and biologic significance of lupus anticoagulant and anticardiolipin antibodies in general obstetric population. Am J Obstet Gynecol 161:369
14. Lockwood CJ, Reece EA, Roberto R, Hobbins JC (1986) Antiphospholipid antibody and pregnancy wastage. Lancet 2:742
15. DeWolf F, Carreras LO, Moerman P, Vermylen J, Van Assche A, Renaer M (1982) Decidual vasculopathy and extensive placental infarction in a patient with thromboembolic accidents. Am J Obstet Gynecol 142:829
16. Sanfelippo MJ, Drayna CJ (1982) Prekallikrein inhibition associated with the lupus anticoagulant: mechanism of thrombosis. Am J Clin Pathol 77:275

17. Dudley DJ, Mitchell MD, Ware Branch D (1990) Pathophysiology of antiphospholipid antibodies: absence of prostaglandin-mediated effects on cultured endothelium. Am J Obstet Gynecol 162:953
18. Clarke GN, Baker HWG (1993) Lack of association between sperm antibodies and recurrent spontaneous abortion. Fertil Steril 59:463–464
19. Hoff C, Peterson RDA (1993) Associations between maternal and fetal serum levels of immune activation markers and fetal growth. Am J Hum Biol (in press)
20. Hoff C, Peevy K, Giattina K, Spinnato JA, Peterson RDA (1992) Maternal-fetal HLA-DR relationships and pregnancy induced hypertension. Obstet Gynecol 80:1007–1012
21. Ho HN, Gill TJ, Nsieh RP, Hsieh HJ, Lee TY (1990) Sharing of human leucocyte antigens in primary and secondary spontaneous abortions. Am J Obstet Gynecol 163:178–188
22. Kilpatrick DC (1992) Cardiolipin antibody levels are not influenced by leucocyte immunotherapy in patients experiencing recurrent spontaneous abortion. Fertil Steril 57:328–330
23. Katz I, Fisch B, Amit S, Ovadia J, Tadir Y (1992) Cutaneous graft-versus-host-like reaction after paternal lymphocyte immunization for prevention of recurrent abortion. Fertil Steril 57:927–992
24. Cunningham DS, Hansen KA, Coddington CC (1992) Changes in T-cell regulation of responses to self antigens in women with pelvic endometriosis. Fertil Steril 58:114–119
25. Halme J, Becker S, Haskill S (1987) Altered maturation and function of peritoneal macrophages: possible role in pathogenesis of endometriosis. Obstet Gynecol 156:783–788
26. Vigano P, Vercellini P, DiBlasio AM, Colombo A, Candiani GB, Vignali M (1991) Deficient antiendometrium lymphocyte-mediated cytotoxicity in patients with endometriosis. Fertil Steril 56:894–899
27. Oosterlynck DJ, Meuleman CV, Waer M, Vandeputte M, Koninckx PR (1992) The natural killer activity of peritoneal fluid lymphocytes in decreased in women with endometriosis. Fertil Steril 58:292–295
28. Gilmore SM, Aksel S, Hoff C, Peterson RDA (1992) In vitro lymphocyte activity in women with endometriosis – an altered immune response? Fertil Steril 58:1148–1152
29. Mahmoud TA, Templeton A (1991) Peritoneal fluid volume and sex steroids in the preovulatory period in mild endometriosis. Br J Obstet Gynecol 98:179–183
30. Badaway SZ, Cuenca V, Marshall L, Munchback R, Rinas AC, Coble DA (1984) Cellular components in peritoneal fluid in infertile patients with and without endometriosis. Fertil Steril 42:704–708
31. Leiva MC, Hasty LA, Pfeifer S, Mastroianni Jr L, Lyttle CR (1993) Increased chemotactic activity of peritoneal fluid in patients with endometriosis. Am J Obstet Gynecol 168:592–598
32. Hammond MG, Oh ST, Anners J, Surrey ES, Halme J (1993) The effect of growth factors on the proliferation of human endometrial stromal cell in culture. Am J Obstet Gynecol 168:1131–1138
33. Petraglia F, Sacerdote P, Cossariza A, Angioni S, Genazzani AD, Franceschi C, Muscettola M, Grasso G (1991) Inhibin and activin modulate human monocyte chemotaxis and human lymphocyte interferon-γ-production. J Clin Endocrinol Metab 72:496–502
34. Oosterlynck DJ, Cornillie FJ, Waer M, Vandeputte M, Koninckx PR (1991) Women with endometriosis show a defect in natural killer activity resulting in a decreased cytotoxicity to autologous endometrium. Fertil Steril 56:45–51
35. Vigano P, Vercellini P, DiBlasio AM, Colombo A, Candiani GB, Vignali M (1991) Deficient antiendometrium lymphocyte-mediated cytotoxicity in patients with endometriosis. Fertil Steril 56:894–899
36. Meyer WR, Lavy G, DeCherney AH, Visintin I, Economy K, Luborsky J (1990) Evidence of gonadal and gonadotropin antibodies in women with suboptimal ovarian response to exogenous gonadotropin. Obstet Gynecol 75:797–799
37. Moncayo H, Moncayo R, Benz R, Wolf A, Lauritzen C (1989) Ovarian failure and autoimmunity: detection of autoantibodies directed against both the unoccupied luteinizing hormone/human chorionic gonadotropin receptor and the hormone receptor complex of bovine corpus luteum. J Clin Invest 84:185–188
38. Kutteh W, Lyda EC, Abraham SM, Wacholtz MC (1993) Association of anticardiolipin antibodies and pregnancy loss in women with systemic lupus erythematosus. Fertil Steril 60:449–455

Hyperprolactinemic Anovulatory Syndrome

H. G. Bohnet

Clinical Manifestation

In practically all appearances hyperprolactinemia is identical to disturbed follicle maturation and disturbed menstrual cycle, it is therefore classified as a type of hyperprolactinemic anovulatory syndrome. The previous classifications depending on the presence or absence of a pituitary adenoma are no longer necessary, since diagnostic and therapeutic proceedings are the same in both cases.

The degree of severity setting limits to ovarian function due to galactemia depends on the extent and period of increased prolactin (PRL) secretion. It comprises a pathophysiological continuum ranging from corpus luteum weakness to amenorrhea. In the course of PRL level normalization, it is not unusual for the different degrees of severity of cycle disturbances to follow an inverse sequence, i.e., from oligomenorrhae or anovulation and corpus luteum weakness affecting the ovulatory (conception) cycle.

Galactorrhea

Although galactorrhea is understood as an indicator of intensified PRL effect on the mammary gland, it is not found in all hyperprolactinemic patients. The incidence of milk secretion classified into different categories ranges from 30- to 50%, depending on the patients. The reason for absence of galactorrhae or rather the biological effect of PRL is not yet clear. An insufficient number of prolactin receptors presumably induced by estrogens might be an explanation for hyperprolactinemia frequently coinciding with low estrogen levels. Another reason is the diversity of the PRL molecule (dimer, polymer) inclined to different biological activities. Various methods of determination do not simultaneously monitor all molecular forms of prolactin. In hypothyreosis, PRL receptors have a higher affinity towards prolactin, therefore having a greater effect on the target organ.

Androgenism

Androgenized women frequently present with (minor) hyperprolactinemia, i.e., up to 40%. Almost one quarter of all hyperprolactinemic patients are androgenised. The question arises and can not definitively be answered whether androgens are only increased due to an adrenal PRL effect or whether they are primarily elevated with peripheral aromatisation into estrogens, finally leading to hyperprolactinemia (resulting in a vicious circle). Hyperthyreosis favors increased adrenal androgen secretion via an increase of PRL receptors of NNR and dehydroepiandrosterone (DHEA, plus sulfate) secretion.

Premenstrual syndrome

Premenstrual syndrome is frequently characterized by hyperprolactinemia and corpus luteum weakness. Disturbed PRL secretion cannot always be attributed to the luteal dysphory complex, but rather reflects a hypothalamic disorder (e.g., disturbance of endorphin secretion) in the sense of a secondary hyperprolactinemia.

Diagnosis and Evaluation of Findings

Reference Intervals

The statement that hyperprolactinemia can be diagnosed when PRL serum levels are pathologically elevated is true, but not very useful in practice, since the literature indicates extremely wide-ranging reference intervals for the lactation hormone. Present findings make it impossible to accept such indefinite reference intervals, given the fact that the parameter of ovulatory cycles are more precise and reliable than they were in the 1970s, when sonographic folliculometries were not carried out on a routine basis. Our reference intervals exclusively consider PRL concentrations in conception cycles of euthyreote women. In conception cycles, basal serum levels never exceed 18 ng/ml either during the ovulatory or during the luteal phase (i.e., the 95th percentile). During the follicular phase, lower PRL concentrations are mostly observed. In cycle monitoring, folliculometries are carried out between the 12th and 14th day of the cycle, usually in combination with determinations of estradiol and luteinizing hormone (LH) serum concentrations and PRL. Alternatively, PRL determination is possible between the 20th and 24th cycle day together with monitoring of the luteal function, i.e., verification of PRL, progesterone and estradiol.

The question of whether the unique determination of basal PRL values justifies a classification into normo- and hyperprolactinemia is partly still a matter of controversy in the literature. If PRL concentrations of more than 18 ng/ml are found, hyperprolactinemia has become manifest. The converse, i.e., classifying PRL concentrations of less than 18 ng/ml as normal PRL secretion, cannot be adopted. Prolactin serum concentrations may be subject to considerable spontaneous fluctuations. Even as many as three to four PRL determinations within 1 h cannot be considered a reliable proof for a representative secretion phase of the lactation hormone. It is no rare observation that during the early follicular phase low to normal and during the late follicular or luteal phase elevated PRL levels occur.

Provocation Tests

Metoclopramide. In order to eliminate uncertainty when determining basal PRL serum concentrations, the application of provocation tests is recommended. In our own patients the metoclopramide stimulation test, proved to be useful. Metoclopramide is currently present as the strongest prolactin stimulator. Prolactin secretion is pharmacologically stimulated by dopamine receptor blocking. The test aims to achieve a strong correlation between metoclopramide-induced prolactin elevations and spontaneous sleep-induced, i.e., physiological, prolactin augmentations. The higher the prolactin increase is under test conditions, the higher prolactin levels spontaneously increase during sleep. An overshooting nocturnal prolactin increase is not necessarily reflected in the baseline secretion of lactotrope hormone. By implementing the metoclopramide test, a nocturnal supraphysiological, i.e., pathological, prolactin increase, able to possibly start a prolactinogenic pathomechanism of ovarian insufficiency, may be documented. This is the latent form of hyperprolactinemia. Normally, metoclopramide induced prolactin increase is significantly higher during the luteal phase than during the follicular phase. Taking these facts into account, it is recommended that this test should preferably be carried out during the luteal phase (22nd day of the cycle) in those infertility patients still having almost regular cycle intervals.

After taking an empty trial 10 mg metoclopramide is slowly injected i.v.; 25 min later another blood test is taken, and the lactation hormone is determined in both samples. They are centrifugalized and the serum is fractionated. Both samples are frozen at 23° and stored for a later radioimmunologic determination of prolactin concentrations.

From clinical experience, we assume manifest hyperprolactinemia in basal serum secretions of more than 20 ng/ml; latent hyperprolactinemia is manifest in a prolactin increase of more than 200 ng/ml in the metoclopramide test.

The actual clinical importance of latent hyperprolactinemia us supported by psychoendocrinological examination results. Latent hyperprolactinemia may be evaluated as an expression of individually increased sensitivity towards stress. Patients concerned rarely talk about their problems and live socially isolated; they easily resign to every day problems.

Thyrotrophin-Releasing Hormone. In order to test the dynamic function of prolactin secretion, the tripeptide thyrotropin-releasing hormone (TRH) test may be implemented instead of the metoclopramide test. The borderline determination between normal and elevated response behavior using i.v. administration of 200 instead of 40 µg is very narrow, since PRL response is submaximum as opposed to metoclopramide response, which is maximum. TRH-stimulated PRL concentrations of more than 40 ng/ml are presumed to be pathological. The incidence of hypothyreosis is twice as high (approximately 20%) in latent (and manifest) hyperprolactinemias than in undisturbed secretion of prolactin hormone. This explains why tests on thyroid function by means of TRH are combined with PRL secretion monitoring.

It should be remembered that, as a rule, dynamic function tests are not appropriate for distinguishing functional from organic hyperprolactinemia.

In oligo- and amenorrhea determination of basal PRL is generally sufficient to prove a PRL-induced cycle disturbance. The higher PRL levels are, the higher the probability of a galactoma causing amenorrhea is. With PRL levels of more than 100 ng/ml, there is a 50% probability of finding a pituitary adenoma, which should be further investigated using a scanning method.

Scanning Methods

Just as computer tomography (CT) has replaced polytomography of the sella turcica (improved resolving, lower exposure to radiation), magnetic resonance imaging (MRI) will probably replace CT examinations. Exposure to radiation is eliminated, and resolving is equally high or even better. The size of the adenoma correlates with the level of basal PRL and is used as a criterion for scaling; an adenoma with a diameter of up to 1 cm, is called a microadenoma, while major tumors, so-called macroadenomas, run the risk of suprasellar extension and injury of nervus opticus, thus requiring visual faculty monitoring.

If proof has been furnished of an intrasellar microadenoma, there is no indication for another MRI 1 or 2 years later, as proposed earlier, except in cases where clinical symptoms become manifest indicating the growth of an adenoma or where annual PRL controls reveal significant increases. However, the diagnosis should be documented prior to a (planned) pregnancy and after delivery. Macroadenomas should be checked at regular intervals.

Degree of Severity of the Prolactinogenic Dysfunction of the Hypothalamo-Pituitary-Ovarian Axis

Hyperprolactinemia is known to correlate with a disturbance of ovarian function. Follicular and luteal steroid secretion will gradually cease, not least due to a decline in hypothalamic gonadotropin-releasing hormone (GnRH)-pulse frequence with consecutive reduction of LH secretion. In the luteal phase, adequate estradiol and progesterone concentrations will be found in at least half of the patients (<12 ng/ml), and in one third anovulation has become manifest (progesterone <3 ng/ml). In the remaining cases amenorrhea is diagnosed. Early follicular estrogen values (>20 and >100 pg/ml) respectively, are rarely lower, being the reason for mostly positive gestagen tests. Follicle-stimulating hormone (FSH) serum concentrations are hardly ever suppressed, reaching similar early follicular concentrations (8–12 m units/ml) as opposed to low LH levels (2–4 m units/ml). Proof of absence of both gonadotropins (>2 m units/ml) leads to the assumption of entire cessation of gonadotropin-releasing pituitary cells. In most cases, an adenoma has shifted or compressed the cells, which can eventually lead to a loss in TSH and adrenocorticotropic hormone (ACTH) secretion.

Therapy Results of Treatment

Medicated therapy of hyperprolactinemia aims to normalize elevated PRL secretion, restoring ovarian function, reducing the size of an adenoma, if present, and eliminating possible ensuing complications such as dysfunction of the pituitary gland or visual field.

Hyperprolactinemia Without Clinical Correlation

Concentrations within the upper reference interval or minor PRL elevations without clinical correlation do not require treatment. An explanation for their existence may be the fact that minor or biologically inactive forms of PRL, e.g., "big PRL" or "big-big", are registered by the respective determination method.

Hyperprolactinemic Anovulatory syndrome

It is a matter of controversy to which extend patients with hyperprolactinemic anovulatory syndrome with or without evidenced microadenoma and no wish for a child should receive PRL-inhibiting therapeutic treatment at all. There is a minor proliferation tendency of prolactinomas, and PRL levels remain constant for many years. Reduced estrogen secretion for several years may, however, provoke decalcification of the bones. Mineral content in hyperprolactinemic women in contrast to cycle-stabilized women of the same age is on average reduced by 20%. Although there is no significantly higher risk of fracture, it would be appropriate to substitute estrogens (and gestagens). Proof has been furnished that neither so-called natural estogens nor ovulation inhibitors have any considerable influence on PRL levels or the size of microadenomas. Monitoring PRL secretion once or twice a year is recommended in order to discover increases or decreases. Decreases might signalize spontaneous regressions due to cell necrosis.

Primary administration of dopaminergics indicate the extent to which hyperprolactinemia responds quickly to therapy and the side effects that may occur. Restoring ovulatory cycles might be of psychological importance to the patient.

Medicated Prolactin Inhibition

If the patient wants a child, medicated PRL inhibition is an alternative. For many years, ergot derivatives have been administered. In Germany we use two primarily dopaminergic substances: bromocriptine and lisuride which have practically no uterotone or vascular side effects. They stimulate the dopamine-2 receptor. Further to its dopaminergic effect metergoline has mainly an antiserotoninergic effect. These substances may reduce PRL with different intensity, but the doses available have similar effects. Bromocriptine and lisuride have almost identical side effects, such as nausea, vomiting, and hypotone circulation weakness. Normal oral doses of two to three tablets of metergoline per day weaken the side effects, thus representing an alternative. Very few side effects will occur if bromocriptine and lisuride are taken with the evening meal. Vaginal administration of bromocriptine is also a favorable alternative with a certain depot effect. Despite increased doses, parenteral administrations of bromocriptine had few side effects. It is preferably administered to patients with macroademonas.

Women suffering from amenorrhea may have higher requirement for PRL inhibitors, depending on the PRL level. PRL inhibition is a continuous basic therapy, i.e., requiring daily administration and not being cycle dependant (even in premenstrual syndrome). In most cases spontaneous menstruation begins 4 weeks later, often followed by conception. If menstruation fails to occur or an early gravidity became manifest, the PRL inhibitor should no longer be administered, although teratogenic damages, have not been described.

All PRL inhibitors available, when appropriately administered, induce reliable PRL depression, while in adenomas they initiate a shrinking of adenoma size, easily shown by MRI. If administration of PRL inhibitors is ceased, PRL levels start to increase again and the adenoma may re-expand. If no ovulatory cycles are achieved despite the administration of PRL inhibitors, perhaps due to intolerance of adequately high doses, supplementary treatment using ovulation-inducing hormones, e.g., human menopausal/chorionic gonadotropin (hMG/hCG) or GnRH may be initiated, if the patient wishes to have children.

A permanent increase of the PRL-inhibiting doses due to clinical symptoms (e.g., insufficient follicle maturation, corpus luteum weakness) is not indicated without monitoring PRL levels, as PRL overdepression may ensue. Permanent serum concentrations below 3 ng/ml may at first normalize the cycle, but then have negative effects on follicle maturation and premature follicle luteinization.

Neurosurgical Intervention

Neurosurgical enucleation of a microadenoma has become of secondary importance in recent years, although two thirds of the patients are considered to be cured after the operation, i.e., PRL secretion has been permanently normalized. Surgical interventions are mainly reserved for infertility patients not tolerating the various PRL inhibitors or refusing administration over a long period of time. Recidivation of a prolactinoma is caused by incomplete removal of the tumor tissue and not by new clonal formation. Due to a relatively long half-life of PRL of approximately half an hour, the decline in PRL serum concentration during the operation is not a reliable indicator. Regression curves allow indirect assumptions to be made of whether or not the adenoma has been completely removed. Prior treatment of hyperprolactinemia by dopaminergics may induce alterations of the tumor tissue, rendering enucleation more difficult.

Hypophyseal Adenoma and Gravidity

A distinction between functional and microadenoma-induced hyperprolactinemia is generally no longer made, since improved scanning methods often revealed microadenomas which had been thought to be a functional disturbance. However, the (historical) importance of adenoma and gravidity will be elucidated here.

The pituitary glands of pregnant women spontaneously increase by half of their size due to hyperplasia of the lactotrope cells stimulated by estrogens.

In rare cases, adenoma growth has been observed during pregnancy. Less than 2% of hyperprolactinemic patients with microadenoma develop symptoms that might indicate tumor progression during pregnancy. Radiologic examinations reveal an asymptomatic tumor growth, in 5% of all women with microadenoma, with exstirpation becoming necessary during gravidity only in isolated cases.

As for macroadenomas, there is clearly a higher probability of an increase in size during gravidity, with a risk of approximately 15%. Headache is the most prominent symptom even before visual impairment commences. Both may become manifest in all trimena. Although bitemporal hemianopsia is a classical visual field defect, other disturbances are possible.

It cannot be predicted which patients are susceptible to tumor growth during pregnancy. For this reason it is necessary to check PRL levels at the beginning of each trimenon even if the women have no complaints. In the case of a significant increase in lactaction hormone compared to the basic values, monthly controls are required as well as a visual field determination. MRI is reserved for special cases.

Should a tumor expansion become manifest, administration of a dopamine agonist is indicated, since this prevents further growth and even reduces tumor size during gravidity. Abortions intended to prevent tumor growth can no longer be accepted. Abortion and malformation rates are not elevated under PRL inhibiting treatment. While maternal and fetal PRL levels decline under medication, intra-amnial PRL content obviously acting as a regulative factor for water and electrolytes and controlled by estrogens and progesterone is not influenced by dopaminergic substances.

Infants may be suckled after delivery without running the risk of stimulating tumor growth. A considerable number of women previously suffering from amenorrhea develop normal menstruation cycles after delivery. The reason for this tumor shrinkage is possibly leading to the regression of the pituitary adenoma.

References

1. Ben-David M, Schenker JG (1983) Transient hyperprolactinemia: a correctable cause of idiopathic female infertility. J Clin Endocrinol Metab 57:442
2. Berg D, Rjosk H-K, Jänicke F, von Werder K (1983) Behandlung der hyperprolaktinämischen Amenorrhoe durch pulsatile Gaben von Gonadotropin Releasing-Hormonen. Geburtshilfe Frauenheilkd 43:686–688
3. Biller BMK, Baum HBA, Rosenthal DI, Saxe VC, Charpie PM, Klibanski A (1992) Progressive trabecular osteopenia in women with hyperprolactinemic amenorrhea. J Clin Endocrinol Metab 75:692–697
4. Bohnet HG (1980) Gelbkörperschwäche als Prolaktin-bedingte Störung des Menstruationszyklus. Fortschr Med 98:1628
5. Bohnet HG (1981) Prolaktin und seine Bedeutung für die Frau. Grosse, Berlin
6. Bohnet HG (1985) Prolaktin und weibliche Sterilität. Leitfaden für die Praxis. Grosse, Berlin
7. Bohnet HG, Aragona C, Friesen HG (1976) Induction of lactogenic receptors in the liver of hypophysectomized female rats. Endocrin Res Commun 3:187
8. Bohnet HG, Dahlen HG, Wuttke W, Schneider HPG (1976) Hyperprolactinemic anovulatory syndrome. J Clin Endocrinol Metab 42:132–143

9. Bohnet HG, Mühlenstedt D, Hanker J, Schneider HPG (1977) Prolactin oversuppression. Arch Gynak 223:173–178
10. Bohnet HG, Kato K (1987) Evaluation of basal hormone levels in hirsute women. Exp Clin Endocrinol 89/1:31–38
11. Corenblum B, Donovan L (1993) The safety of physiological estrogen plus progestin replacement therapy and with oral contraceptive therapy in women with pathological hyperprolactinemia. Fert Steril 59/3:671–673
12. DeWitt W, Coelingh Bennink HJT, Gerards LJ (1984) Prophylactic bromocriptine treatment during pregnancy in women with macroprolactinomas: report of 13 pregnancies. Br J Obstet Gynecol 91:1059
13. Fahlbusch R, Giovanelli MA, Crosignani PG, Faglia G, Rjosk JK, von Werder K (1980) Differential therapy of microprolactinomas: significance of transphenoidal adenomectomy. In: Faglia G, Giovanelli MA, MacLeod RM (eds) Pituitary microadenomas. Academic, London, pp 443–456
14. Fink U, Fink BK, Oeckler R (1990) MRI versus CT imaging. In: Faglia G, Beck-Peccoz P, Ambrosi B, Travaglini P, Spada A (eds) Pituitary adenomas. Excerpta Medica, Amsterdam, pp 229–236 (ICS 961)
15. Gemzell C, Wang CF (1979) Outcome of pregnancy in women with pituitary adenoma. Fertil Steril 31:363–372
16. Holmgren U, Bergstrand G, Hagenfeldt K, Werner S (1986) Women with prolactinoma-effect of pregnancy and lactation on serum prolactin and on tumor growth. Acta Endocrinol 111:452
17. Katznelson L, Alexander JM, Klibanski A (1993) Clinical review 45. Clinically nonfunctioning pituitary adenomas. J Clin Endocrinol Metab 76:1089–1094
18. Krupp P, Monka C (1987) Bromocriptine in pregnancy: safety aspects. Klin Wochenschr 65:823–827
19. Labhart A (1978) Die Adenohypophyse. In: Lebhart A (ed) Klinik der inneren Sekretion. Springer, Berlin Heidelberg New York, p 102
20. Laws ER Jr, Fode NC, Randall RV, Abboud CF, Coulam CB (1983) Pregnancy following transphenoidal resection of prolactin-secreting pituitary tumors. J Neurosurg 58:685–688
21. Lüdecke DK, Quak C, Saeger W (1992) Intraoperative biopsies and prolactin-IRMA in prolactinomas. Endocrin Pathol 3 [Suppl 1]:527
22. Magyar DM, Marshall JR (1978) Pituitary tumors and pregnancy. Am J Obstet Gynecol 132:739–751
23. McNatty KP (1979) Follicular determinants of corpus luteum function in the human ovary. In: Channing CP, Marsh JM (eds) Ovarian follicular and corpus luteum function. Plenum, New York, p 465
24. Molitch ME (1985) Pregnancy and the hyperprolactinemic women. N Engl J Med 312:1362
25. Niemann D (1985) Wechselbeziehungen zwischen der Regulation der Schilddrüsenfunktion und der Prolaktionsekretion und ihre Bedeutung für Frauen mit Infertilität oder Zyklusstörungen. Dissertation, University of Hamburg
26. Rjosk H-K, Fahlbusch R, Huber H, von Werder K (1978) Growth of prolactin-producing pituitary adenomas during pregnancy. In: Fahlbusch R, von Werder K (eds) Treatment of pituitary adenomas. Thieme, Stuttgart, p 395
27. Rjosk H-K, Fahlbusch R, von Werder K (1982) Influence of pregnancies on prolactinomas. Acta Endocrinol (Copenh) 100:337–346
28. Rjosk H-K, Fahlbusch R, von Werder K Spontaneous development of hyperprolactinemia. Acta Endocrinol (Copenh) 100:333–336
29. Ruiz-Velasco V, Tolis G (1984) Pregnancy in hyperprolactinemic women. Fertil Steril 41:793
30. Schlechte J, Walkner L, Kathol M (1992) A longitudinal analysis of premenopausal bone loss in healthy women and women with hyperprolactinemia. J Clin Endocrinol Metab 75:698–703
31. Schneider HPG, Bohnet HG (1977) Hyperprolaktinämische Amenorrhoe and Anovulation. Gynäkologie 10:84
32. Schneider HPG, Bohnet HG (1981) Die hyperprolaktinämische Amenorrhoe und Anovulation. Gynäkologe 14:104
33. Strauß B, Appelt H, Bohnet HG, Quitmann S, Ulrich D (1988) Untersuchungen zur Psychoendokrinologie des Prolaktins. In: Appelt H, Strauß B (eds) Psychoendokrinologische Gynäkologie. Enke, Stuttgart, pp 147–167 (Bücherei des Frauenarztes, vol 18)

34. Tucker HSG, Grubb SR, Wigand JP, Taylor A, Lankford HV, Blackard WG, Becker DP (1981) Galactorrhea-amenorrhea syndrome. Follow-up of forty-five patients after pituitary tumor removal. Ann Intern Med 94:302–307
35. von Werder K, Müller OA, Fink U (1988) Medikamentöse Therapie der Prolaktinome. Akt Endokr Stoffw 9:213–220
36. von Werder K, Müller OA, Fink U, Graef K (1993) Diagnosis and treatment of hyperprolactinemia. In: Comprehensive endocrinology. The pituitary gland, 2nd edn. Raven, New York
37. Willig RP, Bosk A, Lüdecke DK (1992) Prolactin secreting pituitary adenoma: distinct symptoms in the paediatric age group. Acta Endocrinol 126 [Suppl 4]:62

Surgical Therapy of Endometriosis

M. Sillem, C.C. Coddington III, T. Rabe, and B. Runnebaum

Role of Surgery in an Overall Therapeutic Concept

While laparoscopy and/or biopsy must be regarded at present as the gold standard in diagnosing endometriosis, discussing the role of operative interventions in the therapy of this disease entails reporting on a broad range of approaches and opinions. The heterogeneity of patient populations as well as observation and evaluation methods makes comparisons between and general conclusions from published studies extremely difficult. Different staging systems in endometriosis, each of which has its inherent problems, lead to different success rates, even when the same group of patients is evaluated (Rock et al. 1981). The monthly fecundity rate, i.e., number of conceptions divided by the total of person-cycles of exposure, which allows comparison of treatments independent of the lenght of follow-up (Cramer et al. 1979), is calculated only in a minority of publications.

Situations in which surgery is commonly contemplated are: endometriotic lesions that are easily amenable at diagnostic laparoscopy, ovarian cysts, extraperitoneal foci, removal of adhesions and scar tissue in the absence of active disease, failure of medical therapy aimed at either pain or infertility, a patient's request for an aggressive therapeutic approach, recurrent disease or a rapid, definitive solution for the patient no longer desiring fertility. The doubtless advantage of surgical over medical therapy is, that, while often at least as effective (Guzick and Rock 1981; Seiler et al. 1986; Adamson and Pasta 1994), it does not per se impair fertility, thus avoiding time loss in evaluating its success. This seems particularly important for infertile patients over 35 years of age or with longstanding infertility. On the other hand, it should be borne in mind that in a large number of cases, endometriosis is a chronic and recurrent condition and that even the most thorough destruction of foci will not permanently affect the underlying pathophysiological mechanism(s) as long as uterus and ovaries are preserved.

The success of operations that are aimed at pain relief is difficult to assess objectively, and the parameters used to report success rates vary from study to study. However, in approximately 20% of patients, medical attempts to control dysmenorrhea will fail, and in these, a surgical intervention is clearly indicated (Dawood 1985).

The principle of *primum nihil nocere* is particularly important in the management of the asymptomatic, infertile patient. Endometriosis without blockage of both fallopian tubes is not an absolute obstacle to conception and the exact mechanism(s) by which fertility is impaired in these cases is still poorly understood. This means that the success of any therapeutic intervention must be compared to the fertility with expectant management and to the monthly fecundity rates in normal couples. The physiological monthly fecundity rate is estimated to be around 20% in couples who cease to use contraceptive methods. Of these couples, 86% can be expected to achieve a pregnancy within a year; of the remainder, 69% of women will have conceived by the end of the second year without intervention (Leridon and Spira 1984) (Table 1). Table 2 gives an overview of studies reporting "spontaneous" conceptions. More than half of all patients with minimal or mild disease can be expected to conceive without specific treatment within a year, provided additional factors are corrected (Garcia and David 1977; Schenken and Malinak 1982). A monthly fecundity rate of 5.6% in mild and 3.0% in moderate disease has been observed (Olive et al. 1985). In fact, several studies have failed to show an increase in fertility in patients with mild and even moderate disease treated by conservative surgery versus expectant management (Garcia and David 1977; Schenken and Malinak 1982; Olive and Lee 1986; Olive and Haney 1986). Whereas the data do not exclude the possibility that a subgroup of patients with moderate disease and infertility might also benefit from surgery, they stress the importance of identifying and consistently treating other factors compromising the fertility of a couple before recommending a more aggressive surgical approach. Such complicating additional factors are as frequent in patients (couples) with endometriosis as in a general infertility population (Gast et al. 1988). However, in patients with severe disease, surgery seems to improve fertility.

The decision for surgical steps at or after diagnostic laparoscopy should be made in light of a thorough preoperative differential diagnostic workup (Table 3) with respect to the severity of the patient's symptoms, the success of previous therapeutic attempts, and her desires related to childbearing. An

Table 1 Calculated proportion (%) of couples who will conceive within 12 months among couples not yet having conceived at duration *n*, by mean fecundity in the whole population. Fecundity is distributed between couples according to a beta function, with *p* and coefficient of variation of 0.5, and assuming that no couples are totally sterile. (From Leridon and Spira 1984)

No. of months without conception (*n*)	Mean fecundity in the population				
	0.10	0.20	0.25	0.30	0.40
0	66.5	86.0	90.1	92.6	95.0
6	61.1	77.0	80.0	81.3	80.5
12	56.5	69.2	71.0	71.2	68.2
24	48.9	57.0	57.3	56.3	51.5
36	43.1	48.2	47.7	46.3	41.2
48	38.4	41.7	40.8	39.2	34.2
60	34.7	36.7	35.6	33.9	29.3

Table 2 Studies comparing fertility in treated vs untreated patients with endometriosis and no (or treated) other causes for infertility. Figures reflecting spontaneous conception rates are in italics

Author	Study description	Patient group[a]	No.	Pregnancy rate (months of follow-up)	Monthly fecundity rate
Garcia and David 1977	Expectant management	Minimal disease	17	67.4% (21, 10/11 after 12 months)	
Seibel et al. 1982	Expectant vs Danazol, prospective, randomized	Minimal, expectant	14	57% (6 after diagnosis)	
		Minimal, Danazol	11	36% (6 after completion of treatment)	
Schenken and Malinak 1982	Retrospective analysis of CSEL[b] versus expectant management	Mild, expectant	16	75% (≤12, mean 5)	
		Mild, CSEL	29	72.4% (≤12, mean 4)	
Portuondo et al. 1983	Prospective follow-up, timed intercourse only vs AID	Mild, husband fertile, no AID	21	47.6% (18, mean 7.2)	Both groups together: 8.33%
		Mild, husband azoospermic, AID	10	90% (18, mean 3.5)	
Olive et al. 1985	Prospective follow-up, hydrotubation (+) vs no hydrotubation (-)	Mild +	6	83.3%	15.2%
		Mild -	8	50.0%	5.6%
		Moderate +	9	33.3%	3.9%
		Moderate -	31	22.6%	3.0%
		Severe +	1	0	0
		Severe -	15	0	0
Olive and Lee 1986	Retrospective, CSEL[b] (+) vs expectant management (-)	Mild +	11	45.5%	3.9%
		Mild -	34	52.9%	5.7%
		Moderate +	43	51.2%	3.6%
		Moderate -	57	21.1%	2.9%
		Severe +	34	29.4%	1.4%
		Severe -	32	0	0
Thomas and Cooke 1987	Gestrinone vs placebo, randomized double-blind	Asymptomatic + gestrinone	20	25% (12)	
		Asymptomatic + placebo	17	24% (12)	

[a] All studies used the Acosta classification (Acosta et al. 1973) except Seibel et al. (1982), who used Kistner's system (Kistner et al. 1977)
[b] CSEL, Conservative surgery for endometriosis at laparoscopy

open and thorough discussion with the patient is essential to determine the appropriateness and proper timing of surgery for the individual patient.

Table 3 Preoperative diagnostic workup

Symptom/sign	Differential diagnosis	Test
Secondary dysmenorrhea	Leiomyoma uteri Adenomyosis uteri Chronic infection, "frozen pelvis"	Clinical exam., ultrasound, (hysteroscopy) *Chlamydia* culture and serum antibodies
Dysfunctional bleeding	Endometrial hyperplasia, uterine and cervical pathology, PCO, ovarian dysfunction	Endometrial biopsy Pap. smear Luteal phase prolactin and progesterone
Adnexal mass	Functional cyst, ovarian tumor, hydrosalpinx, adjacent organ disease	Clinical exam. Ultrasound (before and after steroid treatment) ESR (Ca-125) Evaluation of other systems as appropriate
Infertility	Ovarian factor	Basal body temperature, luteal phase prolactin and progesterone, TSH, early follicular LH, FSH, estradiol, testosterone, DHEAS, endometrial biopsy, ultrasound
	Tubal and uterine factor	Ultrasound, HSG (hysteroscopy)
	Cervical factor	PCT, Insler score
	Male factor	Semen analysis, PCT, andrological exam.
Dyspareunia	Psychosexual dysfunction vs anatomic disease	Psychosomatic exploration – after indicated evaluations as above
Hematuria	Urinary tract infection, urolithiasis, urinary tract neoplasm	Culture Microscopy Cystoscopy Intravenous urogram, urological consultation
Hematochezia	Chronic inflammatory, bowel disease, diverticulitis, bowel neoplasm	Rectosigmoidoscopy, colonoscopy, barium enema, serial stool samples for blood, microscopy for ova, parasites, culture as needed, gastroenterological consultation

Laparoscopy Versus Laparotomy

Diagnostic laparoscopy is a logical end point in the workup of the patient with infertility and/or pelvic pain. With the improved availability of special instruments and more reproductive surgeons acquiring the technique, operative laparoscopy is increasingly used as an opportunity to initiate surgical treatment.

In this light, laparotomy has almost become a second-line intervention. However, certain situations still make it advisable to prefer laparotomy over the endoscopic approach. Lesions involving the bladder, the bowel, or the peritoneum overlying the ureter or pelvic vessels require extensive experience if they are to be treated laparoscopically (Reich et al. 1991; Nezhat et al. 1992a; Nezhat and Nezhat 1993; Donnez et al. 1995). If difficult endoscopic procedures are not performed routinely, an increase in surgery time and complication rate will result (Smith et al. 1994). A second concern is the opening of a malignant ovarian tumor mistaken for an endometrioma, which may lead to spillage of malignant cells and possibly a deterioration in these patients' prognosis (Sainz de la Cuesta et al. 1994).

An aspect that makes laparoscopy particularly useful in reproductive surgery is the fact that it does not appear to induce de novo adhesion formation to a significant degree. Whereas 51% of patients undergoing open reproductive pelvic surgery showed adhesions in sites not previously affected (Diamond et al. 1987), a similar study showed only 11.8% formation of new adhesions after operative laparoscopy (Operative Laparoscopy Study Group 1991). Only one new adhesion was found at the site of an operative laparoscopic procedure and adhesion scores were significantly reduced at second-look laparoscopy. However, reformation, particularly of dense and cohesive adhesions, was observed in almost all patients (97.1%). Canis and associates (1992) observed a significant decrease in periovarian adhesions at second-look laparoscopy after laparoscopic treatment of large ovarian endometriomas only in patients with initially high adhesion scores.

Two studies proposed treating endometriosis at laparoscopy for IVF egg retrieval (Damewood and Rock 1988) and for GIFT (Corson et al. 1991) in an attempt to increase the chances of conception. The former study reports a 28% pregnancy rate (out of 39 patients) in the 10 months following treatment and the latter showed a trend towards higher success rates of the respective treatment cycle, although this was not significant (77 patients treated).

The approach during a surgical procedure is dependent on several factors to give the best result to the patient while minimizing recovery time and time away from work. First, surgical skill is the cornerstone of a successful procedure, as well as the availability of instrumentation and an organized surgical/anesthesia team. Secondly, good judgement is imperative in making the decision regarding laparoscopy versus laparotomy since every case may present complicating factors which increase the skill level needed to complete the planned surgery. While economic factors are not a primary driving force, they should be part of considerations when plans are developed to provide the optimal level of surgical care. Table 4 summarizes the advantages and disadvantages of the two surgical approaches.

Table 4 Advantages and disadvantages of laparoscopy and laparotomy

	Operative video – laparoscopy	Laparotomy and microsurgery
Equipment cost	200 000 $	100 000 $
Special training	Required	Required
Optimal surgical exposure	Difficult at times	Possible in most instances
Palpation of tissue	Indirect	Direct
Induction of new adhesions	Rare	Frequent
Overnight hospital admission	Not necessary	Necessary
Recovery time	3–5 days	5–8 days

Laser Laparoscopy

The development of laser instruments that can be used through the laparoscope has both simplified existing procedures and opened a range of new possibilities in endoscopic reproductive surgery. While monthly fecundity rates in mild and moderate endometriosis are at the same level as expectant management, medical therapy, and conservative surgery, a significant advantage of laser therapy over these conventional approaches consists in a shorter treatment to pregnancy interval in mild to moderate disease (Fig. 1) and a greatly increased monthly fecundity rate in severe cases (Table 5) (Tulandi et al. 1987; Olive and Martin 1987; Adamson et al. 1988). Although the assessment of "pain relief" using pain scoring on a subjective scale is difficult, and different methods of evaluation have been employed, both laparotomy and laparoscopy seem to be effective. Not surprisingly, success rates decrease with disease severity (Candiani et al. 1986; Davis 1986).

The physical properties of the CO_2 laser (continuous wave, 30 W) allow a controlled destruction of superficial endometriosis implants by vaporization without endangering underlying structures. Tissue destruction (and char formation) can be lessened with the use of the ultrapulse or the swift mode of the CO_2 laser. By having a brief controlled interruption of the laser pulse (ultrapulse) or a permanent rapid movement of the laser beam (swift), there is a decreased depth of penetration, thus minimizing potential for inadvertent injury. However, the CO_2 laser's property of limited tissue penetration necessitates the simultaneous use of electrocautery, argon, or KTP lasers to coagulate major vessels and to cut tissue. Nezhat and Nezhat (1989) have suggested the subperitoneal injection of water to protect underlying structures during laser vaporization. If electrocautery is used, it must be kept in mind that the area of eventual coagulation extends beyond the visible thermal injury for

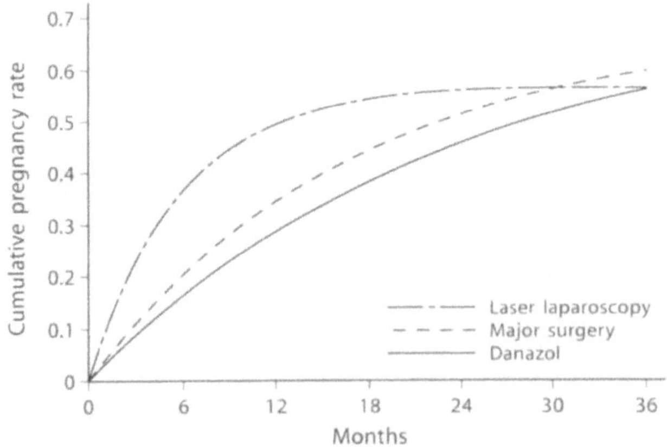

Fig. 1. Comparative cumulative pregnancy curves using the two-parameter exponential model for stage I and II endometriosis patients with no other infertility factors. Data for danazol and major surgery are from Guzick and Rock (1981)

Table 5 Comparison of **a** conservative laparotomy (LAP) and **b** laser laparoscopy (LAS) for the treatment of endometriosis
Table 5 a:

Author	Treatment	Stage	No.	Pregnancy rate (months of follow-up)	Monthly fecundity rate	Pain relief, reoperation rates
Hammond et al. 1976	LAP	Mild[a]	3	66%	n.r.	0 reoperations
		Moderate	7	60%		29% reoperations
		Severe	2	0 (12–144, avg. 35)		50% reoperations
Buttram 1979	LAP	Mild[b]	56	73.2% (15)	n.r.	n.r.
		Moderate	34	55.9% (15)		
		Severe	47	40.4% (15)		
Rock et al. 1981	LAP	Mild[b]	43	67%	2.73%	Overall:
		Moderate	71	49%	1.73%	13.5% reoperations,
		Severe	100	51%	1.57%	30.4% recurrence
Malinak and Wheeler 1985	LAP	Mild[a]	136	57%, 81%[d]		Overall reoperation rate: 13% at 3 years, 32% at 5 years, recurrence at reoperation: 66%
		Moderate	69	54%, 87%[d]		
		Severe	172	36%, 65%[d]		
Candiani et al. 1986	LAP					*Incidence of:* (*preop*≥postop)
		AFS I	23	65.2% (12–72)	n.r.	Dysmenorrhea: 51.4%≥14.3% Dyspareunia: 25.7%≥17.1% Chronic pelvic pain: 4.3%≥11.4%
		AFS II	22	50%		Dysmenorrhea: 69.2%≥15.4% Dyspareunia: 36.5%≥17.3% Chronic pelvic pain: 40%≥13.3%
		AFS III	8	37.5%		Dysmenorrhea: 73.3%≥20% Dyspareunia: 53.3%≥46.7% Chronic pelvic pain: 40%≥13.3%
Singhal et al. 1991	LAP	Mild[c]	16	56% (max. 86)		
		Moderate	10	50%		
		Severe	14	14%		

Table 5 b:

Author	Treatment	Stage	No.	Pregnancy rate (months of follow-up)	Monthly fecundity rate	Pain relief
Nezhat et al. 1986	LAS	AFS I	24	75.1% (18)	n.r.	n.r.
		AFS II	51	62.7%		
		AFS III	19	42.1%		
		AFS IV	8	50.0%		
Davis 1986	LAS					*Patients improved:*
		AFS I–II	31	64.5% (15)		Dysmenorrhea: 90%
						Dyspareunia: 97%
		AFS III	26	57.7%		Dysmenorrhea: 93%
						Dyspareunia: 97%
		AFS IV	7	28.8%		Dysmenorrhea: 95%
						Dyspareunia: 77%
Keye et al. 1987	LAS	AFS I	41	38%		*All patients with pain*
						(Score 0–10): Preop≥postop
		AFS II	10	30%	Average: 2.5%	Dysmenorrhea 8.6≥4.5
						Dyspareunia 6.8≥2.3
		AFS III	5	20%		General pelvic pain 6.8≥2.7
Donnez 1987	LAS	AFS I	42	62% (18)	n.r.	nr.
		AFS II	21	52%		
		AFS III	7	42%		
				includes pts. with additional facotrs	Endometriosis only, laser only	
Olive and Martin 1987	LAS	AFS I	15	39.0%	4.69%	n.r.
		AFS II	8	45.8%	2.13%	
		AFS III	6	50,0%	6.06%	
Gast et al. 1988	LAS	AFS I	122 overall	61%	n.r.	n.r.
		AFS II		47%		
		AFS III		54%		
				(Avg. 10.6, range 2–32), most pts. with additional, corrected factors		
Adamson et al. 1988	LAS		64 overall	Total: 37.5%	6.7%	n.r.
Sutton and Hill 1990	LAS	AFS I	16	94% (12–72)	n.r.	Overall: 70% of pts. pain free or markedly improved, 13.5% relapsed
		AFS II	25	68%		
		AFS III	13	85%		
		AFS IV	2	100%		

pts, patients; n.r., not reported; [a] Acosta classification (Acosta et al. 1973); [b] Buttram classification (Buttram et al. 1977); [c] Classification not specified; [d] Predicted pregnancy rate at 10 years, based on life-table analysis unipolar coagulation. In our experience, contact neodymium-YAG lasers are not advantageous over electrocautery in removing endometriosis implants; nontouch Nd-YAG laser technique may lead to inadvertent deep tissue destruction. For further technical details see Bastert and Wallwiener (1992).

Nezhat et al. (1990) performed second-look laparoscopies after a procedure termed videolaseroscopy and did not find any *de novo* adhesion formation. In a similar study, Sutton (1991) found no recurrence of implants at sites that had previously been lasered, although 18 of 33 patients had a recurrence at different sites. Compared to electrocautery at laparoscopy, lasers are more precise and easier to handle (Sutton 1993); pregnancy rates appear to be in the same order of magnitude.

Removal of Implants and Adhesions

After having diagnosed endometriosis and decided to proceed surgically, the first step is the removal of all amenable implants. Careful examination of the pelvic surface should be performed and lesions noted. An organized approach going over each anatomic structure or area allows for completeness in therapy. By proceeding in this way, there should be minimal confusion between actual areas of disease and petechial spots that occur with tissue manipulation. Nonpigmented lesions might represent more active disease than classical black "powder-burn" implants (Vernon et al. 1986) and should be treated just as vigorously. Cook and Rock (1991) conclude in an extensive review of the literature regarding laparoscopic treatment of endometriosis that "it does not matter how the endometriosis is ablated. The critical issue is the ability of the surgeon to correctly identify endometriosis with its wide range of appearances and to utilize the various treatment modalities correctly to fully treat the disease". If a laparoscopic approach is chosen, this means that at least one additional puncture is needed in order to inspect the pelvic sidewalls underneath the ovaries; most surgeons prefer to operate with three or more puncture sites.

Jansen and Russell (1986) found histological features of endometriosis in two of four subovarian adhesions, which underlines the importance of excising the entire adhesion. However, the high recurrence rate of adhesions, particularly those involving two entire serosal surfaces, has been discussed above. This fact should be weighed against the risks of a dissection, especially if bowel serosa is involved.

Adhesion Prevention

Numerous pharmacological regimens have been proposed to decrease adhesion (re-)formation. Whereas systemic hydrocortisone might be of some value (Jansen 1985), the use of intraperitoneal instillation of dextran or corticosteroids is no longer recommended for localized incisions of the uterus or ovaries. A very promising development is surgical barriers consisting either of oxidized regenerated cellulose (Interceed, Johnson & Johnson) or polytetrafluoroethylene (Gore-Tex, W.L. Gore Co.). All attempts to close peritoneal defects left after surgical ablation of endometriosis either by sutures or by grafts seem to do more harm than good. Spontaneous reepithelization is achieved within several days by the proliferation of little clusters of mesothelial cells on the wound surface rather than from its margins (diZerega 1994). In fact, Nezhat and associates (1990) did not observe any de novo adhesion formation after laser treatment, although denuded peritoneal areas were left to heal without adaptation. Dextran may have value in the prevention of adhesions that are present across several organs. For this type of adhesion, however, it is difficult to prevent some recurrence.

A different approach to adhesion prevention after extensive ablative procedure is to keep ovaries and fallopian tubes from adhering to these structures by means of mechanical suspension. The proximity of the operated organs to each other and the bowel may lead to adhesion formation. These techniques are more frequently performed in America than in Europe. There are three common ways that, although developed at laparotomy, can also be used at laparoscopy:

1. The round ligament may be reduplicated to increase the forward tension on the uterus. This reduplication may be performed with a suture or an endoloop.
2. The round ligaments can be attached to the anterior rectus sheath (Olshausen technique). At laparoscopy, this can be accomplished by suture with intracorporeal stitch or by introducing a Babcock through a lower port (incision) and elevating the round ligament through the incision, fixing it to the rectus sheath.
3. Reduction of the length of the round ligament by the Gilliam technique, where the round ligaments are grasped with an instrument and brought through an aperture in the peritoneum near the internal inguinal ring; this brings each ligament beneath the anterior rectus sheath, where it is fixed with absorbable suture.

Round ligament pain may occur with these procedures but they have not been found to be detrimental to pregnancy. The Olshausen technique may fix the uterus too much to be used if pregnancy is contemplated as it would not allow free uterine growth (Thompson and Rock 1992).

Table 6 provides an overview of the current methods of adhesion prevention.

Table 6 Adhesion prevention: an overview

Drugs	Systemic hydrocortisone (Dextran)
Barriers	Interceed Gore-Tex (lyophilized dura)
Surgical steps	Shortening or fixation of the round ligaments

Removal of Ovarian Endometriomas

Endometriotic cysts of the ovary are thought to develop when comparatively small endometriotic implants on the ovarian surface are invaginated by the mesothelial lining of the ovary (Hughesdon 1957). This hypothesis provides a good explanation for the fact that even large chocolate cysts often contain very little, mostly degenerated, endometriotic tissue when examined morphologically and that their cyst wall is essentially composed of fibrotic tissue (Clement 1987). It furthermore explains their clinical behavior, i.e., relative resistance to hormonal treatment. Larger endometriomas typically cause midcycle adnexal pain or general abdominal discomfort. These observations, together with the necessity of obtaining a biopsy from any adnexal mass that does not dissolve spontaneously or with a short course of exogenous steroids, make surgical intervention the treatment of choice. The influence of ovarian endometriomas on infertility, however, has recently been questioned by Ishimaru and co-workers (1994), who could not detect any difference in biochemical parameters of the peritoneal fluid or the pregnancy rate in endometriosis patients with and without chocolate cysts after treatment with danazol.

In patients with ovarian cysts, a preoperative ultrasound examination is of prime importance. Size of the ovaries, number of cysts, thickness of the cyst wall, and echogenicity of cyst contents should be described. The report should also include a statement regarding the possibility of malignancy. Benign cysts are most likely not to have more than three compartments, smooth cyst walls, no echogenicity, no solid structures and are often unilateral (Mettler et al. 1993). In all patients with ovarian cysts, the serum Ca 12-5 level should be assayed and a malignancy suspected when this is above 200 IU/ml (Kindermann, personal communication).

Smaller endometriomas that are particularly suitable for laparoscopic treatment may not be obvious at first (Candiani et al. 1990), which underlines the importance of diligent mobilization of the ovaries and puncture if they appear enlarged at laparoscopy. In a group of 52 patients with endometriomas, 40 were diagnosed at ultrasound examination, ten after ovarian mobilization and seven after needling the ovary (Wood et al. 1992).

The description of the anatomy of ovarian endometriomas by Hughesdon (1957) (Fig. 2) explains why, in order to decrease recurrence rates, it is necessary to remove the cyst wall by stripping or destroy it by coagulation or vaporization, rather than simply aspirate its contents (Reich and McGlynn 1986; Corson et al. 1988; Hasson 1990). After aspiration, the cyst is opened at a dependent site and the interior of the cyst wall carefully examined. Care also has to be taken to ensure that all contents which may spill into the peritoneal cavity are irrigated with large amounts of lactated Ringer's solution. Bruhat and co-workers (1991) have proposed five criteria to distinguish organic from functional ovarian cysts (Table 7). At this time, a biopsy is taken. Once the cyst wall has been removed or destroyed *in sano*, and hemostasis is achieved by coagulation, the edges are approximated, but sutures are avoided (Martin 1991). The ovarian wound surface can be left open or closed with su-

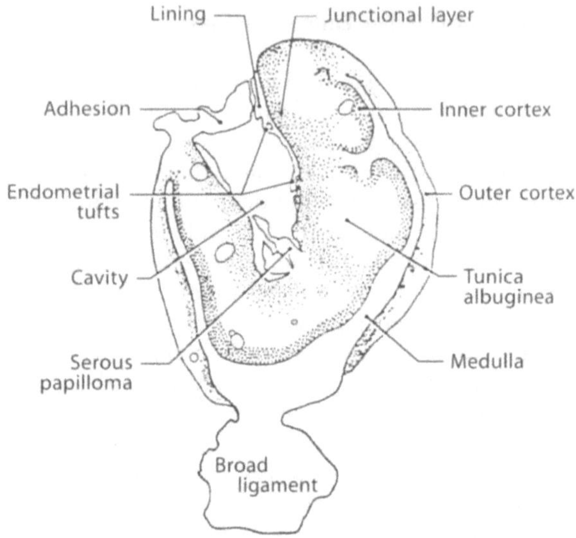

Fig. 2. Schematized diagram of an ovarian endometrioma. (From Hughesdon 1957)

Table 7 Laparoscopic criteria for differentiation between organic and functional ovarian cysts. (From Bruhat et al. 1991)

Criterion	Organic cysts	Functional cysts
Utero-ovarian ligament	Lengthened	Normal
Cyst wall	Thick	Thin
Ovarian vessels	Numerous and regular, starting from the mesovarium	More scanty, coral-like
Cyst fluid	Clear, dark, brown, or dermoid	Saffron yellow
Internal cyst wall appearance	Smooth	Retina-like aspect

Table 8 Success rates of surgical removal of ovarian endometriomas

Author	Method	No.	Recurrence rate	Pregnancies	Pain relief
Reich and McGlynn 1986	Electrocoagulation	23	5	17 in 15 women	
Kojima et al. 1990	Neodymium-YAG laser	30	1	6/16	13/14
Marrs 1991	KTP laser laparoscopy	31	1/31	7/23	
Daniell et al. 1992	CO_2, KTP, and argon laser laparoscopy	47		12/32	
Wood et al. 1992	Laparotomy	27	2	Overall: 26	Overall: 50 of 52 at 1 year
	Laparoscopy (excision, electrocautery, CO_2 laser)	25	3		
Bateman et al. 1994	CO_2 laser				At 1 year:
	Laparotomy	21	19%	46.6%	11/13
	Laparoscopy	36	11%	42%	23/25

tures or fibrin glue. Experience from current suture and adhesion prevention measures suggests that closure will result in more adhesions (Bateman 1994). Adhesion prevention barriers of Interceed or Goretex can be used depending on where one hopes to prevent adhesion formation or reformation. A different approach is to grasp the cyst wall and remove it in a corkscrew-like fashion. Lastly, the cyst wall can be grasped, and, with countertraction from another instrument, hydrodissection can help to remove the capsule completely (Nezhat 1981; Nezhat et al. 1991, 1992a). Some of the published success rates are summarized in Table 8.

Surgical Procedures for Pain Relief

Several procedures have been described that are specifically aimed at the surgical therapy of severe dysmenorrhea and central pelvic pain refractory to medical treatment. The most extensive is presacral neurectomy as described by Cotte (1937, 1949). All operations have in common that they are indicated only in cases of central pelvic pain, and proper patient selection is crucial for their success.

The classical presacral neurectomy must be performed with good visualization and care. One severe complication of damage to the sacral vessels can be avoided and the chance for success maximized. An incision is made in the posterior peritoneal surface after the descending colon has been mobilized to the left side of the abdomen, exposing the hollow of the sacrum. Entry into the peritoneum is made above the iliac vessels with care not to injure them. The peritoneal surface is held and the retroperitoneal tissues are carefully dissected away from the posterior peritoneum. As this is performed, the retroperitoneal tissue may be teased from the area overlying the sacrum. White nerve fibers may be visualized among the fatty retroperitoneal tissue. Kitner clamps with a firm gauze tip may be used to separate the tissues. Hemaclips or suture can be used to secure the ends of the plexus before cutting to remove. Success appears to be dependent on removing nerve fibers which can be seen on pathologic evaluation. The peritoneum can be closed once sufficient tissue between the ureters has been removed. Closure of the abdomen would be in a standard fashion.

Patients with midline dysmenorrhea respond well to presacral neurectomy performed at laparotomy. Success was reported by Tjaden et al. (1990) in 15 of 17 patients after 42 months' follow-up.

Since this approach traditionally required laparotomy, alternatives have been devised. The first endoscopic procedure to relieve pain was laparoscopic uterine nerve ablation (LUNA; Lichten and Bombard 1987). Interruption of uterine autonomous innervation was achieved by electrocoagulation of the uterosacral ligaments with a bipolar forceps. In a randomized, prospective, double-blind study on women without demonstrable somatic or psychiatric disease, these authors compared pain relief after LUNA and after diagnostic laparoscopy. Five of 11 patients who had undergone this procedure reported relief from dysmenorrhea at 1 year of follow-up compared to none in the group with diagnostic laparoscopy only. No complications or side-effects were observed.

Recently, successful methods for laparoscopic presacral neurectomy have been reported (Perez 1990; Nezhat and Nezhat 1992b). While Perez described a method that employed visualization of the presacral nerve through a laparoscope inserted suprapubically, Nezhat and Nezhat used the standard subumbilical trocar. In the group of 25 patients with endometriosis studied by Perez, the mean pain score on a scale from 0 to 10 dropped from 8.71 preoperatively to 2.21 after at least 6 months' follow-up. One patient had to undergo laparotomy for retroperitoneal hemorrhage. Nezhat and Nezhat observed complete pain relief in half of their patients with 92% of patients reporting some relief.

Combination of Medical and Surgical Therapy

Several combinations of medical and surgical therapy of endometriosis have been proposed. Preoperative medical therapy is aimed at reducing the extent of surgery, whereas postoperative ovarian suppression is thought by some authors to reduce recurrence rates. The classical three-step therapy consists of laparoscopic diagnosis and biopsy, followed by 6 months of ovarian suppression, and definitive surgical removal of all accessible lesions at re-laparoscopy immediately subsequent to the suppression therapy (Mettler 1991).

However, considerable disagreement exists concerning the rationale of these regimens (Thomas 1992). One comparative study failed to show a significant advantage of a combined over either medical or surgical therapy alone (Chong et al. 1990). A recent prospective randomized trial in women with severe disease suggested that ovarian suppression with a GnRH agonist after laparotomy was not beneficial with respect to either pain relief or fertility (Parazzini et al. 1994). In the infertile patient, it should be kept in mind that pregnancy rates are highest in the months immediately following an operation (Buttram 1979).

On an individual basis, preoperative ovarian suppression may stabilize a patient who is distressed by pain or hematologically relevant hypermenorrhea. Similarly, careful assessment of the risks involving removal of endometriomas involving delicate structures such as the bowel or ureter may occasionally lead to a decision in favor of postoperative suppression therapy over a radical surgical step.

Summary and Conclusions

The choice of the appropriate therapeutic method for the endometriosis patient depends on the presenting complaints. This may be infertility, pelvic pain, an adnexal mass, or a combination of these. A prerequisite for the treatment of all three problems is a laparoscopic confirmation of the correct diagnosis, preferably including a biopsy. Preoperative ultrasound and determination of the serum Ca 12-5 level are helpful in avoiding inadvertent puncture of a malignant cyst. If values above 200 IU/ml are found, malignancy should be suspected. In patients with bladder or bowel symptoms, cystoscopy or rectoscopy, respectively, is recommended.

Superficial endometriosis implants in the posterior cul-de-sac or on the bladder dome are amenable to electrocautery or laser vaporization. Endometriosis of the fallopian tube wall with its typical appearance of alternating stenoses and dilatations (resembling a pearl necklace) cannot be treated laparoscopically. The same is true for the related clinical entity of *adenomyosis uteri interna*. If ovarian endometriomas with diameters exceeding 1 cm are present, primary cystectomy as described above is advisable since these forms of endometriosis are highly resistant to medical treatments. If extensive disease of the peritoneal cavity is found and an acutely inflammatory aspect prevails, laparoscopic intervention is postponed and a three-step therapy initiated. This means that, after proving the diagnosis (step 1), 6 months of medical therapy is administered, e.g., GnRH analogues (step 2), followed by a re-laparoscopy with removal of all remaining implants. The three-step therapy is also an option in cases where a primary operative laparoscopic treatment is not possible.

Whether or not infertility patients with minimal or mild disease should receive a course of medical therapy after complete laparoscopic removal of all visible implants is still a matter of debate. Here, a comprehensive approach including the treatment of other factors impairing the fertility of the couple is a promising alternative.

If extensive and symptomatic disease of the rectovaginal septum is found, a combined laparoscopic and vaginal approach is preferable. After determining the exact localization, laparotomy and resection of the implants will be necessary in many cases. The patient should be informed that the operation may include bowel surgery and an abdominal surgeon should be available at the time of surgery.

References

Adamson CD, Lu J, Subak LL (1988) Laparoscopic CO_2 laser vaporization of endometriosis compared with traditional treatments. Fertil Steril 50/5:704–710

Adamson GD, Pasta DJ (1994) Surgical treatment of endometriosis-associated infertility: Meta-analysis compared with survival analysis. Am J Obstet Gynecol 171:1488–1505

Bateman BG, Kolp LA, Mills S (1994) Endoscopic vs laparotomy management of endometriomas. Fertil Steril 62:690–695

Bastert G, Wallwiener D (1992) Lasers in gynecology – possibilities and limitations. Springer, Berlin Heidelberg New York

Blackwell RE (1991) Applications of laser surgery in gynecology. Surgical Clin North Am 71/5:1005–1023

Brosens IA (1994a) Is mild endometriosis a progressive disease? Hum Reprod 9/12:2209–2211

Brosens IA (1994b) New principles in the management of endometriosis. Acta Obstet Gynecol Scand 159:8–21

Bruhat MA, Mage G, Chapron C, Pouly JL, Canis M, Wattiez A (1991) Present day endoscopic surgery in gynecology. Eur J Obstet Gynecol Reprod Biol 41/1:4–13

Buttram VC Jr (1979) Conservative surgery for endometriosis in the infertile female: a study of 206 patients with implications for both medical and surgical therapy. Fertil Steril 31/2:117–123
Candiani GB, Fedele L, Vercellini P (1986) Conservative surgical treatment of endometriosis. Acta European Fertilitatis 17/3:173–180
Candiani GB, Vercellini P, Fedele L (1990) Laparoscopic ovarian puncture for correct staging of endometriosis. Fertil Steril 53/6:994–997
Candiani GB, Vercellini B, Fedele L, Bianchi S, Vendola N, Candiani M (1991) Conservative surgical treatment for severe endometriosis in infertile women: are we making progress? Obstet Gynecol Surv 46/7(Suppl):490–498
Canis M, Mage G, Wattiez A, Chapron C, Pouly JL, Bassi S (1992) Second-look laparoscopy after laparoscopic cystectomy of large ovarian endometriomas. Fertil Steril 58/3:617–619
Chong AP, Keene ME, Thornton NL (1990) Comparison of three modes of treatment for infertility patients with minimal endometriosis. Fertil Steril 53/3:497–410
Clement PB (1987) Endometriosis, lesions of the secondary Müllerian system and pelvic mesothelial proliferations. In: Kurman RJ (ed) Blaustein's pathology of the female genital tract. Springer, Berlin Heidelberg New York
Cook AS, Rock JA (1991) The role of laparoscopy in the treatment of endometriosis. Fertil Steril 55/4:663–680
Corson SL, Unger M, Kwa D, Batzer FR, Gocial B (1988) Laparoscopic laser treatment of endometriosis with the Nd:YAG sapphire probe. Am J Obstet Gynecol 718–723
Corson SL, Batzer FR, Gocial B, Daly DC, Eisenberg E, Huppert LS, Maislin G (1991) Surgical treatment of endometriosis at the time of gamete intrafallopian transfer. J Reprod Med 36/4:274–278
Cotte G (1937) Resection of the presacral nerve in the treatment of obstinate dysmenorrhea. Am J Obstet Gynecol 33:1034–1040
Cotte G (1949) Technique of presacral neurectomy. Am J Surg 78:50–53
Cramer DW, Walker AM, Schiff I (1979) Statistical methods in evaluating the outcome of infertility therapy. Fertil Steril 32/1:80–86
Crosignani PG, Vercellini P (1994) New clinical guidelines are needed for the treatment of endometriosis. Hum Reprod 9/12:2205–2206
Damewood MD, Rock JA (1988) Treatment independent pregnancy with operative laparoscopy for endometriosis in an in vitro fertilization program. Fertil Steril 50/3:463–465
Daniell JF, Kurtz BR, Gurley LD (1991) Laser laparoscopic management of large endometriomas. Fertil Steril 55/4:692–695
Davis GD (1986) Management of endometriosis and its associated adhesions with the CO_2 laser laparoscope. Obstet Gynecol 68/3:422–425
Dawood (1985) Dysmenorrhea. J Reprod Med 30/3:154–167
DeCherney AH, Kort H, Barner JB et al. (1980) Increased pregnancy rate with oil soluble hysterosalpingography dye. Fertil Steril 33:407
Diamond MP, Daniell JF, Feste J, Surrey MW, McLaughlin DS, Friedman S, Vaughn WK, Martin DC (1987) Adhesion reformation and de novo adhesion formation after reproductive pelvic surgery. Fertil Steril 47/5:864–866
diZerega GS (1994) Contemporary adhesion prevention. Fertil Steril 61/2:219–235
Donnez J (1987) CO_2 laser laparoscopy in infertile women with endometriosis and women with andexal adhesions. Fertil Steril 48/3:390–394
Donnez J, Nisolle M, Casanas-Roux F, Bassil S, Anaf V (1995) Rectovaginal septum, endometriosis or adenomyosis: laparoscopic management in a series of 231 patients. Hum Reprod 10/2:630–635
Evers JLH (1994) Endometriosis does not exist; all women have endometriosis. Hum-Reprod 9/12:2206–2208
Garcia C-R, David SS (1977) Pelvic endometriosis: infertility and pelvic pain. Am J Obstet Gencol 129/7:740–747
Gast MJ, Tobler T, Strickler RC, Odem R, Pineda J (1988) Laser vaporization of endometriosis in an infertile population: the role of complicating infertility factors. Fertil Steril 49/1:32–36
Guzick DS, Rock JA (1981) Estimation of a model of cumulative pregnancy following infertility therapy. Am J Obstet Gynecol 140/5:573–578
Hammond CB, Rock JA, Parker RT (1976) Conservative treatment of endometriosis: the effects of limited surgery and hormonal pseudopregnancy. Fertil Steril 27/7:756–766

Hasson HM (1979) Electrocoagulation of pelvic endometriotic lesions with laparoscopic control. Am J Obstet Gynecol 135/1:115–121
Hasson HM (1990) Laparoscopic management of ovarian cysts. J Reprod Med 35:863–867
Hughesdon PE (1957) The structure of endometrial cysts of the ovary. J Obstet Gynaecol Br Emp 481–487
Hull ME, Moghissi KS, Magyar DF et al. (1987) Comparison of different treatment modalities of endometriosis in infertile women. Fertil Steril 47:40
Ishimaru T, Masuzaki H, Samejima T, Fujishita A, Nakamura K, Yamabe T (1994) Influence of ovarian endometrioma on fertility. Am J Obstet Gynecol 171/2:541–545
Jansen JPS (1985) Failure of intraperitoneal adjuncts to improve the outcome of pelvic operations in young women. Am J Obstet Gynecol 153:363–371
Jansen JPS, Russel P (1986) Nonpigmented endometriosis: clinical, laparoscopic and pathologic definition. Am J Obstet Gynecol 155/6:1154–1159
Jobson VW, Campion MJ (1991) Vaginal laser surgery. Obstet Gynecol Clin North Am 18/3:511–524
Keye WR Jr, Hansen LW, Astin M, Poulson AM (1987) Argon laser therapy of endometriosis: a review of 92 consecutive patients. Fertil Steril 47/2:208–212
Kojima E, Morita M, Otaka K, Yano Y (1990) Nd:Yag laser laparoscopy for ovarian endometriomas. Obstet Gynecol 35/6:592–596
Koninckx PR (1994) Is mild endometriosis a disease? Is mild endometriosis a condition occurring intermittently in all women? Hum Reprod 9/12:2202–2205
Leridon H, Spira A (1984) Problems in measuring the effectiveness of infertility therapy. Fertil Steril 41/4:580–586
Lichten EM, Bombard J (1987) Surgical treatment of primary dysmenorrhea with laparoscopic uterine nerve ablation. J Reprod Med 32/1:37–42
Marrs RP (1991) The use of potassium-titanyl-phosphate laser for laparoscopic removal of ovarian endometrioma. Am J Obstet Gynecol 164/6/1:1622–1628
Martin DC (1991) Laparoscopic treatment of ovarian endometriomas. Clin Obstet Gynecol 34/2:452–459
Mettler L (1991) Medicosurgical treatment of genital endometriosis focusing on gestagens and antigestagens together with surgical pelviscopy. Ann NY Acad Sci 626:341–366
Mettler L, Caesar G, Neunzling S, Semm K (1993) Stellenwert der endoskopischen Ovar-Chirurgie – Kritische Analyse von 626 pelviskopisch operierten Ovarialzysten an der Universitäts-Frauenklinik Kiel 1990–1991. Geburtsh Frauenheilk 53:253–257
Murphy AA, Green WR, Bobbie D, dela Cruz ZC, Rock JA (1986) Unsuspected endometriosis documented by scanning electron microscopy in visually normal peritoneum. Fertil Steril 46/3:522–524
Nezhat C, Nezhat FR (1989) Safe laser endoscopic excision or vaporization of peritoneal endometriosis. Fertil Steril 52/1:149–151
Nezhat F, Nezhat C (1992a) A clinical and histologic classification of endometriomas: implications for a mechanism of pathogenesis. J Reprod Med 37:771
Nezhat C, Nezhat F (1992b) A simplified method of laparoscopic presacral neurectomy for the treatment of central pelvic pain due to endometriosis. Br J Obstet Gynecol 99:659–663
Nezhat CR, Nezhat FR (1993) Laparoscopic segmental bladder resection for endometriosis: a report of two cases. Obstet Gynecol 81/5:882–884
Nezhat C, Crowgey ST, Garrison CP (1986) Surgical treatment of endometriosis via laser laparoscopy. Fertil Steril 45/6:778–783
Nezhat CR, Nezhat FR , Mether DA, Luciano AA (1990) Adhesion reformation after reproductive surgery by videolaseroscopy. Fertil Steril 53/6:1008–1011
Nezhat C, Silfen S, Nezhat F (1991) Surgery for endometriosis. Curr Opin Obstet Gynecol 3:385
Nezhat C, Nezhat F, Pennington E (1992) Laparoscopic treatment of infiltrative rectosigmoid colon and rectovaginal septum endometriosis by the technique of videolaparoscopy and the CO_2 laser. Br J Obstet Gynecol 99:664–667
Nezhat C, Nezhat F, Nezhat C, Seidman DS (1994) Classification of endometriosis. Improving the classification of endometriotic ovarian cysts. Hum Reprod 9/12:2212–2216
Olive DL, Haney AF (1986) Endometriosis-associated infertility: a critical review of therapeutic approaches. Obstet Gynecol Surv 41:538–555

Olive DL, Lee KL (1986) Analysis of sequential treatment protocols for endometriosis-associated infertility. Am J Obstet Gynecol 154:613
Olive DL, Martin DC (1987) Treatment of endometriosis – associated infertility with CO_2 laser laparoscopy: the use of one- and two-parameter exponential models. Fertil Steril 48/1:18–23
Olive DL, Stohs GF, Metzger DA, Franklin RR (1985) Expectant management and hydrotubations in the treatment of endometriosis-associated infertility. Fertil Steril 44/1:35–41
Operative Laparoscopy Study Group (1991) Postoperative adhesion development after operative laparoscopy: evaluation at early second-look procedures. Fertil Steril 55/4:700–704
Parazzini F, Fedele L, Busacca M, Falsetti L, Pellegrini S, Venturini PL, Stella M (1994) Postsurgical medical treatment of advanced endometriosis: results of a randomized clinical trial. Am J Obstet Gynecol 171:1205–1207
Perez JJ (1990) Laparoscopic presacral neurectomy. Results of the 25 cases. J Reprod Med 35/6:625–630
Portuondo JA, Echanojauregui AD, Herran C, Alijarte I (1983) Early conception in partients with untreated mild endometriosis. Fertil Steril 39/1:22–25
Reich H, McGlynn F (1986) Treatment of ovarian endometriomas using laparoscopic surgical techniques. J Reprod Med 31/7:577–584
Reich H, McGlynn F, Salvat J (1991) Laproscopic treatment of cul-de-sac obliteration secondary to retrocervical deep fibrotic endometriosis. J Reprod Med 7:516–522
Rock JA, Guzick DS, Sengos C, Schweditsch M, Sapp KC, Jones HW (1981) The conservative surgical treatment of endometriosis: evaluation of pregnancy success with respect to the extent of disease as categorized using contemporary classification systems. Fertil Steril 35/2:131–137
Sainz de la Cuesta R, Goff B, Fuller Jr AF, Nikrui N, Eichhorn JH, Rice LW (1994) Prognostic importance of intraoperative rupture of malignant ovarian epithelial neoplasms. Obstet Gynec 84/1:17
Schenken RS, Malinak LR (1982) Conservative surgery versus expectant management for the infertile patient with mild endometriosis. Fertil Steril 37/2:183
Seibel MM, Berger MJ, Weinstein FG, Tamor ML (1982) The effectiveness of danazol on subsequent fertility in minimal endometriosis. Fertil Steril 38/5:534–537
Seiler JC, Gidwani G, Ballard L (1986) Laparoscopic cauterization of endometriosis for fertility: a controlled study. Fertil Steril 46/6:1098–1100
Singhal V, Li TC, Cooke ID (1991) An analysis of factors influencing the outcome of 232 consecutive tubal microsurgery cases. Br J Obstet Gynecol 98:628–636
Smith DC, Donohue LR, Waszak SJ (1994) A hospital review of advanced gynecologic endoscopic procedures. Am J Obstet Gynecol 70/6:1635–1642)
Sutton C (1991) Laser laparoscopy in the treatment of endometriosis. In: Thomas E, Rock JA (eds) Modern approaches to endometriosis. Kluwer, Dordrecht
Sutton C (1993) Lasers in infertility. Hum Reprod 8/1:133–146
Sutton C, Hill D (1990) Laser laparoscopy in the treatment of endometriosis. A 5-year study. Br J Obstet Gynecol 97:181–185
Tjaden B, Schlaff WD, Kimball A (1990) The efficacy of presacral neurectomy for the relief of midline dysmenorrhea. Obstet Gynecol 76:89–91
Thomas EJ (1992) Combined medical and surgical treatment for endometriosis: the best of both worlds? Br J Obstet Gynecol 99(Suppl 7):5–8
Thomas EJ (1993) Endometriosis: still an enigma. Br J Obstet Gynecol 100:615–617
Thomas EJ, Cooke ID (1987) Successful treatment of asymptomatic endometriosis: does it benefit infertile women? Br Med J 294:1117–1119
Thompson JD, Rock JA (1992) TeLinde's operative gynecology, 7th edn.
Tulandi T (1986) Salpingo-ovariolysis: a comparison between laser surgery and electrosurgery. Fertil Steril 45:459
Tulandi T (1987) Adhesion reformation after reproductive surgery with and without the carbon dioxide laser. Fertil Steril 47/4:704–706
Vernon MW, Beard JS, Graves K, Wilson EA (1986) Classification of endometriotic implants by morphologic appearance and capacity to synthesize prostaglandin F. Fertil Steril 46:801–806
Wood C, Maher P, Hill D (1992) Diagnosis and surgical management of endometriomas. Aust NZ J Obstet Gynaecol 32/2:161–163

Hyperandrogenism and Insulin Resistance

T. GÜRGAN and H. YARAH

Introduction

The association between hyperandrogenism and insulin resistance in women has been known since 1921 [1]. This so-called Archard-Thiers syndrome has also been referred to as "diabetes of bearded women". Although these original findings were repeatedly observed [2–5], the cause and effect relationship between hyperandrogenism and hyperinsulinemia has not been clearly delineated. The current literature on the pathophysiology of hyperandrogenism-insulin resistance and the clinical implications of this association are reviewed below.

Does Hyperandrogenism Promote an Insulin-Resistant State?

Several observations allow one to argue that hyperandrogenism per se may promote an insulin-resistant state. Progestogens capable of binding to intracellular androgen receptors have been reported to reduce the number of insulin receptors in animal models [6]. Rarely has the treatment of ovarian hyperandrogenism by medical or surgical means resulted in an apparent improvement in carbohydrate economy. The surgical removal of an androgen-secreting ovarian stromal luteoma resulted in the disappearance of the insulin-resistant state [7]. Similarly, treatment of a patient with polycystic ovary syndrome (PCOS) with insulin resistance and acanthosis nigricans with combination oral contraceptives led to not only a reduction in circulating androgen levels but also a reversal of the attendant insulin resistance [8].

It is, however, generally considered unlikely that hyperandrogenism is the primary event in the genesis of insulin resistance in view of the relatively high circulating androgen levels in men, only a minority of whom have insulin resistance [9]. Moreover, chronic exposure of subhuman primates to high circulating levels of androgens was noted not to alter insulin sensitivity as assessed by glucose tolerance testing [10]. Furthermore, lowering androgen levels in hyperandrogenic hyperinsulinemic patients by medical [11–15] or surgical [16, 17] approaches does not seem to alter insulin sensitivity as assessed by glucose tolerance testing, overall insulin requirements, or in vitro indicators of insulin resistance. Therefore, hyperandrogenism per se does not seem to contribute in a meaningful fashion to the initiation and/or maintenance of insulin resistance and hyperinsulinemia.

Does Insulin Stimulate Ovarian Androgen Production?

Insulin is considered to be a co-gonadotropin stimulating ovarian androgen production. Such an effect of insulin may account for the association between hyperinsulinemia and hyperandrogenism. The human ovary is shown to be a site of insulin action [18–20]. High-affinity low-capacity insulin receptors have been shown to be present on both thecal and stromal cells of the human ovary [18–20]. Physiologic or supraphysiologic concentrations of insulin, acting alone or in concert with pituitary gonadotropins, stimulate ovarian androgen production by theca-interstitial cells of porcine [21], murine [22] and human origin [17–19]. Taken together, these observations suggest that when insulin receptors on thecal and stromal cells are activated by insulin, ovarian androgen biosynthesis is enhanced.

Despite the in vitro studies, the in vivo effect of insulin on ovarian androgen biosynthesis needs to be determined. Acute hyperinsulinemia as induced by the euglycemic glucose clamp technique was noted not to stimulate ovarian androgen production [23]. Acute elevations of circulating levels of insulin therefore may not be sufficient to promote ovarian androgen production.

Chronic hyperinsulinemia in various insulin-resistant states is known to be associated with excessive ovarian androgen production. The insulin-resistant states are a perfect clinical model to evaluate this association. Three types of insulin resistance exist: A, B, and C. In type A defects in insulin receptors (point mutations) exist, whereas in type B circulating anti-insulin-receptor antibodies are present. Post-receptor defect is present in type C insulin resistance. Irrespective of the pathophysiologic mechanisms involved, all three syndromes have been associated with severe hyperandrogenism [24, 25]. Taken together, these observations support the proposition that chronic hyperinsulinemia, either by itself or in concert with pituitary gonadotropins, promotes ovarian hyperandrogenism.

The ability of insulin to promote ovarian hyperandrogenism may also involve a central action in the hypothalamic-pituitary axis. Insulin receptors have been shown to be present in the arcuate nucleus [26]; insulin may therefore stimulate hypothalamic gonadotropin-releasing hormone (GnRH) release. Moreover, insulin has been shown to be synergistic with GnRH in the promotion of anterior pituitary luteinizing hormone (LH) release [27].

Diagnosis of Insulin Resistance

Several tests of different sensitivity may be employed to test insulin sensitivity. These include basal fasting serum insulin levels and testing the response to exogenous or endogenous insulin. Administration of insulin to normal subjects causes an increase in the rate of glucose utilization, a decrease in the rate of hepatic glucose production, and a resultant fall in the level of plasma glucose. Patients with insulin resistance have a quantitatively decreased response to exogenous insulin. Insulin-resistant patients also have inappropriately high glucose levels at glucose tolerance testing. The euglycemic clamp technique, although highly sophisticated and thus not appropriate for routine clinical practice, is the most sensitive method to test insulin sensitivity.

The HA-IR AN Syndrome

The HA-IR AN syndrome is a diagnostic category consisting of three components: hyperandrogenism, insulin resistance, and acanthosis nigricans (AN). AN is an epiphenomenon of insulin resistance and hyperinsulinemia. "Acanthosis nigricans" refers to hyperkeratotic hyperpigmented, occasionally verrucous skin lesions located primarily in intertriginous regions. It most commonly develops on the nape of the neck, in the axillae, beneath the breasts, and on the vulva, and occasionally presents in other body folds. Histologically, AN consists of hyperkeratosis, epidermal papillomatosis and hyperpigmentation. Histochemistry has demonstrated the presence of excess quantities of glycosaminoglycans, especially hyaluronic acid, in the papillary dermis of AN. AN, although highly specific, is not a sensitive marker of insulin resistance.

As many as 5% of hyperandrogenic women have the HA-IR AN syndrome [28]. Virtually any cause of IR and hyperinsulinemia may be associated with hyperandrogenism, as previously discussed. In addition to insulin resistance types A, B, and C, some of the PCOS patients may be categorized as having the HA-IR AN syndrome.

PCOS: New Pathophysiologic Insights

Polycystic ovary syndrome, characterized by chronic anovulation and hyperandrogenism, has been one of the most discussed, controversial, and explored areas in reproductive medicine. The association of insulin resistance and hyperinsulinemia in PCOS has added a new dimension in the elucidation of the pathophysiology of this syndrome.

Women with PCOS have significant insulin resistance and hyperinsulinemia [29–32]. Increased basal circulating levels of insulin are correlated directly with circulating androgen levels, namely testosterone and androstanedione but not dehydroepiandrosterone sulfate [33, 34]. Approximately two-thirds of patients with PCOS are obese and obesity per se promotes an insulin-resistant state. Insulin resistance, however, is not confined to obese PCOS patients; it may also occur in lean patients affected by this syndrome [33–35]. Diminished insulin-stimulated glucose utilization has been demonstrated in PCOS patients, independent of body mass [31, 32]. Obesity and PCOS have a synergistic negative effect on insulin sensitivity so that the prevalence of impaired glucose tolerance or non-insulin-dependent diabetes mellitus (NIDDM) in obese women with PCOS approaches 20% [30, 31]. Given a standard glucose tolerance test, lean PCOS patients appear capable of maintaining a seemingly normal glucose absorption pattern indistinguishable from that of normally cycling controls. However, such a compensated euglycemic state is only possible at the expense of heightened pancreatic insulin output.

Decreases in both insulin sensitivity [32, 36] and responsiveness [32] have been reported in patients with PCOS. However, the cellular mechanisms of insulin resistance remain to be elucidated. Insulin resistance in PCOS apparently involves marked defects in the glucose transport system, mainly the GLUT-4 glucose transporter, without significant alterations in receptor dynamics [37]. A significant decrease in adipocyte GLUT-4 content, independent of body mass and in the absence of metabolic derangement of glucose tolerance, has been shown in in vitro studies on adipocytes from PCOS patients [37]. This unique feature distinguishes it from insulin resistance in obesity and NIDDM, where both receptor and post-receptor defects are involved.

Different pathophysiologic mechanisms of development have also been suggested in obese and lean PCOS patients. Tonically elevated circulating LH levels are the prominent feature of lean PCOS patients whereas insulin resistance and secondary hyperinsulinemia are more common in obese patients affected by the syndrome [38].

How Can Insulin Promote Ovarian Androgen Production in the Face of Systemic Insulin Resistance?

If one assumes insulin resistance to be systemic in nature, it is difficult to rationalize the sparing of the ovary, thereby enabling insulin to act at this locus. However, several hypotheses may be postulated to resolve this issue. These include the presence of a unique ovarian insulin receptor and the existence of alternative receptor sites with which insulin could interact effectively.

Tissue-dependent differences in the structure and/or function of the insulin receptor [39–41] may allow insulin to act at the level of the ovary in the face of systemic insulin resistance. Given that the insulin receptor is a single gene product, we need to assume that insulin receptor variants are derived from post-transcriptional or post-translational modifications. Although attractive, this hypothesis needs to be tested with further studies. Insulin effect in an insulin-resistant state may also be mediated through hybrid insulin-insulin like growth factor-1 (IGF-1) receptors (type 1 receptors).

An alternative solution to this dichotomy is the "specificity spill over" phenomenon [42] which recognizes the similarities and cross-reactions between insulin and IGFs. Although insulin and IGFs bind with high affinity to their own receptors, they can also bind with lower affinity to one or more related receptors. Such a cross-reaction may allow supraphysiologic concentrations of insulin to interact with type-1 IGF receptors (spillover). If insulin may cross-react with type-1 IGF receptors, enhancement of ovarian androgen biosynthesis would require (a) that the type-1 IGF receptors do not undergo down-regulation by cross-reacting insulin [43] and (b) accompanying promotion of androgen production [44]. However, it is also important to recognize that, in some patients, resistance to insulin may coexist with resistance to IGFs [45].

Long-term Risks of Insulin Resistance in PCOS

Metabolic disturbances in PCOS women with insulin resistance include glucose intolerance, hyperinsulinemia, high plasma triglycerides, and low high-density lipoprotein cholesterol [29, 46, 47]. Such metabolic derangements constitute an increased risk for cardiovascular disease and NIDDM in the long term. PCOS should therefore be looked upon not only as a condition with chronic anovulation but also as a metabolic syndrome. In a long-term follow-up study, 33 women aged 40–59 years with ovarian histopathology typical of PCOS at wedge resection performed 22–31 years previously were studied [48]. One hundred and thirty-two age-matched references were taken as controls. The prevalence of both hypertension (39% vs 11%) and NIDDM (15% vs 2.3%) was significantly higher in the PCOS patients compared with controls. In another study, a relative risk of 7.4 for developing myocardial infarction was observed in women with PCOS compared to age-matched references [49].

Medical treatment (e.g., GnRH analogues) does not appear to improve the insulin-resistant state or unfavorable metabolic derangements associated with PCOS [11-15]. Dietary restrictions and weight loss are the only known measures to reverse insulin resistance and the metabolic disturbances associated with it. In obese women with PCOS, even partial weight loss may reduce both androgen excess and glucose-stimulated insulin levels [50]. Whether increased physical activity is also helpful needs to be established.

References

1. Archard C, Thiers J (1921) Le virilisme pilaire et son association a l'insuffisance glycolytique (diabete a femmes de barbe). Bull Acad Natl Med (Paris) 86:51
2. Barbieri RL, Ryan KJ (1983) Hyperandrogenism, insulin resistance and acanthosis nigricans syndrome: a common endocrinopathy and distinct pathophysiologic features. Am J Obstet Gynecol 147:90
3. Chang RJ, Geffner ME (1985) Associated non-ovarian problems of polycystic ovarian disease: insulin resistance. Clin Obstet Gynaecol 12:675
4. Poretsky L, Kalin MF (1987) The gonadotropic function of insulin. Endocr Rev 8:132
5. Barbieri RL, Smith S, Ryan KJ (1988) The role of hyperinsulinemia in the pathogenesis of ovarian hyperandrogenism. Fertil Steril 50:197
6. Krauth MC, Schillinger E (1977) Changes in insulin receptor concentration in rat fat cells following treatment with the gestagens clomegestone acetate and cyproterone acetate. Acta Endocrinol (Copenh) 86:667
7. Tuffier B (1914) Le virilisme surrenal. Bull Acad Natl Med (Paris) 71:726

8. Cole C, Kitabchi AE (1978) Remission of insulin resistance with Orthonovum in a patient with polycystic ovarian disease and acanthosis nigricans. Clin Res 26:412A
9. Pederson O, Hjollund E, Lindskov HO (1982) Insulin binding and action on fat cells from young healthy females and males. Am J Physiol 243, 158
10. Billiar RB, Richardson D, Schwartz R, Posner B, Little B (1987) Effect of chronically elevated androgen or estrogen on the glucose tolerance test and insulin response in female rhesus monkeys. Am J Obstet Gynecol 157, 1297
11. Imperato-McGinley J, Peterson RE; Sturla E, Dawood Y, Bar RS (1978) Primary amenorrhea associated with hirsutism, acanthosis nigricans, dermoid cysts of the ovaries, and a new type of insulin resistance. Am J Med 65:389
12. Geffner ME, Kaplan SA, Bersch N, Golde DW, Landaw EM, Chang RJ (1986) Persistence of insulin resistance in polycystic ovarian disease after inhibition of ovarian steroid secretion. Fertil Steril 45:327
13. Shoupe D, Lobo RA (1984) The influence of androgens in insulin resistance. Fertil Steril 41:385
14. Singer F, Bhargava G, Poretsky L Persistent insulin resistance after normalization of androgen levels in a woman with congenital adrenal hyperplasia. J Reprod Med 6:921
15. Dunaif A, Green G, Futterweit W, Dobrjansky A (1990) Suppression of hyperandrogenism does not improve peripheral or hepatic insulin resistance in the polycystic ovary syndrome. J Clin Endocrinol Metab 70:699
16. Annos T, Taymor ML (1981) Ovarian pathology associated with insulin resistance and acanthosis nigricans. Obstet Gynecol 58:662
17. Scully RE, Mark EJ, McNeely BU (1982) Case records of the Massachusetts General Hospital: case no 25-1982. N Engl J Med 306:1537
18. Poretsky L, Smith D, Seibel M, Pazianos A, Moses AC, Flier JS (1984) Specific insulin binding sites in human ovary. J Clin Endocrinol Metab 59:809
19. Poretsky L, Grigorescu F, Seibel M, Moses AC, Flier JS (1985) Distribution and characterization of insulin and insulin-like growth factor-I receptors in normal human ovary. J Clin Endocrinol Metab 61:728
20. Poretsky L, Bhargava G, Kalin MF, Wolf SA (1988) Regulation of insulin receptors in the human ovary: in vitro studies. J Clin Endocrinol Metab 67:774
21. Barbieri RL, Markris A, Ryan KJ (1983) Effects of insulin on steroidogenesis in cultured porcine ovarian theca. Fertil Steril 40:237
22. Hernandez ER, Resnick CE, Holtzclaw WD, Payne DW, Adashi EY (1988) Insulin as a regulator of androgen biosynthesis by cultured rat ovarian cells: cellular mechanism(s) underlying physiologic and pharmacologic hormonal actions. Endocrinology 122:2034
23. Nestler JE, Clore JN, Strauss JF III, Blackard WG (1987) The effects of hyperinsulinemia on serum testosterone, progesterone, dehydroepiandrosterone sulfate, and cortisol levels in normal women and in women with hyperandrogenism, insulin resistance, and acanthosis nigricans. J Clin Endocrinol Metab 64:180
24. Kahn CR, Flier JS, Bar RS et al (1976) The syndromes of insulin resistance and acanthosis nigricans. N Engl J Med 294:739
25. Flier JS, Eastman RC, Minaker KL, Matteson P, Rowe JW (1985) Acanthosis nigricans in obese women with hyperandrogenism. Diabetes 34:101
26. Van Houten M, Posner BI, Kopriwa BM et al (1980) Insulin binding sites localized to nerve terminals in rat median eminence and arcuate nucleus. Science 207:1081
27. Adashi EY, Hsueh AJW, Yen D (1981) Insulin enhancement of luteinizing hormone and follicle-stimulating hormone release by cultured pituitary cells. Endocrinology 108:1441
28. Barbieri RL (1990) Hyperandrogenic disorders. Clin Onstet Gynecol 33:640
29. Burghen GA, Givens JR, Kitabchi AE (1980) Correlation of hyperandrogenism and hyperinsulinism in polycystic ovarian disease. J Clin Endocrinol Metab 50:113
30. Dunaif A, Graf M, Mandeli J, Laumas V, Dobrjansky A (1987) Characterization of groups of hyperandrogenic women with acanthosis nigricans, impaired glucose tolerance and/or hyperinsulinemia. J Clin Endocrinol Metab 65:499
31. Dunaif A, Segal KR, Futterweit W, Dobrjansky A (1989) Profound peripheral insulin resistance, independent of obesity, in the polycystic ovary syndrome. Diabetes 38:1165
32. Dunaif A, Segal KR, Shelley DR, Green G, Dobrjansky A, Licholai T (1992) Evidence for distinctive and intrinsic defects in insulin action in the polycystic ovary syndrome. Diabetes 41:1257

33. Pasquali R, Casimirri F, Venturoli S et al (1983) Insulin resistance in patients with polycystic ovaries: its relationship to body weight and androgen levels. Acta Endocrinol (Copenh) 104:110
34. Chang RJ, Nakamura RM, Judd HL, Kaplan SA (1983) Insulin resistance in nonobese patients with polycystic ovarian disease. J Clin Endocrinol Metab 57:356
35. Jialal I, Reddi NK, Moodley J, Joubert SM (1987) Evidence for insulin resistance in nonobese patients with polycystic ovarian disease. J Clin Endocrinol Metab 64:1066
36. Ciaraldi TP, El-Roeiy A, Madar Z, Reichart D, Olefsky JM, Yen SSC (1992) Cellular mechanisms of insulin resistance in polycystic ovarian syndrome. J. Clin Endocrinol Metab 75:577
37. Rosenbaum D, Haber RS; Dunaif A (1993) Insulin resistance in polycystic ovary syndrome: decreased expression of GLUT-4 glucose transporters in adipocytes. Am J Physiol (Endocrinol Metab 27):E197
38. Insler V, Shoham Z, Barash A, Koistinen R, Seppala M, Hen M, Lunenfeld B, Zadik Z (1993) Polycystic ovaries in non-obese and obese patients: possible pathophysiological mechanisms based on new interpretation of facts and findings. Hum Reprod 8:379
39. Heidenreich KA; Brandenburg D (1986) Oligosaccharide heterogeneity of insulin receptors: comparison of N-linked glycosylation of insulin receptors in adipocytes and brain. Endocrinology 118:1835
40. Lowe W Jr, Le Roith D (1986) Insulin receptors from guinea pig liver and brain: structural and functional studies. Endocrinology 118:1669
41. Swanson ML, Dudley DT, Walker PS, Boyle TR, Pessin JE (1988) Functional differences in insulin receptors in rat adipocyte and human placental membranes. Endocrinology 122:967
42. Fradkin JE, Eastman RC, Lesniak MA, Roth J (1989) Specificity spillover at the hormone receptor; exploring its role in human disease. N Engl J Med 320:640
43. Poretsky L, Glover B, Laumas V, Kalin M, Dunaif A (1988) The effects of experimental hyperinsulinemia on steroid secretion, ovarian (^{125}I) insulin binding, and ovarian (^{125}I) insulin-like growth factor I binding in the rat. Endocrinology 122:581
44. Hernandez ER, Resnick CE, Svoboda ME, Van Wyk JJ, Payne DW; Adashi EY (1988) Somatomedin-C/insulin-like growth factor I as an enhancer of androgen biosynthesis by cultured rat ovarian cells. Endocrinology 122:1603
45. Massague J, Freidenberg GF, Olefsky JM, Czech MP (1983) Parallel decreases in the expression of receptors for insulin and insulin-like growth factor I in a mutant human fibroblast line. Diabetes 32:541
46. Mattson LA, Cullberg G, Hamberger L, Samsioe G, Silferstope G (1984) Lipid metabolism in women with polycystic ovary syndrome: possible implications for an increased risk of coronary heart disease. Fertil Steril 42:579
47. Rebuffe-Scrive M, Cullberg G, Lundberg PA, Lindstedt G, Bjorntorp P (1989) Anthropometric variables and metabolism in polycystic ovarian disease. Hormone Metab Research 21:391
48. Dahlgren E, Johansson S, Lindstedt G, Knutsson F, Oden A, Janson PO, Mattson LA, Crona N, Lundberg PA (1992) Women with polycystic ovary syndrome wedge resected in 1956 to 1965: a long-term follow-up focusing on natural history and circulating hormones. Fertil Steril 57:505
49. Dahlgren E, Janson PO, Johansson S, Lapidus L, Oden A (1992) Polycystic ovary syndrome and risk for myocardial infarction. Acta Obstet Gynecol Scand 71:599
50. Pasquali R, Antenucci D, Casimirri F, Venturoli S, Paradisi R, Fabbri R et al. (1989) Clinical and hormonal characteristics of obese amenorrheic women before and after weight loss. J Clin Endocrinol Metab 68:173

Gonadotropin Releasing Hormone Treatment

A. Helvacioglu

Introduction

Normal Physiology of Gonadotropin Releasing Hormone (GnRH) Secretion

Gonadotropin releasing hormone is produced by cells in the medial-basal hypothalamus and delivered to the portal circulation via the GnRH-tuberoinfundibular tract. The arcuate nucleus is the central site of action, releasing GnRH into the portal circulation in a pulsatile fashion. Normal gonadotropin secretion requires pulsatile GnRH discharge within a critical range in frequency and amplitude (Knobil 1980). This critical range of GnRH pulsatile secretion is rather narrow, and increased GnRH pulse frequency or dose will eliminate gonadotropin secretion. Decreasing the pulse frequency decreases luteinizing hormone (LH) secretion but increases follicle stimulating hormone (FSH) secretion. Elegant studies by Filicori showed that GnRH pulse frequencies were at every 94, 71, 103, and 216 min in the early follicular, late follicular, early luteal, and late luteal phases of the menstrual cycle (Filicori et al. 1986) respectively. GnRH secretion is regulated by norepinephrine (facilitory) and dopamine (inhibitory). In turn, the catecholamine system can be influenced by endorphins. Furthermore, serotonin and melatonin are also instrumental in this regulation. Since GnRH neurons lack estrogen receptors, estrogen control of GnRH secretion is modulated through neurotransmitters.

Synthetic GnRH and Its Analogs

The hypothalamic decapeptide GnRH was first isolated, characterized, and synthesized in 1971 by Amoss et al. and Schally et al. Its half-life is 2–4 min (Fig. 1). Rapid cleavage of the bonds between amino acids (6–7, 7–8, and 9–10) leads to its rapid metabolism. Substitution of amino acids at the 6- and 10 positions strengthens the bonds, leading to longer half-lives. These amino acid-substituted new synthetic analogs display increased receptor binding and prolonged receptor occupation, resulting in downregulation of receptors. Initial stimulation of gonadotropins during the first few weeks of treatment is called the “flare-up” effect and it is followed by a downregulation and desensitization of the pituitary, leading to hypogonadism. GnRH analogs are destroyed when taken by mouth and must be used parenterally or sprayed through the nasal mucosa. Currently, intramuscular (i.m.) administered depot (long-acting) and daily (short-acting) forms of leuprolide acetate, subcu-

Native GnRH-Decapeptide:

N-TERMINAL								C-TERMINAL	
PYR	HIS	TRP	SER	TYR	**GLY**	LEU	ARG	PRO	GLY --- NH2
1	2	3	4	5	**6**	7	8	9	10

GnRH Agonist-Decapeptide:

N-TERMINAL								C-TERMINAL	
PYR	HIS	TRP	SER	TYR	**D-TRP**	LEU	ARG	PRO	GLY --- NH2
1	2	3	4	5	**6**	7	8	9	10

Goserelin (Zoladex^{TM}):

N-TERMINAL								C-TERMINAL	
PYR	HIS	TRP	SER	TYR	**D-SER (BU^{t})**	LEU	ARG	PRO	**AZA-GLY** --- NH2
1	2	3	4	5	**6**	7	8	9	**10**

Nafareline (Synarel^{TM}):

N-TERMINAL								C-TERMINAL	
PYR	HIS	TRP	SER	TYR	**D-NAL (2)**	LEU	ARG	PRO	GLY --- NH2
1	2	3	4	5	**6**	7	8	9	10

GnRH Agonist-Nonapeptide:
Leuprolide (Lupron^{TM})

N-TERMINAL								C-TERMINAL
PYR	HIS	TRP	SER	TYR	**D-LEU**	LEU	ARG	PRO-EA
1	2	3	4	5	**6**	7	8	9

GnRH Antagonists-Decapeptide:

N-TERMINAL								C-TERMINAL	
X	X	X	SER	TYR	**X**	LEU	ARG	PRO	X --- NH2
1	2	3	4	5	**6**	7	8	9	10

Fig. 1. GnRH, its analogs and antagonists. The highly potent analogs all share a similar N-terminal sequence, which is identical with the GnRH 1–5 pentapeptide. Substitution of amino acids at the 6 and 10 positions increases the receptor affinity of these peptides and enhances their resistance to peptidases (analog). However, amino acid subsitutions in positions 1–3 result in antagonistic activiy. Further substitutions at 6 and 10 enhance this antagonistic potency; X denotes amino acid subsitutions

taneously (s. c.) administered sustained release pellets, goserelin acetate and the nasal spray form of nafareline acetate are the available preparations for clinical use in the United States. GnRH analogs induce a hypoestrogenic state that is comparable to oophorectomy. During suppression, serum concentrations of estradiol, FSH, LH, and progesterone decrease significantly, serum testosterone decreases slightly, and serum prolactin concentrations are not affected. Amenorrhea occurs in all patients 1–2 months after the start of treatment and menses return 57–102 days after the last depot injection (Helvacioglu et al. 1993).

Subsitution of amino acids in position 1, 2, 3, 6, or 10 results in an antagonistic analog. Since the new synthetic peptides are very different from the native decapeptide, receptor occupation leads to an immediate antagonistic response, resulting in hypogonadism. However, antagonists are not widely used in the current clinical practice due to their side-effects (histamine release) and poor potency. Recently, new potent and safer third-generation GnRH antagonists have become available for research use. Cetrorelix (SB-75; [Ac-D-Nal(2)^{1}, D-Phe(4Cl)“, D-Pal(3)^{3}, D-Cit^{6}, D-Ala10] GnRH) is one of these third generation antagonists and has been promising in research to delay LH surge with a single injection given in the late follicular phase (Leroy et al. 1994).

Clinical Applications

GnRH Analogs

Endometriosis. In the conservative management of endometriosis, GnRH analogs can be used to suppress the symptoms and the growth of this disease in the perimenopausal woman until the patient goes through natural menopause, thus avoiding major surgery in some women. When fertility is of concern, analogs can be used to suppress the disease prior to infertility treatment, alone or combined with the conservative surgery. There have been no convincing data to show that combined therapy improves the outcome with respect to pain or pregnancy. However, in severe (American Fertility Society stage III or IV) pelvic endometriosis, 2 months of preoperative GnRH analog suppression of ovarian function makes the surgery technically easier in some cases. In severe cases, when complete resection of endometriosis is not possible, postoperative analog suppression may be helpful in pain management. As conservative management of endometriosis, analogs have been found to be as effective as danocrine in randomized, prospective studies (Henzl et al. 1988) with respect to post-treatment pregnancy rates. Currently, chronic use of analogs has no place in the treatment of symptomatic endometriosis in women who are not interested in fertility and who have many years to reach the age of menopause. This is due to its prohibitive cost and the side-effects related to hypoestrogenism such as proposed increased mortality secondary to increased cardiovascular disease risk and osteoporosis after its protracted use (Dlugi et al. 1988; Uemura et al. 1994).

Leiomyomas. Controlled studies have shown that uterine fibroids will have decreased in size by an average of 68.4%–74.9% following 3 months of analog suppression. After discontinuation of treatment, however, fibroids have been reported to return to their previous size within 2 months (Healy et al. 1986). According to this author's experience, shelling of myomas usually becomes more difficult due to the less defined surgical planes after GnRH analog suppression. Preoperative administration of GnRH analogs in patients with a uterus of 14–18 weeks' size increased the use of vaginal hysterectomy, decreased intraoperative blood loss, and shortened hospital stay and convalescence in one prospective, randomized study (Stovall et al. 1994). For these purposes GnRH analog should be used for 2 months prior to surgery.

Controlled Ovarian Hyperstimulation. Premature or "escape" ovulations occur in over 30% of the controlled ovarian hyperstimulation cycles with human menopausal gonadotropins (hMGs) (Fleming and Coutts 1986). To prevent pre-human chorionic gonadotropin (pre-hCG) luteinization. GnRH analogs have been successfully used in combination with hMGs in assisted reproductive technologies (ART), including in vitro fertilization (IVF) and gamete intrafallopian transfer (GIFT). In our institution, we use two different protocols for analog use in controlled ovarian hyperstimulation. According to the first protocol, leuprolide acetate 0.5 mg twice a day (b.i.d.), i.m. injections begin in the mid-luteal phase to continue for 10 days. After 10 days, the dose is decreased to 0.5 mg and hMG stimulation begins. Both medications are continued until the desired follicular size is reached. According to the second protocol, the patient is given oral contraceptives the month before she is scheduled for an IVF cycle. Four days before the last contraceptive pill, the patient is started on leuprolide 0.5 mg b.i.d. for a total of 8 days. On day 1 or 2 of menses, ovarian stimulation begins. Efficiency of controlled ovarian hyperstimulation and pregnancy rates improve with GnRH analog use (Gagliardi et al. 1991; Weise et al. 1988). GnRH analogs have also been used as an effective alternative to hCG for inducing ovulation in stimulated cycles in women who are at risk for developing ovarian hyperstimulation syndrome (Lanzone et al. 1994). To trigger ovulation, 200 g of s.c. buserelin acetate was used instead of 5000 IU of hCG in women who did not have GnRH analog downregulation. Pregnancy rates remained comparable in the two groups, while ovarian enlargement in the luteal phase was lower in the GnRH analog group. Another use for GnRH analogs in IVF cycles is to control the cycle timing to accommodate the social needs of the IVF team and to group the patients in satellite programs.

Premenstrual Syndrome (PMS). Recent research has shown significant improvement in the symptoms of women with PMS when GnRH analogs are administered chronically along with low-dose estrogen. However, the high cost of the medication is currently a prohibiting factor in the long-term management of the disease. Women with intractable PMS, who are relieved from their symptoms during a minimum of 6 monhts of GnRH analog suppression, may be good candidates for surgical castration (GnRH analog test). A shorter duration of GnRH analog suppression for this purpose is not recommended due to the significant placebo effect seen in PMS patients (Helvacioglu et al. 1993).

Polycystic Ovary Syndrome and Ovarian Androgen Excess. Long-term administration of GnRH analogs leads to ovarian suppression with consequent androgen reduction (Steingold et al. 1987). Nafarelin (Andreyko et al. (1986), buserelin (Faure and Lemay 1987), leuprolide (Rittmaster 1988), tryptorelin (Couzinet et al. 1986), and goserelin (Rademaker et al. 1991) have been used for the treatment of ovarian hirsutism with varying success. Additional estrogen during the long-term use of GnRH analogs prevents side-effects due to hypoestrogenism. However, this does not potentiate the therapeutic effect of GnRH analogs on hirsutism (Tiitinen et al. 1994). The high cost of the analogs prohibits their long-term use in treating ovarian androgen excess. Short-term (3–6 months) GnRH analog challenge could be used as a diagnostic test in the differential diagnosis of functional ovarian tumors from other nonneoplastic causes of ovarian hyperandrogenism.

Control of Menstrual Bleeding. GnRH analog treatment in dysfunctional uterine bleeding or menorrhagia in association with fibroids or bleeding disorders, and suppression of menses in aplastic anemias, should be limited to a short duration just long enough to stabilize the patient. Treatment should continue until the patient is ready for surgery to allow increases in iron stores and hemoglobin in case of fibroids.

Contraception. Antiprogesterone mifepristone (RU-486) has been the only new major contribution of the armament of contraceptives since the introduction of oral contraceptive pills in 1957. GnRH analogs can disrupt cyclic function when given either continuously or intermittently. They have only weak effects when administered for a short period during the follicular phase. They are rather unreliable in suppressing the corpus luteum and placental function during pregnancy. GnRH antagonists can readily suppress follicular development but high doses may be required to block ovulation if administration is delayed until the late follicular phase. The antagonists may be luteolytic at any stage of the luteal phase. Therefore more research is needed on this subject to verify the efficacy of antagonists as a postcoital contraceptive. Continuous administration of GnRH analogs currently remains the simplest and most reliable approach to analog contraception and may be a potential, novel contraceptive method in the near future. GnRH antagonists have potential as a method of contraception in lactating women without affecting the postnatal rise in testosterone in male infants. Data on the marmoset monkey have shown the efficacy of the antagonist as a postpartum contraceptive (Fraser et al. 1994). However, human research is needed to establish the safety and the efficacy of the GnRH anatagonist as a postpartum contraceptive during lactation. Research on GnRH antagonist use as a male contraceptive is less promising. Addition of antagonists to high-dose testosterone treatment has not proven to be successful in suppressing spermatogenesis any more than does testosterone alone.

Precocious Puberty. The effectiveness of GnRH analogs for the suppression of idiopathic central precocious puberty is well established (Kaplan and Grumbach 1990), although the question, "Do GnRH analogs improve final height?" remained unanswered until recently. The man final height of 34 untreated girls with idiopathic central precocious puberty was 153.5 cm with a range of 135.8–171.5 cm (Sigurjonsdottir and Hayles 1968). Some girls with true precocious puberty and poor adult height prediction who are treated with GnRH analogs achieve an adult height more comparable to their target height. However, the lack of effect on height in girls with predicted height at the onset of therapy similar to their target height, and preservation of the growth potential in the slow evolutive forms, suggest that these forms might not require immediate therapy. Careful follow-up before therapy may be a better way of evaluating their natural course. Some forms of idiopathic central precocious puberty may not necessitate analog therapy (Brauner e al. 1994). In older girls with idiopathic central precocious puberty, it seems that final adult height may be slightly improved with GnRH analog treatment but it remains nearly 1 SD below the mean target height (Oerter et al. 1993). An excellent review of the published and submitted data has indicated that treatment with GnRH analogs does not significantly after the final adult height of girls with idiopathic central precocious puberty whose age at diagnosis is greater than 6 years. The treatment of girls whose age at diagnosis is less than 6 years may improve final height by 2%–4% (Kletter and Kelch 1994).

Other Uses. Recently, GnRH analogs have been used, tested, or proposed for use in the treatment of cyclic auditory dysfunction, dysfunctional uterine bleeding in women after liver transplantation, dysfunctional uterine bleeding in women during aplastic anemia crisis, prostate cancer, breast cancer, ovarian epithelial cancer, hidradenitis suppurativa, and the management of catamenial pneumothorax, in addition to their many other conventional indications.

Breast cancer. GnRH analog use has been associated with some favorable responses of breast cancer in postmenopausal patients (Manni et al. 1986; Nicholson et al. 1986). GnRH analogs have been shown to have a growth inhibitory effect on certain breast cancer cell lines (Miller et al. 1985), although currently there has been no approved use of GnRH analogs in the management of breast cancer.

Prostate Cancer. Leuprolide acetate is the only GnRH analog approved by the Food and Drug Administration for clinical use in the palliative treatment of advanced prostate cancer.

Ovarian Caner. A favorable response to treatment with GnRH agonists has been reported in some patients with refractory ovarian epithelial cancer (Kavanagh et al. 1989). Recent research has suggested that the leuprolide acetate effect on ovarian cancer cell proliferation is independent of pituitary gonadotropin and steroid, that it involves a cell cycle regulatory event, and that the duration of benefit observed in vivo for some patients may be related to total tumor volume at the time of treatment (Thompson et al. 1991).

Hidradenitis Suppurativa. In chronic, severe, recurrent, resistant cases of hidradenitis suppurativa, GnRH agonist suppression has been successfully used to predict the outcome of surgical castration prior to the scheduled surgery (Bogers et al. 1992). This "GnRH agonist test" could be used to differentiate the cases which will benefit from surgical castration.

Menstrual Asthma. The successful treatment of cyclic severe attacks of bronchial asthma during ovulation and menstrual periods by means of GnRH analogs has been described (Blumenfeld et al. 1994a).

Catamenial Pneumothorax. Resistant catamenial pneumothorax can be successfully managed with GnRH analogs. With an estrogen "add-back" regimen, long-term successful suppression of disease without side-effects has been reported (Garris et al. 1994).

GnRH

Diagnostic Testing

GnRH Test of Predict Fertility After Varicocelectomy. In men, to predict fertility after varicocelectomy, "GnRH challenge test" has been proposed. After 100 µg intravenous (i.v.) bolus of GnRH, patients are sampled for LH and FSH at 0, 15, 30, 60, and 120 min. The pregnancy group ($n=5$) had a significant decrease in LH levels at 30 min compared to a nonpregnancy group (Masato et al. 1994).

GnRH Test of Hypothalamic – Pituitary Function. In general the magnitude of the LH response to GnRH reflects the severity of the hypothalamic disorder. In anorexia nervosa, the sicker the patient gets, the lower is the LH response to the GnRH test (Nillius and Wide 1977). The GnRH test still has a place in research to assess the pituitary gonadotropin reserve, although for diagnostic purposes it is of very dubious value.

Ovulation Induction. For the past 10 years, pulsatile GnRH has been used to induce ovulation in clinical practice. This technique has been proven to be an effective and safe therapeutic tool in the management of anovulatory infertility. Absence of ovarian hyperstimulation and the low incidence of multiple pregnancies are particularly advantageous for outpatient treatment. Poor patient compliance, however, has made pulsatile GnRH treatment a less popular choice in ovulation induction compared to daily hMG injections. The clinical success rate of GnRH ovulation induction is comparable to that of hMG ovulation induction and the price of monitoring is lower. Pulsatile GnRH should be the treatment of first choice after clomiphene citrate failure in the management of anovulatory infertility in motivated patients. A microchip-controlled peristaltic pump that can deliver 25 or 50-µl boluses of GnRH solution at 90 or 12-min intervals is used to administer the drug i.v. or s.c. A GnRH dose/bolus of 2.5 µg every 60 min i.v. is fully capable of restoring ovulation in hypogonadotropic hypogonadism (Filicori et al. 1991). At present, the most popular starting GnRH dose per bolus is 5 µg i.v. to be increased to 10–20 µg/bolus when no response occurs within 10–15 days. A 60-min pulse interval is the most commonly used frequency since the clinical response of the patients has been the most favorable. Native GnRH has been used to trigger ovulation, instead of hCG or GnRH analogs, in women with polycystic ovarian disease, hoping to prevent the development of ovarian hyperstimulation syndrome. However, the incidence of severe ovarian hyperstimulation syndrome has remained the same (Blumenfeld et al. 1994b).

Idiopathic Hypogonadotropic Hypogonadism. Subjects with idiopathic hypogonadotropic hypogonadism have an isolated deficiency of GnRH secretion which prevents them from undergoing puberty. Other endocrine functions are normal and their hypogonadism can be reversed with long-term GnRH treatment. Such treatment in men with idiopathic hypogonadotropic hypogonadism produces pituitary-gonadal activity similar to that observed in normal pubertal and adult subjects (Spratt et al. 1989).

Adverse Effects of GnRH Analog Use

The main side-effects noted with the use of GnRH analogs are those associated with hypoestrogenism, and the severity appears to be related to the degree of ovarian suppression. Besides the symptoms of menopausal vasomotor unstability, the main health concerns focus on osteoporosis and cardiovascular risk arising from prolonged hypoestrogenism.

Cardiovascular Risk. Protracted use of GnRH analogs increased total serum cholesterol, HDL-C, and LDL-C, with no statistical significance in one study (Lemay et al. 1988). Another study (Dlugi et al. 1988) showed an increase in LDL-C in 6 months but no effect on HDL-C levels. Two other studies with nafarelin and goserelin showed no change in serum lipid profiles (Henzl et al. 1988; Gardner et al. 1988).

Osteoporosis. Studies have shown a significant decrease in bone mineral density (BMD) after 6 months of GnRH analog suppression. Reduction in BMD was greater in women younger than 33 years of age after 24 weeks of treatment ($n=12$ controls and 7 patients). However this bone loss recovered to pretreatment levels in the next 24 weeks once the treatment had been stopped (Uemura et al. 1994).

Angina and Myocardial Infarction. Use of leuprolide acetate has been associated with angina in men undergoing prostate cancer treatment. Recently, angina and subsequent myocardial infarction were reported in a woman with a strong family history of heart disease 1 month after the first leuprolide injection (McCoy 1994). When cardiac function in healthy young women was evaluated by Doppler echocardiography performed before and 3 weeks after initiation of GnRH analog treatment, significant decreases in peak aortic flow velocity, cardiac index, and mean acceleration were observed (Eckstein et al. 1993). This issue must be thoroughly discussed with those patients who have a strong family history of heart disease.

Failure to Suppress Ovarian Function

Incomplete suppression of ovarian function by some depot GnRH analogs is seen occasionally. Filicori et al. (1993) have shown that in adult women, while immunoreactive-LH was suppressed in the 3rd month with all GnRH analogs tested, FSH suppression with depot GnRH analogs was less marked than that with high-dose short-acting s.c. buserelin. This condition will manifest itself with the signs of incomplete suppression during the 3rd month of depot GnRH analog administration, particularly when goserelin is employed.

References

Amoss M, Burgus R, Blackwell R, Vale W, Fellows R, Guillemin R (1971) Purification, amino acid composition and N-terminus of the hypothalamic luteinizing hormone-releasing factor (LRF) of bovine origin. Biochem Biophys Res Commun 44:205–208

Andreyko JL, Monroe SE, Jaffe RB (1986) Treatment of hirsutism with a gonadotropin-releasing hormone agonist (nafarelin). J Clin Endocrincol Metab 63:854–859

Blumenfeld Z, Bentur L, Yoffe N, Alroy G, Rubin AHE (1994a) Menstrual asthma: use of gonadotropin-releasing hormone analogue for the treatment of cyclic aggravation of bronchial asthma. Fertil Steril 62:197–200

Blumenfeld Z, Lang N, Amit A, Kahana L, Yoffe N (1994b) Native gonadotropin-releasing hormone for triggering follicular maturation in polycystic ovary syndrome patients undergoing human menopausal gonadotropin ovulation induction. Fertil Steril 62:456–460

Brauner R, Adan L, Malandry F, Zantleifer D (1994) Adult height in girls with idiopathic true precocious puberty. J Clin Endocrinol Metab 79:415–420

Bogers JW, Minderhoud-Bassie W, Huikeshoven FJM (1992) A case of hidradenitis suppurativa treated with gonadotropin-releasing hormone agonist and by total abdominal hysterectomy with bilateral salpingooophorectomy. Am J Obstet Gynecol 167:517–518

Couzinet B, Le Strat N, Brailly S, Schaison G (1986) Comparative effects of cyproterone acetate or a long-acting gonadotropin-releasing hormone agonist in polycystic ovarian disease. J Clin Endocrinol Metab 63:1031–1035

Dlugi AM, Rufo S, D'Amico JF et al (1988) A comparison of the effects of buserelin versus danazol on plasma lipoproteins during treatment of pelvic endometriosis. Fertil Steril 49:913–916

Eckstein N, Pines A, Fisman EZ, Fisch B, Limor R, Vagman I, Barnan R, Ayalon D (1993) The effect of hypoestrogenic state, induced by gonadotropin-releasing hormone agonist, on Doppler-derived parameters of aortic flow. J Clin Endocrinol Metab 77:910–912

Faure N, Lemay A (1987) Ovarian suppression in polycystic ovarian disease during 6 month administration of a luteinizing hormone-releasing hormone (LH-RH) agonist. Clin Endocrinol (Oxf) 27:703–713

Filicori M, Santoro N, Merriam Gr, Crowley WF Jr (1986) Characterization of the physiological pattern of episodic gonadotropin secretion throughout the human menstrual cycle. J Clin Endocrinol Metab 62:1136–1139

Filicori M, Flamigni C, Meriggiola MC, Ferrari P, Michellacci L, Campaniello E, Valdiserri A, Cognigni G (1991) Endocrine response determines the clinical outcome of pulsatile gonadotropin-releasing hormone ovulation induction in different ovulatory disorders. J Clin Endocrinol Metab 72:965–972

Filicori M, Flamigni C, Cognigni G, Dellai P, Arnone R, Falbo A, Capelli M (1993) Comparison of the suppressive capacity of different gonadotropin-releasing hormone analogs in women. J Cin Endocrinol Metab 77:130–133

Fleming R, Coutts JRT (1986) Induction of multiple follicular growth in normally menstruating women with endogenous gonadotropin suppression. Fertil Steril 45:226–230

Fraser HM, Recio R, Conn MP, Lunn SF (1994) Gonadotropin-releasing hormone antagonist for postpartum contraception: outcome for the mother and male offspring in the marmoset. J Clin Endocrinol Metab 78:121–125
Gagliardi CL, Emmi AM, Weiss G, Schmidt CL (1991) Gonadotropin-releasing hormone agonist improves the efficiency of controlled ovarian hyperstimulation/intrauterine insemination. Fertil Steril 55:939-943
Garris PD, Sokol MS, Kelly K, Whitman GF, Plouffe L (1994) Leuprolide acetate treatment of catamenial pneumothorax. Fertil Steril 61:173–174
Gardner RI, Crook D, Shaw RW (1988) A preliminary study of the serum lipid profiles of patients undergoing therapy for endometriosis. Br J Obstet Gynecol 95:725
Healy DL, Lawson FR, Abbott M, Baird DT (1986) Toward removing uterine fibroids without surgery: subcutaneous infusion of luteinizing hormone-releasing hormone agonist commencing in the luteal phase. J Clin Endocrinol Metab 63:619–625
Henzl MR, Corson SL, Moghissi K et al (1988) Administration of nasal nafarelin as compared with oral danazol for endometriosis. N Engl J Med 318:485–488
Helvacioglu A, Yeoman RR, Hazelton JM ,Aksel S (1993) Premenstrual syndrome and related hormonal changes: long-acting gonadotropin releasing hormone agonist treatment. J Reprod Med 38:864–870
Kaplan SL, Grumbach MM (1990) Pathogenesis of sexual precocity. In: Grumbach MM, Sizonenko PC, Aubert ML (eds) Control of the onset of puberty. Williams and Wilkins, Baltimore, pp 620–662
Kavanagh JJ, Roberts W, Townsend P, Hewitt S (1989) Leuprolide acetate in the treatment of refractory or persistent eptihelial ovarian cancer. J Clin Oncol 7:115–118
Kletter GB, Kelch RP (1994) Clinical review 60: effects of gonadotropin-releasing hormone analog therapy on adult stature in precocious puberty. J Clin Endocrinol Metab 79:331–334
Knobil E (1980) The neuroendocrine control of the menstrual cycle. Recent Prog Horm Res 36:53–57
Lanzone A, Fulghesu AM, Villa P, Guida C, Guido M, Nicoletti MC, Caruso A, Mancuso S (1994) Gonadotropin-releasing hormone agonist versus human chorionic gonadotropin as a trigger of ovulation in polycystic ovarian disease gonadotropin hyperstimulated cycles. Fertil Steril 62:35–41
Lemay A, Sandow J, Bureau M et al (1988) Prevention of follicular maturation in endometriosis by subcutaneous infusion of luteinizing hormone-releasing hormone agonist started in the luteal phase. Fertil Steril 49:410
Leroy I, d'Acremont MF, Brailly-Tabard S, Frydman R, de Mouzon J, Bouchard P (1994) A single injection of a gonadotropin-releasing hormone (GnRH) antagonist (Cetrorelix) postpones the luteinizing hormone (LH) surge: further evidence for the role of GnRH during the LH surge. J Clin Endocrinol Metab 62:461–467
Manni A ,Santen R, Harvey H, Lipton A, Max D (1986) Treatment of breast cancer with gonadotropin releasing hormone. Endocrine Rev 7:89–94
Masato F, Hayashi A, Imanishi O, Tanaka H, Okada H, Matsumoto O, Kamidono S (1994) The significance of gonadotropin-releasing hormone test for predicting fertility after varicocelectomy. Fertil Steril 61:779–782
McCoy MJ (1994) Angina and myocardial infection with use of leuprolide acetate. Am J Obstet Gynecol 171:275–276
Miller WR, Scott WN, Morris R, Frase HM, Sharpe RM (1985) Growth of human breast cancer cells inhibited by a luteinizing hormone-releasing agonist. Nature 313-231-233
Nicholson RI, Walker KJ, Turkes A, Dyas J, Gotting KE, Plowman PN, Williams M, Elston CW, Blamey RW (1986) The British experience with the LHRH agonist Zoladex (ICI 118630) in the treatment of breast cancer. In: Klijn JGM, Paridaens R, Foekens JA (eds) Hormonal manipulation of cancer: peptides, growth factors and new (anti) steroidal agents. Raven, New York, pp 331-342
Nillius SJ, Wide L (1977) The pituitary responsiveness to acute and chronic administration of gonadotropin-releasing hormone in acute and recovery stages of anorexia nervosa. In: Vigersky RA (ed) Anorexia nervosa. Raven, New York, pp 225–241
Oerter Ke, Manasco PK, Barnes KM, Jones J, Hill S, Cutler Jr GB (1993) Effects of luteinizing hormone-releasing hormone agonists on final height in luteinizing hormone-dependent precocious puberty. Acta Paediatr 388 (Suppl):62–68
Rademaker M, Simpson NB, Gudmunsson J, Bonduelle M, Fleming R, Coutts JRT (1991) Effect of the gonadotropin-releasing hormone analogue, goserelin, and oes-

tradiol replacement of sebum excretion rates and hair size in mildly hirsute women. J Dermatol Treat 1:289–292
Rittmaster RS (1988) Differential suppression of testosterone and estradiol in hirsute women with the superactive gonadotropin-releasing hormone agonsit leuprolide. J Clin Endocrinol Metab 67:651–654
Schally AV, Arimura A, Baba Y, Nair RM, Matsuo H, Redding TW, Debeljuk L (1971) Isolation and properties of the FSH and LH-releasing hormone. Biochem Biophys Res Commun 43:393–398
Sigurjonsdottir TJ, Hayles AB (1968) Precocious puberty. Am J Dis Child 115:309–321
Spratt DI, Finkelstein JS, O'Dea LStL, Rao PN, Crowley WF (1989) Pulsatile gonadotropin-releasing hormone (GnRH) treatment of men with idiopathic hypogonadotropic hypogonadism: a model for studies of the neuroendocrine control of sexual maturation. In: Shaw RW, Marshall JC (eds) LHRH and its analogues: their use in gynaecological practice. Butterworth, London, pp 113–125
Steingold K, de Ziegler D, Cedars M et al (1987) Clinical and hormonal effects of chronic gonadotropin-releasing hormone agonist treatment in polycystic ovarian disease. J Clin Endocrinol Metab 65:773–778
Stovall TG, Summit RL, Washburn SA, Ling FW (1994) Gonadotropin-releasing hormone agonist use before hysterectomy. Am J Obstet Gynecol 170:1744–1751
Thompson MA, Adelson MD, Kaufman LM (1991) Lupron retards proliferation of ovarian epithelial tumor cells cultured in serum-free medium. J Clin Endocrinol Metab 72:1036–1041
Tiitinen A, Simberg N, Stenman UH, Ylikorkala O (1994) Estrogen replacement does not potentiate gonadotropin-releasing hormone agonist-induced androgen suppression in treatment of hirsutism. J Clin Endocrinol Metab 79:447–451
Uemura T, Mohri J, Osada H, Suzuki N, Katagiri N, Minaguchi H (1994) Effect of gonadotropin releasing agonist on the bone mineral density of patients with endometriosis. Fertil Steril 62:246–250
Weise HC, Fiedler K, Kato K (1988) Buserelin suppression of endogenous gonadotropin secretion in infertile women with ovarian feedback disorders given human menopausal/human chorionic gonadotropin treatment. Fertil Steril 49.:399-403

Ovarian Hyperstimulation Syndrome

C. De Geyter

Definition

The ovarian hyperstimulation syndrome is a serious iatrogenic complication of reinforcement of ovarian function by drug administration that becomes clinically manifest only in the luteal phase under the influence of exogenous and endogenous reproductive hormones. In severe ovarian hyperstimulation exudate massively penetrates the extravascular room with ensuing ascites, hydrothorax and general edema. The fluid shift is caused by increased capillary permeability with simultaneous decrease of blood pressure. This shift of fluid components results in a hemoconcentration which may lead to thromboembolic phenomena and acute renal insufficiency becoming threatening to life.

Classification

Ovarian hyperstimulation is no uniform clinical entity. According to its characteristic features different gradings are described, with the intensity of treatment varying accordingly. The classification of the ovarian hyperstimulation syndrome has been defined over the course of many years in conformity with prevailing diagnostic possibilities and by meeting the requirements of treatment schemes in reproductive medicine. The first, chiefly clinical classification, was proposed by Rabau et al. (1967) and was later modified by Schenker and Weinstein (1978). The classification by Rabau is mainly based on the clinical parameters (vaginal examination, abdominal distention, nausea, vomiting, dyspnea) and laboratory findings (urinary estrogen and pregnanediol excretion, hemoconcentration). With the use of sonography a more precise classification was established which became the WHO standardized grading system comprising grades I, II, and III. Grade I of the hyperstimulation syndrome is characterized by ovarian enlargement measuring less than 6 cm in diameter while grade II shows enlarged ovaries measuring 6–12 cm in diameter. Characteristics of hyperstimulation syndrome grade III are enlarged ovaries more than 12 cm in diameter accompanied by ascites or hydrothorax and signs of hemoconcentration. Only grade III of the ovarian hyperstimulation syndrome is clinically relevant, requiring clinical treatment. However, the gradings I, II, and III have now become obsolete due to pro-

Table 1 Criteria of ovarian hyperstimulation syndrome (according to Navot et al. 1992)

Imminent hyperstimulation	Critical hyperstimulation
Ovaries >12 cm	Ovaries >12 cm
Ascites	Massive ascites and dyspnea
Hydrothorax facultative	Hydrothorax, vulvar edema
Hemoconcentration >45%	Hemoconcentration >55%
Leukocytosis >15 000 mm^3	Leukocytosis >25 000 mm^3
Oliguria	Oliguria
Creatinine within normal limit	Creatinine rising
Elevated liver enzymes	Renal insufficiency
	Imminent thromboembolic phenomena

gress in assisted fertilization and the common use of transvaginal ultrasonographically guided aspiration of follicles. Oocyte retrieval often produces a blood-tinted ascites without further symptoms of ovarian hyperstimulation. In such cases the new classification by Navot provides better criteria for the differentiation of the clinically relevant hyperstimulation syndrome grade III (Navot et al. 1992). It sets down the definition on an imminent (hemoconcentration>45%) and critical (hemoconcentration>55%) hyperstimulation syndrome (Table 1).

Pathogenesis

In cases where gonadotropin is administered in ovarian stimulation treatment to achieve a mono- or oligofollicular reaction of the ovaries, e.g., for ovulation induction required in insemination therapy, the ovarian hyperstimulation syndrome is hardly ever seen and it is even more rare in Clomid-induced cycles (Hammerstein 1967). However, it appears to be a relatively common consequence of intentional hyperstimulation serving the purpose of in vitro fertilization and embryo transfer, and in this context was first described by Friedman et al. (1984). The frequency of the severe hyperstimulation syndrome in in vitro fertilization and embryo transfer varies at present between 1.6% (Smitz et al. 1990) and 2.4% (our own patients). The single aspiration of almost as many follicles as possible in the oocyte retrieval for in vitro fertilization and embryo transfer by no means reduces the incidence of severe hyperstimulation syndrome.

The pathogenesis of the ovarian hyperstimulation syndrome is unknown so far. The intrinsic characteristic of this syndrome is a generalized vasodilatation with increased capillary permeability (Balasch et al. 1991), the genesis of which has not yet been identified. These vessel alterations result in massive transudation into the abdomen, subcutaneous tissue, and pleura. Experiments on animals have shown that ascites is not primarily generated on the ovarian surface but the entire abdominal serosa (Yarali et al. 1993). The reduced circulatory volume gradually activates vasoconstrictive defense mechanisms: adrenaline→leukocytes; renin-angiotensin system→reduced blood supply of the kidneys (Navot et al. 1992); hypersecretion of the antidiuretic hormone→a subjectively uncomfortable feeling of thirst, prostaglandins for maintenance of renal perfusion (Balasch et al. 1991). Alterations in the hemoconcentration, clinically evidenced by the hematocrit value, only become manifest after a significant loss of liquid from the circulation. Reduced arteriolar perfusion of the kidneys may cause acute insufficiency of the renal function. Hemoconcentration representing a concentration of blood coagulation factors may induce thromboembolic phenomena, rated as the most prominent cause of death in this syndrome. Liver function is hampered by metabolism of superelevated estrogen levels as well as by the hepatotoxic effect of liver parenchymal edema. Cholestase has occasionally been observed, causing pruritus (Younis et al. 1988). This complication, however, has a favorable prognosis. In contrast to liver dysfunction, the adult respiratory distress syndrome (ARDS) is serious complication of the ovarian hyperstimulation syndrome affecting pulmonary function through exudate in the pulmonary parenchyma (Schenker 1993).

Risk Factors

While the ovarian hyperstimulation syndrome only becomes clinically manifest in the luteal phase, it is mainly caused by the intensity of stimulation treatment during the follicular phase of the menstruation cycle. Monitorings during stimulation treatment comprise the determination of serum estradiol concentrations as well as sonographic examinations; yet the role of these two parameters is the subject of controversy to this day. During the follicular phase estrogen levels in the serum have been found to correlate positively with later development of an ovarian hyperstimulation syndrome (Haning et al. 1983). However, hyperstimulation syndromes may also occur in the presence of low estradiol levels, whereas not every patient showing superelevated estradiol levels develops a hyperstimulation syndrome. Moreover, the number of smaller follicles developing in addition to graafian follicles is decisive in the incidence of ovarian hyperstimulation syndrome (Blankstein et al. 1987). With regard to the risk evaluation of ovarian hyperstimulation syndrome, prior to treatment it is important to sonographically identify the ovarian necklace sign that is pathognomonic for the syndrome of polycystic ovaries (Adams et al. 1985). After desensitization of the adenohypophysis induced by GnRH analogues of long efficacy ovarian stimulation favours the recruitment of a greater number of follicles and as such this combination scheme represents an additional risk factor (Golan et al. 1988). Presently, direct effects of GnRH on the ovary in the development of ovarian hyperstimulation syndrome are also postulated (Mordel and Schenker 1993). The formation of a great number of secondary follicles during the follicular phase concomitant with a rapid increase of the serum-estradiol concentration may possibly herald ovarian hyperstimulation syndrome.

Although hyperandrogenemic metabolism represents a risk factor, it is extremely difficult to evaluate the risk of ovarian hyperstimulation syndrome using endocrinologic routine diagnosis as the sole parameter (DeGeyter et

Table 2 Risk factors in ovarian hyperstimulation syndrome (according to Navot et al. 1992)

Hyperstimulation eventual	Hyperstimulation improbable
Age <35 years	Age >36 years
Hyperandrogenemia	Hypergonadotropinemia
Asthenic body structure	Strong body structure
"High ovarian responder"	"Low responder"
Necklace sign of the ovary	Resting ovary
Pregnancy	No pregnancy
HCG administration during luteal phase	Progesterone administration during luteal phase
Application of GnRH-analogues	Clomiphene or hMG stimulation alone

al. 1993). Elevated serum levels of androstendione and sex hormone binding globulin are the only predictors of a later hyperstimulation syndrome (Gustafson et al. 1992).

The risk factors are summarized in Table 2.

Prophylaxis

Restricted administration of exogenous gonadotropins in the stimulation of follicle maturation is considered the most effective means of avoiding hyperstimulation. This may reduce the incidence of ovarian hyperstimulation syndrome but cannot completely eliminate it. What seems paradoxical is the fact that patients requiring only low doses of gonadotropins for follicle maturation are inclined to the hyperstimulation syndrome (DeGeyter et al. 1993). An extraordinarily high pregnancy rate in these patients aggravates the therapeutic dilemma; in our own patients we diagnosed a pregnancy in 12 out of 20 women (60%) who received in patient treatment for severe hyperstimulation syndromes.

Since the ovarian hyperstimulation syndrome only becomes manifest at efficient hCG levels, the endogenous preovulatory LH peak has been induced by GnRH instead of hCG in cases of either superelevated serum estradiol concentrations or a surplus of mature follicles (Emperaire and Ruffie 1991; Imoedemhe et al. 1991), thus almost entirely avoiding the development of a hyperstimulation syndrome. Furthermore, possibilities of cryopreservation of fertilized oocytes or embryos in a potentially hyperstimulated cycle with delayed transfer during a nontreated or estrogen-gestagen supplemented cycle have also been discussed (Salat-Baroux et al. 1990; Wada et al. 1992). In patients with severe ovarian hyperstimulation syndrome, massive cystic structures frequently develop in both ovaries after ovulation induction with hCG and follicle aspiration, which led us to proceed to repeated transvaginal aspirations (under sonographic guidance) of these luteal cysts even before embryo transfer (Amit et al. 1993). This admittedly highly invasive method permitted reduction of the frequency of later ovarian hyperstimulation syndrome and the duration of clinical hospitalization.

Therapeutics

In the absence of knowledge of the exact pathogenesis of ovarian hyperstimulation syndrome, therapeutic approaches are symptomatic and empiric. The leading parameter in present therapeutic efforts is the estimation of the hematocrit value, which corresponds well to the degree of severity of the syndrome. In patient treatment is indicated when hematocrit estimation exceeds 45%; a hematocrit>55% is life threatening. Under close in patient observation the patient's fluid input/output must be recorded with additional daily controls of hematocrit, electrolyte balance, renal function, liver enzymes, bilirubin, and plasma coagulation. Daily determination of abdominal distention and weight increase should also be carried out. Hemoconcentration can be influenced by adequate fluid administration (minimum 2 l/day) and normal human albumin. Although heparin may increase the risk of intraabdominal bleeding in the event of a cyst rupture, the danger of thromboembolic phenomena, which causes most of the fatalities occurring in the ovarian hyperstimulation syndrome, should be reduced by low-dosed heparinization. The appearance of oligo-anuresis, which is symptomatic for imminent renal insufficiency, justifies the administration of diuretic agents (e.g., 20 mg furosemide after previous administration of 100 g normal human albumin 20% i.v.) in an intact pregnancy. The application of diuretics as described should, however, only be commenced after initiation of infusion therapy to eliminate hemoconcentration. Reduced oncotic pressure (e.g., requiring administration of a dextran solution), hyponatremia (requiring 5% NaCl i.v.) and hypercalcemia (therefore no Ringer's lactate solution) require careful treatment. Renal function may be improved by intravascular administration of dopamine (4.32 mg/kg/24 h) with the specific aim of increasing the renal blood supply (Ferraretti et al. 1992).

A causal medical treatment for severe ovarian hyperstimulation syndrome does not yet exist. Based on the identification of special pathologies considered to be related to the development of ovarian hyperstimulation syndrome, several therapeutic methods have been tested. In most cases, indomethacin, a synthetic inhibitor of prostaglandins, has been applied to reduce the increased secretion of prostaglandins (Schenker and Polishuk 1976). Prostaglandins, however, ensure adequate renal blood supply. Therefore, indomethacin is no longer recommended (Balasch et al. 1990). Different treatment schemes, partially based on experiment on animals, have been applied in the treatment of ovarian hyperstimulation syndrome, e.g., antihistamines (Knox 1974) and angiotensin converting enzyme inhibitors (Schenker 1993). Prospective comparative studies proving or disproving the efficacy of these substances are not yet available. In a prospective study, absence of efficacy in the treatment of ovarian hyperstimulation syndrome has been proven solely for cortisone (Tan et al. 1992).

Alternatively, paracentesis of ascites has proved an extremely helpful tool, leading to prompt subjective alleviation of symptoms. Under sonographic control transabdominal (Borenstein et al. 1989) as well as transvaginal (Aboulghar et al. 1990) access is possible. It may be necessary to repeat these aspirations more than once (up to six times in our own patients). In the presence of dyspnea caused by hydrothorax, fast alleviation can be obtained by means of pleurocentesis. Mainly in cases where renal insufficiency is pronounced, the aspiration of ascites is highly efficient, supplemented with intensive protein substitution by infusions (Aboulghar et al. 1993). In an intact pregnancy the hyperstimulation syndrome may, however, last up to 3 weeks. When a severe hyperstimulation syndrome is diagnosed the possibility of early pregnancy (perhaps multiple pregnancy) must be taken into consideration; therefore it is very important not only to know the hematocrit value but also to initiate serial determination of the hCG concentration in the serum.

References

Aboulghar MA, Mansour RT, Serour GI, Amin YM (1990) Ultrasonically guided vaginal aspiration of ascites in the treatment of severe ovarian hyperstimulation syndrome. Fertil Steril 53:933–935

Aboulghar MA, Mansour RT, Serour GI, Sattar MA, Amin YM, Elattar I (1993) Management of severe hyperstimulation syndrome by ascitic fluid aspiration and intensive intravenous fluid therapy. Obstet Gynecol 81:108–111

Adams J, Polson DW, Abdulwahid N, Morris DV, Franks S, Mason HD, Tucker M, Price J (1995) Multifollicular ovaries: clinical and endocrine features and response to pulsatile gonadotropin releasing hormone. Lancet II:1376–1378

Amit A, Yaron Y, Yovel I, Peyser MR, David MP, Botchan A, Lessing JB (1993) Repeated aspiration of ovarian follicles and early corpus luteum cysts in an in-vitro fertilization programme reduces the risk of ovarian hyperstimulation syndrome in high responders. Hum Reprod 8:1184–1186

Balasch J, Carmona F, Llach J, Arroyo V, Jové I, Vanrell JA (1990) Acute prerenal failure and liver dysfunction in a patient with severe ovarian hyperstimulation syndrome. Hum Reprod 5:348–351

Balasch J, Arroy V, Carmona F, Llach J, Jiménez W, Paré JC, Vanrell JA (1991) Severe ovarian hyperstimulation syndrome: role of peripheral vasodilation. Fertil Steril 56:1077–1083

Blankstein J, Shalev J, Saadon T, Kukia EE, Rabinovici J, Pariente C, Lunenfeld B, Serr DM, Mashiah S (1987) Ovarian hyperstimulation syndrome: prediction by number and size of preovulatory ovarian follicles. Fertil Steril 47:597–601

Borenstein R, Elhalah U, Lunenfeld B, Schwartz ZS (1989) Severe ovarian hyperstimulation syndrome: a reevaluated therapeutic approach. Fertil Steril 51:791–795

DeGeyter Ch, DeGeyter M, Castro E, Bals-Pratsch M, Hanker JP, Schlegel W, Nieschlag E, Schneider HPG (1993) Predictive parameters for ovarian response to hyperstimulation with exogenous gonadotropins after suppression of gonadotropin secretion of the pituitary using a long-acting GnRH agonist. Eur J Obstet Gynec Reprod Biol 51:139–147

Emperaire JC, Ruffie A (1991) Triggering ovulation with endogenous luteinizing hormone may prevent the ovarian hyperstimulation syndrome. Hum Reprod 6:506–510

Ferraretti AP, Gianaroli L, Diotallevi L, Festi C, Trounson A (1992) Dopamine treatment for severe hyperstimulation syndrome. Hum Reprod 7:180–183

Friedman CH, Schmidt GE, Chang FE, Kim MH (1984) Severe ovarian hyperstimulation syndrome following follicular aspiration. Am J Obstet Gynecol 150:436–437

Golan A, Ron-El R, Herman A, Weinraub Z, Soffer Y, Caspi E (1988) Ovarian hyperstimulation syndrome following D-Trp-6 luteinizing hormone-releasing hormone microcapsules and menotropin for in vitro fertilization. Fertil Steril 50:912–916

Gustafson O, Carlström K, Nylund L (1992) Androstenedione as a predictor of ovarian hyperstimulation syndrome. Hum Reprod 7:918–921

Hammerstein J (1967) Gefahren der ovariellen Überstimulierung bei Anwendung von Clomiphen und Gonadotropinen zur Ovulationsauslösung. Geburtsh Frauenh 12:1125–1251

Haning JR RV, Austin CW, Carlson IH, Kuzma DL, Shapiro SS, Zweibel WJ (1983) Plasma estradiol is superior to ultrasound and urinary estriol glucuronide as a predictor of ovarian hyperstimulation during induction of ovulation with menotropins. Fertil Steril 40:31–36

Imoedemhe DAG, Chan RCW, Sigue AB, Pacpaco ELA, Olazo AB (1991) A new approach to the management of patients at risk of ovarian hyperstimulation in an in-vitro fertilization programme. Hum Reprod 6:1988–1091

Knox GE (1994) Antihistamine blockade of the ovarian hyperstimulation syndrome. Am J Obstet Gynecol 118:992–994

Mordel N, Schenker JG (1993) Gonadotrophin-releasing hormone agonist and ovarian hyperstimulation syndrome in assisted reproduction. Hum Reprod 8:2009–2014

Navot D, Margalioth EJ, Laufer N, Birkenfeld A, Relou A, Rosler A, Schenker JG (1987) Direct correlation between plasma renin activity and severity of the ovarian hyperstimulation syndrome. Fertil Steril 48:57–61

Navot D, Bergh PA, Laufer N (1992) Ovarian hyperstimulation syndrome in novel reproductive technologies: prevention and treatment. Fertil Steril 58:249–261

Salat-Baroux J, Alvarez S, Antoine JM, Cornet D, Tibi Ch, Plachot M, Mandelbaum J (1990) Treatment of hyperstimulation during in-vitro fertilization. Hum Reprod 5:36–39

Scham et al. 1994

Schenker JG, Polishuk WZ (1976) The role of prostaglandins in ovarian hyperstimulation syndrome. Eur J Obstet Gynec Reprod Biol 6:47–52

Schenker JG, Weinstein D (1978) Ovarian hyperstimulation syndrome: a current survey. Fertil Steril 30:255–268

Schenker JG (1991) Prevention and treatment of ovarian hyperstimulation. Hum Reprod 8:653–659

Smitz J, Camus M, Devroey P, Erard P, Wisanto A, Van Steirteghem AC (1990) Incidence of severe ovarian hyperstimulation syndrome after GnRH agonist/HMG superovulation for in-vitro fertilization. Hum Reprod 5:933–937

Tan SL, Balen A, El Hussein E, Campbell S, Jacobs HS (1992) The administration of glucocorticoids for the prevention of ovarian hyperstimulation syndrome in in-vitro fertilization: a prospective randomized study. Fertil Steril 58:378–383

Wada I, Matson PL, Troup SA, Hughes S, Buck P, Lieberman BA (1992) Outcome of treatment subsequent to the elective cryopreservation of all embryos from women at risk of the ovarian hyperstimulation syndrome. Hum Reprod 7:962–966

Yarali H, Fleige-Zahradka BG, Yuen BH, McComb PF (1993) The ascites in the ovarian hyperstimulation syndrome does not originate from the ovary. Fertil Steril 59:657–661

Younis JS, Zeevi D, Rabinovicz R, Laufer N, Schenker JG (1988) Transient liver function test abnormalities in ovarian hyperstimulation syndrome. Fertil Steril 50:176–178

Operative Diagnosis Therapy

Hysterosalpingosonography

R. Turanli, K.H. Broer, and I. Turanli

Methods most frequently applied in the verification of cavity and tube factor in the evaluation of infertility are hysterosalpingography, i.e. the radiographic visualization of the cervical canal, uterine cavity and fallopian tubes after the injection of contrast material, which allows precise identification of the uterus, the tubes and the ovaries, and laparoscopy, for the inspection of the peritoneal cavity. Details on the uterine cavity and the tubes may also be obtained from hysteroscopy. Some years ago vaginal sonography was introduced as a method of ultrasonic diagnosis for the determination of tubal patency and the monitoring of the uterine cavity. Evaluations of the tube and cavity factors are of major importance in infertility diagnosis since facts on tubal patency decisively influence the prognosis and treatment of infertile couples. Therefore, any method that is less invasive is of great interest. Hysterosalpingography, laparoscopy, hysteroscopy and pertubation of the tubes are highly invasive examinations which in recent years we have been trying to replace at our clinic by ultrasonic diagnosis, with the aim of applying it in a greater number of patients. Transvaginal ultrasonography allows visualization of the uterus, uterine cavity, tubes and ovaries. A comparison with established methods revealed high conformity and sensitivity with the advantage of reduced invasiveness. Hysterosalpingosonography can be performed in the physician's office; it is well tolerated and accepted by patients since exposure to radiation is avoided, as are expensive operative methods performed under anaesthesia during hospitalisation.

Hysterosalpingosonography is conducted using a normal ultrasound apparatus equipped with a vaginal sound perceptor of 5 MHz. No anaesthesia is required. For the visualization of the tubes, either physiological salt solutions or contrast agents are used (e.g. Echovist and Schering). This contrast agent is a solution containing microcystiferous galactose with no side-effects and causing no pain. When the fluids are retrieved in the pouch of Douglas the tube factor is considered positive. Reproduction of the diagnosis is possible using video documentation. If no exact assessment (approx. 20%) is obtained, it is recommended that the patency of the fallopian tube be investigated by hysterosalpingography or, preferably, by laparoscopy.

The new procedure of hysterosalpingosonography using NaCl or Echovist achieves a diagnostic score of more than 80%, which is a sufficiently positive argument to justify the replacement of established but far more complicated methods dating back to the early times of sterility diagnosis. Other authors such as Deichert (1989) and Sauter (1990) have achieved diagnostic scores of 75%–90% with exclusive application of Echovist.

All working teams using the new examination technique have reported similarly high scores in the vaginal sonographically assisted determination of tubal adhesions. The contrast agent Echovist proves to be highly advantageous since it allows a precise side-location of the tubal adhesion which is not achieved with physiological salt solution, though the latter is undeniably less expensive. In their reports on the application of physiological salt solution, Marulis (1991) confirmed that peritubal conditions could be diagnosed, but our investigations and findings do not confirm these results in all respects. Among the alternative examination techniques, laparoscopy seems to have by far the best success rate.

From our experience and studies we conclude that for the evaluation of the uterine cavity, quite good visualization of the inner tube can be achieved by using physiological salt solution as opposed to contrast agents. For visualizing the pouch of Douglas, however, contrast agents have proved to be more efficient. Alternatively a combined procedure should be considered, initially monitoring the uterine cavity using physiological salt solution followed by administration of contrast agent for better visualization and side-location of the fallopian tubes.

The application of Echovist may be advantageous when using Doppler ultrasound systems: Schlief and Deichert (1991) have already reported positive results under Doppler ultrasound guidance. Nevertheless, its relatively high cost might at present hinder its routine use.

The high diagnostic score in respect of tube and cavity factors achieved by the new ultrasound examination technique indicates it to be a method that allows out-patient evaluation of the cavity and tube factor in the diagnosis of sterility, thus avoiding the immediate introduction of invasive procedures such as laparoscopy. By eliminating invasive methods and exposure to radiation it constitutes an important diagnostic technique in those with sterility.

It may be concluded that with a positive result from vaginal hysterosalpingosonography of the tubes there is a high certitude of neither a tubal obstruction nor a negative tube factor. A negative result from hysterosalpingosonography necessitates further investigations such as laparoscopy or hysteroscopy. Hysterosalpingosonography is recommended as a less invasive method with only a few side-effects; it can be easily carried out in an office setting at a favourable cost benefit ratio. Ultrasound-guided examination techniques should be used for early inspections of the uterine cavity and tube factor in the diagnosis of sterility, thus offering a further alternative in the investigation of female sterility.

References

Broer KH, Turanli R (1991) Patency of the cavum uteri and the fallopian tube investigated by vagino-abdominal ultrasound. First World Congress of Ultrasound in Obstetrics and Gynecology, London. Ultrasound in Obstetrics and Gynecology, Book of abstracts, vol 1. Parthenon, London

Broer KH, Diekman H, Klinghammer J, Turanli I (1991) Hystero-salpingo-vaginal-sonography for the assessment of fallopian tube patency XII. World Congress of Gynecology and Obstetrics. Intern J Obstet Gynecol 2:194

Broer KH, Turanli I, Freund I (1990) Investigation of tubal patency by a new ultrasound procedure. VII World Congress of Human Reproduction, Helsinki, Handbook of abstracts 86

Deichert U, Schlief R, van de Sandt M, Juhnke I (1989) Transvaginal hysterosalpingo-contrast sonography (HyCoSy) compared with conventional tubal diagnostic. Hum Reprod 4:418

Henkel B, Schlief R (1987) Transvaginal contrast-sonographic assessment of fallopian tube patency. In: Euroson 87, Proceedings of the Sixth Congress of the European Federation of Societies for Ultrasound in Medicine and Biology, Helsinki, June 14–18, p 223

Maroulis GB, Parsons AK, Yeko T (1991) Transvaginal ultrasonographic diagnosis of pelvic structures using a fluid contrast technique. Fertil Steril. The American Fertility Society

Nicolini UM, Belloti B, Bonazzi D, Zamberletti GB, Candiani (1987) Can ultrasound be used to screen uterine malformations? Fertil Steril 47(1):89

Randolph JR, Kang Ying Y, Maier DB, Schmidt CL, Ricklick DH (1986) Comparison of real time ultrasonography, hysterosalpingography and laparoscopy/hysteroscopy in the evaluation of uterine abnormalities and tubal patency. Fertil Steril 46(5):828

Richman TS, Viscomi GN, DeCherney A, Polan ML, Olson Alcebo L (1984) Fallopian tubal patency assessed by ultrasound following fluid injection. Radiology 152:507

Sautter T (1990) Transvaginal-Sonographie (1990) Lehrbuch und Lehratlas. Hippokrates, Stuttgart

Schlief R, Deichert U, Schürman R (1991) Assessment of fallopian tube patency by hysterosalpingo-contrast-sonography. First World Congress of Ultrasound in Obstetrics and Gynecology, London. Ultrasound in obstetrics and gynecology, book of abstracts. Parthenon, London

Schürman R, Schlief R, Niendorf HP (1991) Tubal patency and uterine malformations assessed by contrast sonography. XIII. World Congress of Gynecology annd Obstetrics. Int J Gynecol Obstet 2:154

Role of Hysterosalpingography in the Diagnosis of Sterility

K.H. Broer and D. Beyer

The first method of imaging of the uterine cavity and tube was roentgen hysterosalpingography. Although modern techniques that do not require radiation exposure, such as hysteroscopy, laparoscopy, and hysterosalpingosonography, have tended to usurp the place of hysterosalpingography (HSG), there are still some situations in which HSG is indicated. For certain diagnostic purposes, such as precise localization of uterine tube blockages, or imaging of the uterine cavity in cases of uterine change or anomalies, HSG can give valuable diagnostic information.

The new digital radiographic techniques in particular, which allow a further considerable reduction of the radiation dose, mean that HSG still has a place, especially when the results of the non-radiographic techniques referred to above are inconclusive. In 25 patients studied using the conventional radiographic technique, Ott and Fayez found that the mean X-ray exposure time in HSG was only 0.93 min (range 0.5–2.5 min), and on average only two radiographs were made. The calculated radiation dose to the ovaries was 0.25–0.15 rad. Today, it may be assumed that the use of digital radiography reduces the dose by a further 20–30%.

Indications for HSG

Uterine Cavity

Even after the advent of hysteroscopy, HSG has continued in special cases to have a role to play in the diagnosis of anomalies of the uterine cavity. HSG allows precise delineation of the type and extent of any deformation of the

Table 1 Indications for hysterosalpingography (HSG) in patients with changes of the uterine cavity

Suspected maldevelopment or malformation of the uterus
Suspected impairment of the uterine cavity due to intramural or submucous myomas
Suspected tuberculous endometritis (rare)
Habitual abortion with insufficiency of the internal orifice of the cervix uteri
Requirement for examination for cervical changes after a cesarean section

Table 2 Indications for HSG in patients with changes of the uterine tube

Primary and secondary sterility *after* sonographic and other examinations
Follow-up after microsurgical dilatation of an occlusion of the uterine tube

cavity. Occasionally, the differential diagnosis between endometrial polyps and submucous myomas may be difficult, and in such cases hysteroscopy can give additional diagnostic information. Combination with transvaginal uterine ultrasonography allows a comprehensive, minimally invasive diagnostic study of the uterine cavity. Table 1 shows the diagnostic alternatives in cases of changes in the uterine cavity.

Uterine Tube

HSG also has a place in up-to-date fertility diagnostics, in investigation of the tube factor, although a more exact diagnosis will be obtained by laparoscopy and chromohydrotubation of the fallopian tubes. If the tubes are radiolucent, peritubal adhesions accompanied by motility disturbances, or limited changes to the fimbria that disturb the mechanism of reception of the ovum, cannot be appreciated radiographically. For this reason, HSG needs to be combined with laparoscopy, and possibly also tubal endoscopy, for a complete diagnosis.

The usefulness of HSG is also undisputed in cases where laparoscopy is contraindicated, as when a general anaesthetic is undesirable, or in a patient who has already undergone several laparotomies with suspected intestinal fixation, or other medical contraindications. It is also an established screening technique in the performance of induction of ovulation by gonadotropins in the first stage of tube factor diagnosis.

Examination Technique

The technique of HSG has been described in many places and has many variants. At the start of the procedure, a portio adaptor is placed; various flexible and rigid instruments are available for this. Plastic vacuum adaptors, balloon catheters, vacuum intrauterine probes, and the widely successful Schulze adapter are all used.

After fixation of the instrument, the patient is moved on the X-ray table from the lithotomy position into normal supine lying, and 5–8 ml water soluble contrast medium, which is quickly reabsorbed and is tolerated by the tube epithelium, is slowly injected. (In nulliparae, often only 3–4 ml is given, while for patients with a large uterine cavity or with hydrosalpinx, 100 ml or more may be used). During the injection, very brief control films are made.

Once the uterine cavity has filled, the contrast medium passes into the tube and, in normal cases, into the abdominal cavity. After 10–15 min, if required, a delayed film can be taken showing the distribution of the contrast agent in the peritoneal cavity.

Contraindications

Pregnancy and any acute or chronic inflammatory process of the abdomen are absolute contraindications against HSG.

Complications and Diagnostic Errors

Complications such as salpingitis occur in about 1–3% of cases and may be seen even when every aseptic precaution against an ascending infection is taken.

Rarely, the passage of contrast agent into the abdominal cavity causes peritoneal irritation with cramp-like pain and possibly fever.

In the case of the uterine tube, a mistaken diagnosis may be caused by technical faults, errors in interpretation, and tube spasm, which mimics isthmic occlusion. Painful spasms are especially to be expected if the procedure is carried out without sedation or local anaesthesia. A misleading appearance of isthmic occlusion is more frequently seen by HSG than by only chromohydrotubation viewed endoscopically. Moreover, radiography may show intramural obliteration of the tube where at operation isthmic occlusion is revealed, which requires a different operative technique.

Summary

Even with the advent of modern non-radiological diagnostic techniques such as the various ultrasonographic techniques and endoscopic procedures, the use of new digital radiographic apparatus and improved contrast agents means that there is undoubtedly still a place for hysterosalpingography. Combining all the diagnostic techniques together is often the only way to achieve a complete investigation of the cavity and tube factors.

However, HSG alone is an insufficient basis on which to decide whether microsurgical fertilisation procedures or other procedures such as IVF or ICSI are indicated.

HSG can often be a useful technique to assess tube function postoperatively, e.g. to assess the success of microsurgical dilatation of an isolated tube occlusion.

References

Broer KH (1981) Diagnostic und Therapie zervikaler Sterilitätsursachen. In: Kaiser R, Schumacher GFB (eds) Menschliche Fortpflanzung. Thieme, Stuttgart

Fochem K (1984) Röntgendiagnostik in der Gynäkologie-Hysterosalpingographie. In: Schinz (ed) Radiologische Diagnostik in Klinik und Praxis, vol IV. Thieme, Stuttgart, pp 364–378

Frangenheim (1977) Die Laparoskopie in der Gynäkologie, Chirurgie und Pädiatrie, 3rd edn. Thieme, Stuttgart

Leidenberger F (1995) Diagnostik der gestörten Tubarfunktion und anatomische Veränderungen des Uterus und des kleinen Beckens. In: Schirren C, Leidenberger F et al (eds) Unerfüllter Kinderwunsch. Deutscher Ärzteverlag, Cologne, p 119
Ott JD, Fayez JA (1991) Hysterosalpingography. A Text and Atlas. Urban and Schwarzenberg, Baltimore
Semm (1969) Prüfung der Tubardurchgängigkeit. In: Käser O, Friedberg V, Ober KG, Thomsen K, Zander J (eds) Gynäkologie und Geburtshilfe, vol I. Thieme, Stuttgart
Stumpf PG, March CM (1980) Febrile morbidity following hysterosalpingography. Fertil Steril 33:487

Hysteroscopic Surgery

Y. Karaman

Introduction

Over past decades, the developments in respect of fiberoptics, light sources, high-resolution lenses, and endoscopic surgical instrumentation have led hysteroscopy to become an important diagnostic and therapeutic tool in patients with intrauterine disease. Diagnostic hysteroscopy, which was first performed in 1969, has found a place in routine office practice and allows the gynecologist to diagnose and treat abnormal uterine bleeding (secondary to polyps, leiomyomas, endometritis, and hyperplasia), to identify and remove intrauterine foreign bodies, and to diagnose intrauterine causes of infertility. As conservation of the uterus is increasingly being demanded by women who have abnormal bleeding, operative hysteroscopy has to become a routine surgical technique in the hands of gynecologists.

Instruments

Hysteroscopic instruments are manufactured by many companies. The hysteroscope assembly consists of a telescope 4–6 mm in diameter with 30° views (available with 0°, 15°, and 70° views) and an external stainless steel sheath approximately 5 mm in diameter for panoramic office hysteroscopy and 7–9 mm in diameter for operative hysteroscopy.

Diagnostic hysteroscopy can be done using three types of hysteroscope: the panoramic hysteroscope, the microcolpohysteroscope, and the contact hysteroscope.

The rigid panoramic hysteroscope is the most frequently used instrument. Flexible hysteroscopes can be easily used for tubal cannulation and when the abnormalities in the uterine cavity prevent access by rigid instruments, but operating channels of the flexible hysteroscope only permit the passage of extremely small and delicate instruments and do not provide the opportunity to carry out most operative hysteroscopic procedures.

Hamun's microcolpohysteroscope combines the panoramic and contact modes of hysteroscopy. It offers distant panoramic vision as well as very close contact vision with different magnification, ranging to 150×. In fact, the high magnification process allows direct observation of vitally stained living cells of suspicious areas of tissue.

The contact hysteroscope, which is used without an external light source and without expansion of the intrauterine cavity, is performed with the objective lens of the telescope in contact with the structure under observation. It cannot give a panoramic view of the intrauterine cavity, which limits its usefulness.

Instruments for Operative Hysteroscopy

Generally operative sheaths provide an operating channel for instruments and a part for inflow of distending medium. Recently many hysteroscope sheaths have become available with a separate part for outflow of fluid. Fluid enters throught the inner channel and is removed through a separate channel in the outer sleeve by using a suction pump or drainage by gravity.

Different operating instruments such as scissors, grasping forceps, unipolar coagulation electrodes, or laser fibers can be introduced through the operating channel. The Stors sheath also incorporates a movable bridge, which can aid in directing flexible instruments.

Fiber lasers such as the Nd:YAG, argon, and KTP-532 lasers can be used for hysteroscopic surgery. Because the laser energy is delivered through a flexible fiberglass fiber and because of the level of laser energy, they readily penetrate through liquid, making them suitable for hysteroscopic use. As the CO_2 laser does not have these advantages, its use for hysteroscopic surgery is not practical.

The laser most commonly used in the uterine cavity is the Nd:YAG laser, which has a wavelength of 1064 nm and which can penetrate deeply into tissues (4–6 mm). It can be used to cut when the fiber is placed in contact with the tissue.

Another hysteroscopic surgical instrument is the resectoscope, which consists of a working element including a 4-mm telescope (hysteroscope) on the inside and a finger-controlled mechanism to hold and manipulate an electrode. The shapes and sizes of electrodes vary. Loop electrodes are used for the resection of myomas, polyps, and endometrium, and roller-bar or roller-ball electrodes are available for coagulation of the endometrium. The double-channeled sheath is designed to allow inflow of a liquid medium and outflow through small openings at the outer end of the outer sheath.

Finally operative hysteroscopy is usually done by placing a good video camera in the telescope and watching the image on a video monitor. This allows greater comfort for the operator and provides a magnified view.

Uterine Distention

Both diagnostic and operative hysteroscopy need adequate distention of the uterine cavity. The most commonly used distention media are carbon dioxide gas, low viscosity fluid (e.g., dextrose, glycine, sorbitol, mannitol, and saline) and high-viscosity fluid (e.g., dextran 70).

Carbon dioxide is used widely for diagnostic hysteroscopy. It can be insufflated by a special insufflator for hysteroscopy with a maximum pressure of usually not more than 100 mmHg. It is not easy to perform most hysteroscopic operations using carbon dioxide because of the bleeding, the difficulty of adequate visualization, and the risk of fatal gas embolus.

Most surgeons prefer a liquid medium for operative hysteroscopy. The low-viscosity fluids are the most popular distention media for intrauterine laser surgery; they include dextrose (5% or 10%), saline (NaCl 0.9%), glycine 1.5%, and sorbitol/mannitol.

High-viscosity fluids, such as 32% dextran-70 in 10% glucose (Hyskon), have superb optical qualities and do not mix with blood, but caramelization during resectoscopy or Nd:YAG laser surgery can damage the instruments. Intravascular absorption has been linked to anaphylactic shock [1, 13]. Absorption of these solutions into the systemic circulation can cause serious complications, including electrolyte imbalance, fluid overload, and pulmonary or cerebral edema.

There are several pumps designed to control the flow and intrauterine pressure of liquid, which has to be 60–75 mmHg [14]. It seems prudent to keep intrauterine pressure as low as possible in order to provide good visualization of the intrauterine cavity.

Indications and Surgical Techniques

Abnormal Uterine Bleeding

Abnormal uterine bleeding in the latter part of a woman's reproductive years is one of the most important indications for hysterectomy. Once malignancy or another organic lesion has been ruled out, dysfunctional uterine bleeding is diagnosed.

Endometrial ablation was designed to control menorrhagia by destroying the endometrium. It requires the destruction of the endometrium through the basalis to decrease flow or create amenorrhea. The ND:YAG laser (because of its superior penetrating ability) and the hysteroscopic resectoscope with a roller-ball electrode have been advocated for this procedure.

Patients are usually treated preoperatively to thin the endometrium. This is done to facilitate ablation of the endometrial basalis layer. Some authors use danazol [5, 7] and others use GnRH analogues.

There are two techniques of endometrial ablation by means of the Nd:YAG laser. The first was described by Goldrath and used a power setting of 55 W and a 600-μm fiber which was dragged against the endometrium (touch or dragging technique) [4]. This touch technique destroys the endometrium and the superficial layers of the myometrium by vaporization and necrosis. Subsequently a nontouch or blanching technique was described which needs a power setting of 70 W and decreases the risk of bleeding and fluid intravasation [9]. In this technique, the fiber is held as close and as perpendicular to the surface of the endometrium as possible in order to achieve sufficient destruction of the endometrium. It is easy to blanch the fundus and upper portion of the uterus but not the lower uterine segment; for this reason, combination with a touch technique is needed for the lower uterine segment. Daniell et al. have used a nontouch technique with the Nd:YAG laser at the area of the tubal ostia and a roller-ball electrode for the rest of the procedure [2]. Their results showed amenorrhea to occur in 29% of patients, hypomenorrhea in 34%, and failure in 10%.

We use a technique similar to that of Daniell et al., employing the touch technique with the Nd:YAG laser at the area of the tubal ostia and the resectoscope with a wire loop electrode for the rest of the procedure. In 100 cases where we performed endometrial ablation, from 1990 to 1992, amenorrhea was observed in 25% of patients, hypomenorrhea in 59%, normal menses in 10%, and failure in 6%.

Myomectomy

Submucosal myomas or combined localization of intramural and submucosal myomas can cause menorrhagia, infertility, or recurrent abortion. Office hysteroscopy is necessary to establish the precise location of myomas. Preoperative medication is not necessary for a pediculated myoma. However, if more than 50% of the surface of the myoma is in an intramural location or if the diameter is 4–5 cm or more, preoperative treatment by means of a GnRH agonist for 4–8 weeks is necessary. This treatment can reduce the volume and the vascularization of the myoma, which can facilitate the operative procedure. After transection of the base of the myoma by Nd:YAG laser fiber, the myoma is manipulated with the end of the laser fiber (which is used as an écarteur); the cleavage area is thereby easily found and transected using the laser fiber. If the myoma is big, as much as possible is removed and the residual myoma is vaporized by multiple entry points as perpendicular as possible to the myoma (myolysis). The tissue is allowed to slough out. Second-look hysteroscopy is necessary in these cases to manage any residual tissue that might protrude into the uterine cavity [3]. Among our personal cases, 88 myomectomies have been performed by Nd:YAG laser; 81 of these cases had complete myomectomy and seven had partial myomectomy and myolysis. Second-look hysteroscopy was performed and in five cases a second myomectomy was undertaken. In two cases residual myoma completely disappeared, with complete necrosis and resorption. Of the 88 patients, eight had an infertility problem and four of these subsequently.

Excision of Uterine Septum

The mechanism by which the septate uterus causes pregnancy loss is not clear. However, this loss is due to poor implantation dynamics because of reduced blood supply to the septum and the ability of the half cavity to enlarge and distend without the irritability leading to premature labor. The association of incompetent cervix and uterine septum is another cause of pregnancy loss.

The diagnosis is usually made by hysterosalpingography and by hysteroscopy. Ultrasonography by the vaginal route can also make the diagnosis of uterine septum and clarify whether it is associated with bicornuate uterus.

But the usual method of diagnosis is combined hysteroscopy and laparoscopic examination.

Surgery is indicated if poor reproductive performance and pregnancy loss are due to the septum. A transection technique is used with a fiber of the Nd:YAG laser or with the resectoscope's electrode or scissors. The incision between the anterior and posterior walls proceeds from the apex of the septum to the fundus but not into the fundal myometrium. Arterial bleeding usually signifies entry into the myometrium. Concomitant laparoscopy is generally done to verify tubo-ovarian pathology in infertile women and the presence of a septate rather than a bicornuate uterus. Because of the avascular aspect of the septum, it will not heal together, and therefore the use of an intrauterine device is not necessary. The use of estrogen treatment after the operation is debatable and not of proven benefit.

Office hysteroscopy is necessary after 1 or 3 months. A review of patients managed by hysteroscopic surgery showed an increase of surviving infants from 3.7% to 78.4% [6, 8]. Our personal data using the Nd:YAG laser on 18 patients showed 13 pregnancies (72%) and ten term deliveries (57%). Excluding three patients with severe andrologic problems, these rates are 87% and 67% respectively.

Intrauterine Synechiae

Intrauterine synechiae can be managed by hysteroscopic surgery. Vigorous curettage, endometritis, intrauterine infection after an abortion, and intrauterine devices are the common causes of synechiae. Intrauterine adhesions can also be observed after metropasty, submucosal myomectomy, and endometrial tuberculosis. The diagnosis is made with hysterosalpingography and hysteroscopy because of infertility or pregnancy wastage.

There are many classification schemes for this clinical entity. Sugimato and March and also the American Fertility Society proposed an intrauterine classification of synechiae [10, 12].

Our personal data using the Nd:YAG laser and 100 μg ethynylestradiol per day for 6 weeks following the surgery showed 16 term pregnancies in 37 patients (43%). The pregnancy rates in patients with mild (n=12), moderate (n=16), and severe (n=3) synechiae were 50%, 56%, and 11% respectively.

In conclusion, with the development of new laser techniques, optics, light sources, and sophisticated video cameras, hysteroscopy, which is one of the oldest gynecologic endoscopic procedures, is becoming an essential tool in the diagnosis and management of intrauterine problems.

References

1. Ahmet M, Falcone T, Tulandi T, Houle G (1991) Anaphylactic reaction because of intra-uterine 32% dextran-70 instilation. Fertil Steril 55:1014–1016
2. Daniell JF, Kurtz BR, Ker RW (1992) Hysteroscopic endometrial ablation using the rollerball electrode. Obstet Gynecol 80:329 pp
3. Donnez J, Gillerot S, Bourgonjon D, Clercks F, Nisolle M (1990) Nd:YAG laser hysteroscopy in large submucoses fibroids. Fertil Steril 54:999
4. Goldrath MH, Fuller TA, Segal S (1981) Laser photo-vaporisation of endometrium for the treatment of menorrhagia. Am J Obstet Gyn 140:14

5. Goldrath MH (1990) Use of danazol in hysteroscopic surgery for menorrhagia. J Reprod Med 35:91
6. Hassiakos DK, Zourcas PA (1990) Transcervical division of uterine septa. Obstet Gynecol Surv 45:165
7. Loffler FP (1987) Hysteroscopic endometrial ablation with the Nd:YAG laser using a non-touch technique. Obstet Gynecol 69:679
8. Loffer FD (1992) Hysteroscopic laser surgery. Clin Obstet Gynecol 35:242
9. Lomano JM (1988) Dragging technique versus blanching technique for endometrial ablation with the Nd:YAG laser in the treatment of chronic menorrhagia. Am J Obstet Gynecol 159:152
10. March CM, Israel R, March AD (1978) Hysteroscopic management of intra-uterine adhesions. Am J Obstet Gynecol 130:653
11. Suginoto O (1978) Diagnostic and therapeutic hysteroscopy for traumatic intra-uterine adhesions. Am J Obstet Gynecol 131:539
12. The American Fertility Society (1988) The American Fertility Society Classifications of adnexal adhesions, distal tubal occlusion, tubal occlusion secondary to tubal ligation, tubal pregnancies, müllerian anomalies and intra-uterine adhesions. Fertil Steril 49:944
13. Trimbos-Kemper TCM, Veering BT (1989) Anaphylactic shock from intra-cavitary 32% dextran 70 during hysteroscopy. Fertil Steril 51:1053–1054
14. Vulgarapulos SP, Haley LC, Hulka JF (1991) Intra-uterine pressure and fluid absorption during continuous flow hysteroscopy. Am J Obstet Gynecol 167:386–391

Diagnostic Laparoscopy in the Infertile Woman

H. Hassa

Introduction

The basic principle of executing in infertility workup is to individualize the diagnostic tests and perform them as rapidly, inexpensively and noninvasively as possible. This approach helps to reduce frustration and stress for the affected couple as well as costs and possible complications that may be associated with certain procedures. In this context, more invasive tests such as laparoscopy and hysteroscopy should be reserved for later parts of the infertility workup and only after preliminary basic investigations have failed to disclose abnormalities that may be responsible for the couple's infertility.

Investigation of the infertile should be initiated with a thorough history and physical and pelvic examination. Semen analysis should be undertaken as the first diagnostic test. When performed correctly, it should give a rough idea regarding the fertility potential of the male.

Investigation of the female should establish the presence and quality of ovulation and patency of the fallopian tubes. Presence of ovulation can be established relatively reliably with luteal phase serum progesterone measurements.

Hysterosalpingography (HSG) should be the initial test for investigation of the uterine cavity and the fallopian tubes. Other tests of controversial value include timed endometrial biopsies, postcoital test, and determination of antisperm antibodies in either or both partners. Hormone analysis is performed when indicated. Ultrasound can be incorporated into the infertility workup if necessary.

Laparoscopy is the endoscopic visualization of the intraperitoneal pelvic structures and is indicated in the presence of an abnormal HSG or when the rest of the infertility examination fails to disclose an abnormality. Laparoscopy may be performed earlier during the diagnostic workup in cases with advanced age, clinical suspicion of pelvic adhesive disease, pelvic mass, or endometriosis. It is generally agreed that an infertility workup cannot be finalized without laparoscopy. In addition to its excellent diagnostic capabilities, laparoscopy also permits operative procedures during the same session. Laparoscopy has also been an integral part of certain assisted reproductive techniques such as gamete intrafallopian transfer (GIFT) and zygote intrafallopian transfer (ZIFT) (Gomel et al. 1986; Cohen 1970; Hassa 1987; Frangenheim 1991; Steptoe 1976).

Table 1 Indications for diagnostic laparoscopy in infertility (modified from Hassa 1987)

A. Assessment of the fallopian tubes:
1. Assessment or confirmation of tubal patency
2. Evaluation of fimbrial-ovarian relationship
3. Confirmation of distal tubal occlusion and its operability
4. Evaluation of functional proximal tubal occlusion encountered during a prior HSG (i.e., tubal spasm)
5. Evaluation of proximal tubal occlusive and nonocclusive pathological lesions (i.e., salpingitis isthmica nodosa, endometriosis, tuberculous salpingitis)
6. Evaluation of the proximal and distal tubal segments for suitability of a microsurgical reversal operation
7. Second-look evaluation of the fallopian tubes following microsurgery or laparoscopic surgery
B. Assessment of the ovaries:
1. Confirmation of ovulation with the observation of the ovulatory stigma
2. Assessment of patients with presumed luteinized unruptured follicle syndrome
3. Assessment of the ovaries for the presence of superficial and deep endometriosis (endometriomas)
4. Assessment of the ovaries and ovarian biopsy in patients with ovarian failure and chromosomal abnormalities. Laparoscopy for this latter indication is, however, controversial and rarely used.
C. Assessment of the uterus:
1. Diagnosis and treatment of uterine fibroids
2. Diagnosis of müllerian anomalies
3. Differential diagnosis of the septate and bicornuate uterus
D. Assessment of the peritoneal surfaces:
1. Diagnosis and staging of endometriosis
2. Diagnosis and treatment of pelvic adhesions
3. Evaluation and sampling of peritoneal fluid

Another important application of laparoscopy is to assess the treatment results following fertility-promoting procedures, following procedures that may potentially cause adhesions and following adjunctive treatment for gynecological cancer.

Indications for diagnostic laparoscopy in infertility are outlined in Table 1.

Indications for and Timing of Laparoscopy in Infertile Couples

The indications for and timing of laparoscopy differ in certain groups of infertile couples (Hassa 1987; Taylor and Gomel 1986; Portuondo and Irdala 1984):

Group 1. Couples with an Otherwise Normal Infertility Workup

This group includes patients with an otherwise normal infertility examination and a negative history for pelvic inflammatory disease, adhesions, pelvic pain, or endometriosis. The etiology of infertility has not been revealed through tests performed prior to a laparoscopy. The crucial aspects that determine the timing of laparoscopy in these patients are the age of the female partner and duration of infertility.

Fecundity demonstrates a clear relationship with the age of the woman. In women 20–25 years of age, mean duration to conception is 6 months, whereas in women over 30 this period is significantly prolonged. In women less than 30 years of age, laparoscopy should be performed at least 6 months after the completion of other diagnostic tests that yield no abnormalities. During this period the couple should be given a change for spontaneous conception. Empirical treatment aimed at improving cycle fecundity can also be instituted prior to laparoscopy. In women above 30, laparoscopy can be performed at an earlier period.

Group 2. Infertile Women with a Suspicious History

This group includes women with a history of:

a) Pulmonary tuberculosis
b) Unproven pelvic inflammatory disease
c) Prior use of an intrauterine device
d) Abdominal surgery for a nongynecologic indication (i.e., appendectomy)
e) Severe dysmenorrhea or pelvic pain.

The timing of laparoscopy in this group is determined according to the findings at HSG. When HSG is suspicious or clearly abnormal, laparoscopy should be undertaken immediately. It should be noted that HSG can give false-positive or false-negative results. The incidence of such findings may be as high as 23% and 76% respectively. When HSG and laparoscopy were compared, the correlation between the two tests was 59% in our patients (Hassa and Karacadağ 1981). It should be emphasized that HSG should be performed properly, with strict adherence to established techniques. A poorly performed HSG has little or no value from the diagnostic point of view. During the course of an infertility examination HSG and laparoscopy should not be regarded as competitive but rather complementary procedures. A concomitant hysteroscopy is necessary only if an abnormality in the uterine cavity has been observed in a previously obtained HSG and/or an ultrasound scan (Snowden and Jorett 1984).

In women with a suspicious history but a normal HSG, indications for laparoscopy are similar to those for group 1 patients.

Group 3. Women with a Positive History for Tubal or Peritoneal Disease

a) Women hospitalized for pelvic inflammatory disease
b) Women who had their IUD removed for pelvic inflammatory disease
c) Women with a history of endometrial or peritoneal tuberculosis
d) Women with a history of perforated appendicitis or peritonitis
e) Women diagnosed with endometriosis in a prior laparoscopy or laparotomy
f) Women with a history of pelvic surgery.

In this group of women, the conventional waiting period of 12 months is unwarranted. In women with normal HSG, laparoscopy should be performed immediately when HSG is suspicious or abnormal. In certain subjects, HSG may be bypassed, favoring a laparoscopy concomitant with a hysteroscopy. A properly timed laparoscopy dictates the future mode of management (tubal reconstruction vs IVP) in this group of women.

Group 4. Women Suspected of Having Pelvic Endometriosis

a) Women with otherwise normal infertility examinations. The incidence of pelvic endometriosis may reach up to 70% in couples with unexplained infertility (Hassa 1987).
b) Women with a history of pelvic pain or severe dysmenorrhea unresponsive to medical treatment.
c) Women with otherwise unexplained pelvic pain elicited during pelvic examination (Jansen and Russell 1986).
d) Women with other symptoms of pelvic endometriosis such as secondary dysmenorrhea, premenstrual spotting, rectal pain and tenesmus, pollakiuria, and hematuria.
e) Women with a previous history of endometriosis.

In women with unexplained infertility, the timing of laparoscopy is determined as in group 1. In others, laparoscopy should be initiated as early as possible and concomitant with other infertility tests when feasible.

Group 5. Anovulatory Patients Failing to Conceive Following Six Cycles of Ovulation Induction with First Line Agents (i.e., Clomiphene Citrate, Bromocriptine, Dexamethasone)

Laparoscopy is not indicated in anovulatory patients with a history and HSG findings negative for tubal or peritoneal disease. Ovulation induction should be commenced with first-line agents following evaluation of the male partner. However, assessment of the fallopian tubes and the pelvis should be undertaken when conception does not occur despite six ovulatory treatment cycles.

Group 6. Patients Failing to Conceive Following four to six Cycles of Artificial Insemination from Husband or Donor

Timing of indications for laparoscopy are similar to group 5.

Group 7. Prior to and Following Tubal Microsurgery

Laparoscopy is essential prior to tubal reconstructive surgery. In tubal factor infertility, the prognosis associated with reconstructive surgery is significantly dependent upon the nature and extent of adhesions, which are best assessed by laparoscopy. Principal indications for tubal microsurgery by laparotomy include tubocornual anastomosis for occlusive and nonocclusive proximal tubal pathologies, and tubotubal anastomosis for reversal of sterilization. In the former group, laparoscopy is necessary to differentiate cornual spasm during HSG from true intraluminal pathologies. It also permits the assessment of the remainder of the tubes and observation of any additional pathologies in the pelvis. In the latter, evaluation in the distal tube and its suitability for anastomosis should be considered. Not infrequently findings are at variance from what is expected from the operative report of previous sterilization. Laparoscopy may also be considered for a second-look following failed tubal reconstruction by laparotomy. This indication is, however, debatable as referral of patient to IVF appears to be a more rational approach.

Group 8. Infertility Scheduled to be treated by Assisted Reproductive Technologies such as IVF, GIFT, and ZIFT

The role of laparoscopy in this group of patients is both diagnostic and interventional. In the case of IVF, laparoscopy is not an essential procedure, particularly if IVF is being undertaken for male indications. Accessibility to the ovaries is not an indication for laparoscopy since the advent of transvaginal ultrasonographic follicular aspiration. Laparoscopy may be performed to evaluate the fallopian tubes in women planned to undergo GIFT of ZIFT.

Timing of Laparoscopy in Relation to the Menstrual Cycle

Laparoscopy may be performed any time during the menstrual cycle (Taylor and Gomel 1986). Performance during the luteal phase allows visualization of the corpus luteum and its stigma, and procurement of endometrial biopsy. However, when hysteroscopy is scheduled with it, the combined procedure is best timed in the follicular phase to enable better assessment of the uterine cavity. If an operative laparoscopy is to be done it should be planned in the follicular phase so that a corpus luteum does not complicate surgery on the involved ovary. Bleeding from the corpus luteum may be troublesome and is best avoided simply with timing. Endometriotic implants may be more visible during the luteal phase of the cycle. In the presence of ovarian endometriomas, timing of laparoscopy in the follicular phase will prevent the differential diagnosis of corpus luteum. Moreover bleeding from the corpus luteum in an ovary with an endometrioma will also be avoided. Laparoscopy is no longer considered to be an indication for diagnosis of the luteinized unruptured follicle syndrome. Laparoscopy performed for differential diagnosis of cornual spasm and true intraluminal tubal pathology should be scheduled during the follicular phase. There are two reasons for this: the follicular phase is preferred in case a hysteroscopy is needed and when transcervical tubal catheterization is performed, and lush luteal endometrium may preclude the passage of the tubal catheter into the proximal tube. It is best to avoid laparoscopy during menstruation because of the concern that dissemination of endometrial fragments may occur with chromopertubation.

The Conduct of Laparoscopy in Infertile Women

Laparoscopy in infertile women should be conducted in a systematic fashion (Hassa 1987; Semm 1977). It should begin with the inspection of the trocar entry to recognize early any inadvertent injury to intraabdominal structures. In the inspection of the upper abdominal cavity, adhesions between the diaphragm and the liver capsule suggest previous pelvic inflammatory disease with perihepatitis (Fitz-Hugh-Curtis syndrome). The gynecologic surgeon will occasionally be called upon to make differential diagnosis in the patient presenting with an acute abdomen of undefined etiology. In this setting visualization of the appendix gains importance.

For a detailed inspection of the genital organs, manipulation of the uterus with a uterine cannula and the Trendelenburg position are essential. A panoramic view of the uterus and the adnexae is obtained. It should be remembered that the objects under vision are smaller than they actually are when the telescope is withdrawn and get larger as the telescope is advanced. A suprapubic trocar is then advanced into the peritoneal cavity for insertion of the manipulation probe. Care should be exercised not to cause an inadvertent injury to the bladder or bowel during insertion of the trocar. The bladder is best emptied prior to initiation of the procedure.

Inspection of the Uterus and Neighboring Structures

Inspection of the Uterus. Most commonly the operator is expected to make the differential diagnosis between a septate and a bicornuate uterus. The fundis is flat and widened in the former while two distinct uterine horns can be observed in the latter. The location and size of the fibroids should be noted. Adhesions may be encountered between the uterus and the adnexal structures and between the uterus and the bowel or omentum. Occasionally the pelvis is totally obliterated with adhesions precluding visualization of the uterus and the adnexae.

Inspection of the Vesicouterine Pouch. The uterus is retroverted with the aid of the uterine cannula and vesicouterine pouch is inspected under close vision. This area can harbor adhesions and/or endometriotic implants. The vesicouterine pouch is also referred to as the starting point of the alpha (α) inspection of the pelvis. Following inspection of the vesicouterine pouch, the pouch of Douglas is evaluated and the procedure is continued with the uterus and adnexae.

Inspection of the Rectouterine Pouch (Pouch of Douglas). The uterus is anteverted with the aid of the uterine cannula. For this maneuver to be performed effectively, the buttocks of the patient should be at least 4–5 cm beyond the edge of the operating table. The presence and nature of fluid accumulation in the pelvis is noted and samples are withdrawn when indicated (i.e., cultures when PID, cytology when malignancy is suspected). Blood-tinged peritoneal fluid suggests the presence of retrograde menstruation, endometriosis, cyst rupture, or ectopic pregnancy.

Inspection of the Ovaries and the Fallopian Tubes

Inspection of the Ovaries. All surfaces of the ovaries should be inspected carefully. The ovaries should be flipped with the aid of a manipulating probe. The ovaries are the site of adhesions, functional cysts, benign and malignant neoplasia, and endometriosis. The posterior aspect of the ovary that lies in the ovarian fossa may harbor a corpus luteum or minimal endometriotic lesions. Ovarian cysts should be carefully inspected and gently manipulated if there is suspicion of malignancy. Papillary overgrowths on the cyst capsule, bilateral cysts, and presence of ascites may indicate malignancy. If the cyst is deemed benign, aspiration and biopsy could be undertaken. Adhesions may distort the normal tubo-ovarian relationship or encapsulate the ovaries. Laparoscopic adhesiolysis should be performed in such cases when feasible and safe.

Inspection of the Fallopian Tubes. According to the alpha system of inspection the right tube is evaluated first. The tubocornual portion of the tubes should be inspected carefully and palpated with the manipulating probe. Occlusive and nonocclusive lesions of the tubocornual segment should be defined. Salpingitis isthmica nodosa, endometriosis, tuberculous salpingitis and nonspecific inflammation and fibrosis are some of the more common lesions that may be responsible for proximal intraluminal tubal pathology. These lesions commonly present with fusiform enlargements of the tubocornual region. The fimbrial end of the tube should be inspected en face in order to gain maximum information regarding anatomical integrity and free flow of dye. Agglutination of the fimbria, fimbrial phimosis, and distal tubal occlusion are the most common lesions in the distal ampulla and infundibulum. Occasionally the tube may be constricted or obstructed a few centimeters proximal to the fimbrial end, which is termed prefimbrial phimosis or occlusion. Distal tubal pathologies are not infrequently accompanied by adhesions between the tubes and neighboring structures, most commonly the ovary. Information obtained regarding the extent and tenacity of the adhesions and the thickness and diameter of the tubal wall will dictate the mode of further management. IVF should be preferred over reconstructive surgery in unfavorable cases.

Following the inspection, the fallopian tubes should be palpated with the probe throughout its full length. Chromopertubation is the last step in evaluation of the tubes at laparoscopy. The dye (methylene blue or indigo carmine) should be injected very slowly with little pressure in order to avoid spasm of the cornual tubal segment. Free spill of the dye should be noted from the distal end of the tube. Localized collections of dye in the tube may be due to physiologic contractions of the tube or intraluminal pathologies.

Documentation of Laparoscopic Findings

Laparoscopic findings should be documented immediately after the procedure. Sketching the findings in a diagram is very useful. Video documentation and storage may be preferred (Brooks 1993).

References

Brooks PG (1993) Documentation in laparoscopy. In: Saderstrom RM (ed) Operative laparoscopy. Raven, New York

Cohen MR (1970) Endoscopy at the infertile female. In: Cohen MR (ed) Laparoscopy, culdoscopy and gynecography. Saunders, Philadelphia

Frangenheim H (1991) Laparoskopie. In: Turanli IS, Broer KH (eds) Sterilite ve IVF (Tüp Bebek) Tedavisi. Önel, Cologne (in Turkish)

Gomel V, Taylor PJ, Yuzpe AA (1986) Indication, contraindication and complications. In: Gomel V, Taylor PJ, Yuzpe AA, Rioux JE (eds) Laparoscopy and hysteroscopy in gynecologic practice. Year Book Medical, Chicago

Hassa H (1987) Gynecological Laparoscopy. Anadolu Universiti, Basimevi, Eskisehir (in Turkish)

Hassa H, Karacadağ O (1981) Infertil olgularda tubal faktörün dêgerlendirilmesi (Turkish). Anadolu, Tip Dergisi. 3:405–409

Portuondo JA, Irdala JP (1984) Clinical selection of infertile patients for laparoscopy. Int J Fertil 29:234–239

Semm K (1977) The technique of gynecologic laparoscopy. In: Semm K (ed) Atlas of gynecologic laparoscopy and hysteroscopy. Saunders, Philadelphia

Snowden EU, Jorett JC (1984) Comparison of diagnostic accuracy of laparoscopy, hysteroscopy and hysterosalpingography in evaluation of female infertility. Fertil Steril 41:709–712

Steptoe P (1976) Laparoscopy for infertility and fertility. In: Steptoe P (ed) Endoscopy. Appleton, New York

Taylor PJ, Gomel V (1986) Endoscopy in the infertile patient. In: Gomel V, Taylor PJ, Yuzpe AA, Rioux JE (eds) Laparoscopy and hysteroscopy in gynecologic practice. Year Book Medical, Chicago

Management of Tubal Infertility: In Vitro Fertilization Versus Reconstructive Surgery

V. Gomel and P.J. Taylor

Introduction

Reconstructive surgery was the only therapeutic option for women with tubal infertility until the introduction of in vitro fertilization and embryo transfer (IVF). The wide clinical application of IVF and assisted reproductive techniques offers such women a realistic alternative.

In vitro fertilization and embryo transfer replaces the reproductive function of the fallopian tube. Indeed, tubal factor infertility remains a principal indication for IVF [12].

In the last decade and a half operative laparoscopy has been increasingly used in the treatment of tubal and peritoneal infertility [3, 4]. This approach permits the undertaking of a reconstructive procedure during the initial diagnostic laparoscopy without significantly increasing the risk of the intervention. Additional advantages are the elimination of a laparotomy incision resulting in less postoperative discomfort, reduced requirements for postoperative analgesia, a shorter convalescence and a quicker return to normal activity [3–5].

During the same interval a vast body of experience has been gained in IVF procedures worldwide. While IVF techniques continue to require precision and remain labour-intensive, they have been progressively simplified. Oocyte recovery is now almost exclusively performed through the vaginal route under ultrasonographic control and local anaesthesia; laboratory procedures, embryo transfer and support of the luteal phase have been largely standardized. All of these developments have transformed IVF into an ambulatory procedure. There has been gradual improvement in results.

In the face of these developments in IVF, is there still a place for reconstructive tubal surgery? This chapter will attempt to address this question and to elucidate the place of each treatment option.

The goals for an infertile couple should be either a live birth or the ability to feel that they have exhausted all reasonable attempts to achieve a pregnancy. If the latter is to be the outcome, the two persons are more likely to resolve the conflict if they have been actively involved in the decision-making process [6].

As is evident from the preceding, the infertile woman with tubal damage has two therapeutic options to achieve a pregnancy: reconstructive surgery or IVF. However, surgery and IVF must not be regarded as competitive but rather as complementary options to achieve the desired goal. The choice of treatment will be influenced by various considerations, both technical and non-technical [6].

Technical Considerations

In vitro fertilization is obviously the only treatment option for those with inoperable fallopian tubes and tubal disease coincident with another important fertility factor [7]. For those to whom reconstructive tubal surgery offers a greater chance of success, the logical sequence of treatment would be tubal surgery first, reserving IVF for those to whom the former proves to be unsuccessful.

The provision of accurate information regarding both IVF and tubal surgery is essential in the decision-making process of the couple. The live birth rate per cycle of IVF and the cumulative rate after multiple cycles of treatment must be given, along with information on potential complications of the procedure, multiple pregnancy, abortion and ectopic pregnancy rates. In addition, the effect of frozen embryo replacement upon the cumulative pregnancy rate must be considered in the analysis. Similar information must also be provided regarding reconstructive tubal surgery. It is imperative that such figures reflect local experience, which may be better or worse than reported international data [6]. However, in this chapter, figures derived from the world literature will be used.

In Vitro Fertilization

The Society for Assisted Reproductive Technology recently published assisted reproductive technology results for the year 1992 [8]. They were 29404 initiated cycles of IVF, of which 24996 led to retrieval of oocytes. This represents voluntary reporting by 249 programs in the United States and Canada. The yield in terms of deliveries per retrieval was 16.8%. While most registries now report pregnancy and delivery rates per oocyte pick-up cycles, the treated couple is interested to know rates based upon cycles initiated. Considering the cancellation rate was 15.4%, the delivery rate per cycle initiated would be approximately 14.3%. French data have shown that the pregnancy rate remains relatively constant in successive cycles [9]. Based upon this finding and the preceding figure of 14.3%, a cumulative delivery rate of 46% would be expected after four cycles of treatment. However, recent data have shown a steady decline in the success rate with successive failed IVF attempts [10]. The cumulative pregnancy rate was 13% after one IVF cycle, 19% after two, 24% after three and 27% after four. The decline in pregnancy appears to affect women in advanced reproductive age and those with polycystic ovarian disease and couples with male factor infertility. Whereas the cumulative pregnancy rate after four cycles of treatment was 43% in women 35 years of age or younger, among those between 36 to 40 this rate was only 29% [10].

While the delivery rate may be improved by replacement of frozen embryos, the net effect would be limited because not all cycles provide spare embryos nor would all the frozen embryos withstand the thawing process. Transfer of cryopreserved embryos yields a delivery rate of approximately 11.5% [8].

In vitro fertilization and embryo transfer is not risk-free, especially in stimulated cycles. Although uncommon, ovarian hyperstimulation, bleeding and infection occur [11, 12]. Pregnancies resulting from IVF have an abortion rate of 20%–25%. The overall tubal pregnancy rate is 5%–6% of clinical pregnancies [2, 8, 9]. In a study from our centre, the rate of tubal pregnancy among patients without tubal factor infertility was only 2.6% of clinical pregnancies. However, this rate was 12% in patients with prior tubal disease, the very patients who must choose between IVF and tubal surgery [13]. The twin pregnancy rate is around 25%. Four percent of pregnancies are triplets or a high order of multiples [8]. The Caesarean section rate is over 35% and approximately one-quarter of the births are premature. It is significant that more than 10% of monofoetal births are preterm. This rate is obviously significantly greater among twins, triplets or more. The perinatal mortality is high, approximately 30 per 1000. This rate is also increased among singletons (approximately 19 per 1000 [14].

Reconstructive Surgery

The overall risks of reconstructive tubal surgery, performed either laparoscopically or by laparotomy, are small and include recognized complications of anaesthesia and surgery. Surgery, if successful, will offer multiple cycles in which to achieve conception and the opportunity to have more than one pregnancy. The abortion rate subsequent to reconstructive tubal surgery is not increased over that of a normal population. The live birth and ectopic pregnancy rates are dependent upon the specific nature of the tubal disease and the extent of tubal damage [15].

Non-technical Considerations

The non-technical considerations include age, cost and the wishes of the couple. Female fecundity is adversely affected by age. This becomes more evident after 40 years of age.

A viable birth rate of 45% has been reported after reversal of sterilization in women 40 years of age or more. In this series the anastomosed tube(s) had a minimum length of 4 cm and the follow-up period was at least 1 year [16]. The comparable figures for IVF (per oocyte recovery cycle) are 8.3% at the ages of 40 and 41 and 2.4% thereafter [1]. In women of advanced reproductive age, the marked decline of fecundity rate per cycle of IVF must be weighed against the fact that reconstructive surgery offers multiple cycles during which conception may occur. Therefore, while the younger woman may consider surgery first and IVF thereafter (if this becomes necessary), those between 37 and 40 years of age may be advised to consider IVF first.

The effect of cost, depending on the jurisdiction and means of the couple will also play an important role in the decision-making process.

Investigation

Thorough investigation of both the male and female partner will aid in the selection of therapeutic options.

Hysterosalpingography (HSG) and laparoscopy are complementary methods of assessing tubal and peritoneal factors. A well-performed preliminary HSG is most useful. It will provide invaluable information about the uterus including the presence of congenital anomalies, synechiae, endometrial polyps, submucous fibroids and even a forgotten IUD. It will reveal proximal tubal occlusion, non-occlusive proximal tubal disease, distal tubal occlusion and the nature of the intratubal architecture. These findings will greatly influence the subsequent investigation and treatment [4, 17]. With those seeking a sterilization reversal, initial review of the operative and pathology reports of the sterilization will frequently yield information regarding the length and region of tube removed or destroyed and thus give an indication regarding reversibility and prognosis [4, 18].

The presence of severe semen abnormalities in addition to tubal factor infertility will favour IVF as primary treatment, although the success rate in these circumstances is lower.

Selection

Periadnexal adhesive disease may be the only apparent lesion or may be present in addition to tubal occlusion. The tubes may be occluded at their outer end or proximally as the final result of pathological processes, or may have been interrupted by a previous sterilization.

If periadnexal adhesive disease is the sole lesion, laparoscopic salpingo-ovariolysis, performed preferably at the time of the initial diagnostic laparoscopy, is the approach of choice. There is a live birth rate of approximately 50%–60% and an ectopic pregnancy rate of 5% among patients who have undergone this procedure. Agglutination of the fimbriae (fimbrial phimosis) will necessitate a fimbrioplasty which may also be performed laparoscopically. This condition frequently coexists with periadnexal adhesions, which are dealt with first. The live birth rate after fimbrioplasty is between 40% and 48% and the rate of ectopic is 5%–6% [19–24].

Distal tubal occlusion (hydrosalpinx) may be treated surgically. In major published series the live birth rate following microsurgical salpingostomy varies between 19% and 35%, and the ectopic rate between 5% and 18%. The improvement in results yielded by microsurgical salpingostomy is much less impressive than that attained using other tubal procedures [15, 25–28]. Furthermore salpingostomy, performed laparoscopically, in appropriately selected cases, yields almost similar results [21, 23, 29–32].

The factors that affect the outcome of salpingostomy include: (1) distal ampullary diameter, (2) tubal wall thickness, (3) nature of the tubal endothelium at the neostomy site, (4) extent of adhesions and (5) type of adhesions. These factors have been quantified in a numerical scoring system which permits estimation of the surgical outcome [33]. In cases deemed favourable (mild), the reported live birth rates after microsurgical salpingostomy vary between 50% and 70%. This rate drops to less than 20% in those scored as unfavourable (severe) [28, 34]. In such cases IVF may be the initial treatment of choice. If surgery appears to be the initial treatment of choice, whether to proceed with an immediate laparoscopic salpingostomy or to undertake reconstructive microsurgery must depend upon local experience and success rates with both approaches.

In cases of proximal tubal occlusion, selective salpingography and/or transcervical fallopian tube cannulation may be useful in elucidating false-positive results obtained by hysterosalpingography and in overcoming obstruction associated with a mucous plug or cornual synechiae (35]. True pathological tubal occlusion resulting from salpingitis isthmica nodosa, endometriosis and extensive postinflammatory fibrosis may be treated by microsurgical tubocornual anastomosis. The reported live birth rates after such procedures vary between 37% and 58% and ectopic pregnancy rates between 5% and 7% [15, 26, 36, 37]. On the basis of the results obtained in our centre, in such cases we offer microsurgical correction as the first line of treatment.

Laparoscopic tubotubal anastomosis to reconstruct a previous tubal sterilization and segmental tubal excision (i.e. for ectopic pregnancy) are currently under exploration. However, these techniques, for the present, must be viewed as experimental. These, like other microsurgical reconstructive tubal procedures, are now performed through a mini-laparotomy incision and on a short (24 h or less) hospital stay basis [38, 39]. Furthermore, microsurgery excels in tubotubal anastomosis and produces excellent results which are principally dependent upon the length of the reconstructed tube. Live birth rates of 60%–80% can be achieved provided the reconstructed tube is longer than 4 cm and the ampullary portion more than 1 cm [15, 18, 26, 40, 41]. The tubal pregnancy rates are usually low. Microsurgical reconstruction offers the opportunity to conceive more than once. This and the impressive results would favour the choice of this approach over IVF.

Surgical correction of a Kroener (fimbriectomy) sterilization is possible but the outcome is dependent upon the remaining ampullary length. Live birth rates of approximately 30% have been reported when more than 50% of the ampulla has been preserved [15, 26]. The remaining tubal length can be determined by hysterosalpingography, and if sufficient ampulla is not present IVF should be recommended as initial treatment.

Conclusion

The development of operative laparoscopy, tubal microsurgery and IVF in the last 20 years has significantly improved the outlook of couples suffering from tubal infertility. These are complementary approaches which may be used singly or in combination.

The choice of the primary and any subsequent treatment is dependent upon a careful consideration of both non-technical and technical factors. These must be individualized to the circumstances of the patients. Information about success and complication rates of the available treatment options must accurately reflect local experience. Active involvement of the couple in the decision-making process is more likely to result in resolution of the conflict of infertility if treatment should prove unsuccessful [6].

References

1. FIVNAT 1989 et bilan general 1986–1989 (1990) Contrib Fertil Sexual 18:588–600
2. Medical Research International, Society for Assisted Reproductive Technology, The American Fertility Society (1991). In vitro fertilization-embryo transfer (IVF-ET) in the United States: 1989 results from the IVF-ET registry. Fertil Steril 55:14–23
3. Gomel V (1995) From microsurgery to laparoscopic surgery: a progress. Fertil Steril 63:464–468
4. Gomel V, Taylor PJ (1995) Diagnostic and operative gynecologic laparoscopy. Mosby, St. Louis
5. Gomel V (1989) Operative laparoscopy: time for acceptance. Fertil Steril 52:1–11
6. Gomel V, Taylor PJ (1992) In vitro fertilization versus reconstructive tubal surgery. J Assist Reprod Genet 9:306–309
7. Gomel V (1983) Microsurgery in female infertility. Little Brown and Co., Boston, pp 129–134
8. Assisted reproductive technology in the United States and Canada: 1992 results generated from the American Fertility Society/Society for Assisted Reproductive Technology Registry (1994). Fertil Steril 62:1121–1128
9. Cohen J (1991) The efficiency and efficacy of IVF and GIFT. Hum Reprod 6:613–618
10. Lurie D, Check JH, Callan C, Baker A, Benfer K (1993) IVF success rate declines with each failed attempt. Presented at the Pacific Coast Infertility Society Meeting, 1993
11. Tureck RW, Garcia C-R, Blasco L, Mastroianni L Jr (1993) Perioperative complications arising after transvaginal oocyte retrieval. Obstet Gynecol 81:590–593
12. Dicker D, Ashkenazi J, Feldberg D, Levy T, Dekel A, Ben-Rafael Z (1993) Severe abdominal complications after transvaginal ultrasonographically guided retrieval of oocytes for in vitro fertilization and embryo transfer. Fertil Steril 59:1313–1315
13. Zouves C, Erenus M, Gomel V (1991) Tubal ectopic pregnancy after in vitro fertilization and embryo transfer: A role for proximal occlusion or salpingectomy after failed distal tubal surgery? Fertil Steril 56:691–695
14. Rufat P, Olivennes F, deMouzon J, Dehan M, Frydman R (1994) Task force report on the outcome of pregnancies and children conceived by in vitro fertilization (France: 1987 to 1989). Fertil Steril 61:324–330
15. Gomel V (1983) Microsurgery in female infertility. Little, Brown and Co., Boston, pp 225–244
16. Trimbos-Kemper TCM (1990) Reversal of sterilization in women over 40 years of age: a multicenter survey in the Netherlands. Fertil Steril 53:575–577
17. Gomel V, Taylor PJ, Yuzpe AA, Rioux JE (1986) Laparoscopy and hysteroscopy in gynecologic practice. Year Book Medical Publishers, Chicago, pp 77–79
18. Gomel V (1980) Microsurgical reversal of female sterilization: a reappraisal. Fertil Steril 33:587–597
19. Gomel V (1975) Laparoscopic tubal surgery in infertility. Obstet Gynecol 46:47–48
20. Gomel V (1983) Salpingo-ovariolysis by laparoscopy in infertility. Fertil Steril 340:607–610
21. Gomel V (1983) Microsurgery in female infertility. Little, Brown and Co., Boston, pp 143–144

22. Bruhat MA, Mage G, Manhes H et al (1983) Laparoscopy procedures to promote fertility: ovariolysis and salpingolysis results of 93 selected cases. Acta Eur Fertil 14:476–479
23. Dubuisson JB, Borquet deJoliniere J, Aubriot FX et al (1990) Terminal tuboplasties by laparoscopy: 65 consecutive cases. Fertil Steril 54:401–403
24. Fayez JA (1983) An assessment of the role of operative laparoscopy in tuboplasty. Fertil Steril 39:476–479
25. Gomel V (1978) Salpingostomy by microsurgery. Fertil Steril 29:387–389
26. Gomel V (1980) Clinical results of infertility microsurgery. In: Crosignani PG, Rubin BL (eds) Microsurgery in female infertility. Academic Press, London
27. Gomel V, Swolin K (1980) Salpingostomy: microsurgical technique and results. Clin Obstet Gynecol 23:1243–1258
28. Boer-Meisel ME, te Velde ER, Habbema JDF, Kardaun JWPF (1986) Predicting the pregnancy outcome in patients treated for hydrosalpinx: a prospective study. Fertil Steril 45:23–29
29. Gomel V (1977) Salpingostomy by laparoscopy. J Reprod Med 18:265–268
30. Canis M, Mage G, Pouly JL, Manhes H, Wattiez A, Bruhat MA (1991) Laparoscopic distal tuboplasty: report of 87 cases and a 4-yeare experience. Fertil Steril 56:616–621
31. Daniell JF, Herbert CM (1984) Laparoscopic salpingostomy utilizing to CO_2. Fertil Steril 41:558–563
32. McComb P, Paleoulogou A (1991) The intussusception salpingostomy technique for the therapy of distal ovoductal occlusion at laparoscopy. Obstet Gynecol 78:443–447
33. Gomel V (1988) Distal tubal occlusion. Fertil Steril 49:946–948
34. Gomel V, Erenus M (1990) Prognostic value of the American Fertility Society's Classification for Distal Tubal Occlusion. Fertil Steril (Suppl) 54:S106
35. Kerin JF, Surrey ES, Williams DB, Daykhovsky L, Grundfest WS (1991) Falloposcopic observations of endotubal isthmic plugs as a cause of reversible obstruction and their histological characterization. J Laparoendosc Surg 1:103–110
36. Donnez J, Casanas-Roux F (1986) Prognostic factors influencing the pregnancy rate after microsurgical cornual anastomosis. Fertil Steril 46:1089–1092
37. McComb P (1986) Microsurgical tubocornual anastomosis for occlusive cornual disease: reproducible results without the need for tubouterine implantation. Fertil Steril 46:571–577
38. Gomel V, Taylor PJ (1993) Reconstructive tubal surgery in the female. In: Insler V, Lunenfeld B (eds) Infertility, male and female. Churchill Livingstone, Edinburgh, pp 481–503
39. Gomel V, Rowe TC (1995) Microsurgical tubal reconstruction and reversal of sterilization. In: Wallach EE, Zacur HA (eds) Reproductive medicine and surgery. Mosby, St. Louis, pp 1074–1092
40. Gomel V (1977) Tubal reanastomosis by microsurgery. Fertil Steril 28:59–65
41. Pie Xue, Yuen-Yu Fa (1989) Microsurgical reversal of female sterilization. J Reprod Med 34:451–455

Complications of Laparoscopic Examinations

H. FRANGENHEIM

Introduction

In general laparoscopic-pelviscopic examinations are considered to be a reliable tool, simple in handling and available to any operator. Experience, however, reveals the contrary, i.e., with any invasive examination specific complications may arise, and laparoscopy is no exception. At any phase of laparoscopy complications may occur, and numerous statistics are available detailing the essential ones.

Statistics

It is questionable how far statistics dating back to the mid-1970 s are still significant. Preliminary statistics compiled by internist [6] cannot be projected to the gynecological situation. Patients of internists have worse conditions, and the techniques applied and the technical equipment are different.

French statistics [4, 9] reveal similarities. A majority of cardiorespiratory complications and deaths resulted from different intraperitoneal pressures and methods of positioning the patients. Preliminary German statistics report analogous results comprising complications arising from the development of the laparoscopic technique and equipment (optics, insufflation and coagulation equipment, forceps, supporting tools, etc.). Statistics reported in 1978 by Chamberlain [3], annual data of the American Society of Gynecological Laparoscopy (AAGL) [12, 13, 14], and the findings by Semm [15, 16] et al. commencing in the mid-1970 s reflected the situation at that time. Since then, laparoscopy has become an internationally recognized clinical procedure.

In an essay [contribution to manual 5–8] as well as in numerous publications, Fragenheim has described complications arising from laparoscopy and repeatedly submitted proposals for their possible prevention. Borten [2] has authored a book entitled "Laparoscopic Complication, Prevention and Management" which comprehensively covers the subject, though without any significantly new aspects. Minimally invasive surgery in gynecology and the use of surgery in combination with different types of laser have generated new and different kinds of complications on which there is still a relative lack of information. Laparoscopy has been adopted by numerous general surgeons for new indications, and this will yield more data on the complications of surgical laparoscopy.

Frequency of Complications

Recent statistics indicate a mortality of 1 in 100 000 laparoscopies. Emphysema occurs in approximately 5% of cases, abdominal lesions (mainly coagulation damage) in 1%–3%, cardiorespiratory disturbances in 0.5% and other complications in approximately 1%. Complications necessitated laparotomy in ca. 1%.

To prevent complications, the safety prescriptions for the equipment must be met, and patients must be carefully selected to exclude those susceptible to complications.

Information

Patients must be informed about laparoscopy and the possible complications that might necessitate laparotomy. Written consent to the operation should be obtained. If a laparoscopic tubal sterilization is planned, the husband's consent is not required. However, to avoid any problems that might arise from civil law it is recommended that the partner's consent is obtained.

Technical Implementation of Laparoscopy

Before starting the laparoscopic examination the good function of all optics and auxiliary equipment must be guaranteed! The anesthetist decides on the method of anesthesia to be applied, which may be total anesthesia, intubation, or local anesthesia, and is responsible for the necessary examinations prior to anesthesia.

Although anesthetists are not always available, their presence should be ensured if a long micro-invasive operation is to be performed. Their experience reduces the risk of complications since they can promptly and properly react using appropriate equipment, should the need arise. In routine laparoscopies primary complications of anaesthesia, e.g., cardiocirculatory collapses, rarely occur (approx. 0.5%); nevertheless, EKG monitoring is recommended. In long operations with permanent automatic refill of CO_2 an undercooling of the patient may happen. When starting anaesthesia the abdomen may be erroneously distended. After the introduction of a stomach tube the air escapes, avoiding gastric perforation. A stomach tube must not be introduced routinely.

Preparation

The bladder should be emptied by spontaneous micturition with repeated catheterization if a long time has elapsed before the commencement of laparoscopy. Occasionally a filled bladder is punctured since urinary reflux may provoke inflammatory complications. If the microinvasive operation is expected to last long, a catheter should be introduced. Vagina and abdomen should be disinfected (although omphalitis occurs relatively seldom). The patient is placed on the operation table in a position with the head lowered (15%–20%) according to Trendelenburg. An extreme lowering of the head by 45% – as recommended in former times – is not necessary since cardiorespiratory disturbances may result. A gynecological examination aims at excluding inflammatory processes and eliminating secondary laparoscopic complications and ascending infections.

Application of Pneumoperitoneum and Introduction of the Laparoscopic Trocar

Most serious incidents due to laparoscopic examinations occur during the application of the pneumoperitoneum and the introduction of the laparoscopic trocar. The appropriate placement of the pneumoperitoneum, leaving sufficient distance between the posterior abdomen and abdominal organs, is the decisive factor in a successful laparoscopy. Insertion points of the insufflation needle are the lower umbilical cavity or approximately 4 cm left of or above the umbilicus (at these points normally no adhesions are to be expected); insertion may be performed through the posterior vaginal fornix in adipose patients or, in the case of repeated operations, by mid-incision on the left-hand side in the lower third of the conjugate spina iliaca anterior to the umbilicus. When inserting the Veress needle to install the pneumoperitoneum the abdominal cutis should be lifted either by hand or by skin clip. Slowly the Veress or a similar needle is moved forward at 45°. Cutis, panniculus adiposus, and peritoneum are penetrated. As soon as the needle reaches the abdominal cavity, insufflation is commenced at 1 l CO_2 per minute, and constantly increased to 2–3 l per minute. Approximately 1 l CO_2 is resorbed per minute, which leads to a reduced insufflation period if 2–3 l is introduced. Intraperitoneal pressure must be measured continuously.

The value of so-called secruity tests, e.g., aspiration after injection of liquid or the needle test, is controversial. In my opinion they should not be carried outh. If *emphysema* is generated during the insufflation of gas, a period of 10 min should be allowed to elapse so that resorption can occur; thereafter vision will be clear again. In the event of extensive intraperitoneal or subcutaneous emphysema becoming evident in the abdomen or neck, or pericardial emphysema, a longer pause may be required, or the operation should be postponed to eliminate any risk.

The formation of aeroembolisms is rarely observed if small vessels are incidentally punctured. After measurements according to Lindemann, carbonic acid is bound to the alkali reserve of the blood and resorbed to a certain degree. The structure of the body and relaxation of the patient determine the volume of gas to be insufflated. Intraperitoneal pressure should be measured and not exceed 15–200 mmHg. Previous data on higher pressures are no longer valid. As soon as a sufficient pneumoperitoneum is installed, the laparoscopic trocar is introduced by incision in the lower umbilical cavity. The abdomen should be lifted either by hand or by two towel forceps. Alternatively the fascia is lifted and pierced with the tip of the three-cornered trocar. Conical trocars must be pushed forward at a different pressure, most often by rotation. I consider them more dangerous since the pressure of the conical trocars might cause injuries, given the short distance (approximately 2 cm) between the posterior abdomen and major vessels.

Introduction of the Trocar and Start of Laparoscopy

The introduction of the trocar represents one of the most dangerous moments. The danger of perforating a distended abdomen has been described. A lesion must be stitched immediately either microsurgically or by extending the small median section and drawing forth the stomach. If an enterocentesis has incidentally occurred a malodorous gas escapes from the trocar husk, a situation whereby the trocar husk should remain in situ. The patient must be laparotomized, and the perforation must be found and stitched. If the bladder has been injured it is recommended that a suprapubic permanent catheter be introduced. Careful postoperative stationary treatment and appropriate administration of antibiotics must be ensured. When introduced according to the Z-stitch method the laparoscopic trocar has to be shifted 4–5 cm to the right as soon as it has passed the epidermis to be continued in the vertical direction parallel to the axis. It has been reported that a number of major, but unrecognized lesions of the ascending colon have occurred with this Z-method, causing severe complications. Therefore, this method should no longer be applied.

Lesions of vessels require an approach guided by different aspects. Lesions of reticular vessels are characterized by profuse bleeding from between the reticular leaves or on the reticulum. In most cases they can only be stopped by laparotomy.

Lesions of major vessles caused by either the insufflation cannula or the laparoscopic trocar generally provoke a further circular rupture of the vessel wall, regardless of the size of the lesion. The entire vessel volume has thus been opended, resulting in massive bleeding. Such bleeding from iliac vessels, the aorta, and the vena cava generally extends retroperitoneally. Lesions of major vessels cause a loss of blood in the range of 1 l within 20 s. Vasovagal reflexes impede the introduction of infusion cannulas for transfusions to stabilize blood circulation. As a safety measure it is recommended that cannulas be introduced before the operation begins.

In the case of a lesion of the aorta, attention must be paid to the bifurcation which lies on the level of the incision site of the laparoscopic trocar, i.e., inferior to the umbilicus. Anatomic variations are, however, possible, being known as superior or inferior bifurcation. Less experienced operators are once again advised to introduce the trocars approximately 4 cm below the umbilicus. This will help to minimize vasal lesions which are hardly recognized by the operator since the blood does not pour into the abdominal cavity, as might be assumed, but rather extends retroperitoneally from the renal pelvis into the small pelvis. The anaesthetist is the first to recognize the fall of blood pressure and the collapse. By compression of the aorta and infusions, time is gained until a vasal surgeon can intervene. Such a very severe and in most cases lethal complication explains why laparoscopies should be performed in a surgery room. An immediate emergency operation requires adequate preconditions with an experienced anaesthetist not only trained for normal gynecological operations.

Electrosurgical Operations – Complications

Any electrosurgical operation requires preliminary comprehensive information on the various coagulation methods, i.e., monopolar or bipolar high frequency current and thermocoagulation, and their specific complications. Any operator using laser technolgoy should have adequate knowledge about its specific properties and fields of application. Different lasers are still being tested and cannot yet be commented on.

Most prominent are complications arising from laparoscopic tubal sterilizations. Too extensive tubal coagulations may cause insufficient blood supply to the ovaries, leading to disturbances of the menstrual cycle and precocious menopause.

If the intestine is erroneously touched by a tool not yet cooled down, necroses occur, becoming manifest 24 h later in diffuse lower abdominal complaints. Depending on the degree of coagulation the small intestine will perforate after 2–7 days, initiated by a local pelviperitonitis which may rupture and lead to a diffuse peritonitis with all its symptoms. The death of a patient caused by an endotoxic shock cannot be excluded depending on the kind of exciter. Not commonly known is the fact that at the end of a tubal sterilization the coagulated tubal tissue reaches a temperature of 120°C; this temperature is maintained for ca. 20 s and cools to 80°C 40 s later. In the course of a further coagulation of the tubal parts on the opposite side the intestine may erroneously be touched and injured by the heat, as can also occur due to direct contact with the coagulation forceps. The consequences are similar to the disease described above. Therefore, the cooling down phase should be restricted to approximately 20 s if possible.

Adhesiolyses where scissors cannot be utilized demand a careful approach under coagulation since the colon, which is frequently drawn forward, might also be injured by the heat. It is recommended that a reserved attitude be adopted towards adhesiolyses; only a small number of adhesions cause pain.

Laparoscopic Tubal Sterilizations – Complications

Mechanical coagulating techniques for laparoscopic tubal sterilizations may provoke characteristic complications. Apart from complications arising during the technical procedure of laparoscopy, the clips or rings used in mechanical tubal sterilizations may be rejected shortly afterwards. The tube may then recanalize, as is frequently observed in post-partum sterilizations. Some clips do not surround the entire tube, leading to the assumption that the tubal lumen has been only partly retrieved. The disadvantage of Tantalon clips was that they could not be pressed together strongly enough with the consequence that tubal lumen was not impenetrable, as shwon by x-ray. Extremely elastic tubal muscles tore such clips apart. So far (1994) no proof has been furnished that Filshie clips still on sale are safer, owing to the lack of specific research. With regard to possible pregnancies, Yoon rings and Silastic ribbons are most reliable. Increased postoperative complaints, have only occasionally been reported, this increase being due to contusion of nerves in the mesosalpinx.

The founders of laparoscopic sterilization and other authors have reported spontaneous recanalizations after a period of 3 years following coagulation by monopolar high-frequency current for vast tubal destruction. Bipolar and thermal coagulation involves the danger of carbonizing tissue if coagulation is applied for too long and at too high temperatures, thus gluing the forceps to the tissue. The opening and removal of the forceps may delacerate the tubal wall, reaching as far as the mesosalpinx and causing tearing. The two most frequent sterilization methods are bipolar coagulation on the one hand and application of Yoon rings on the other.

Dissection of the tubes does not offer greater safety with regard to possible pregnancies. A tubual biopsy taken from the coagulated area merely serves to prove proper coagulation if legal problems arise.

Sterility Diagnosis – Complications

Diagnosis of sterility often requires the detachment of unexpected adhesions to enable an efficient survey of the genital organs. In penetration tests pressure increases during CO_2 insufflation and hydropertubation for exploding adhesive fimbriae do not make sense. At best small doses of CO_2 may enter the blood path, with consequent extravasation of the blue solution during hydropertubation. Details on electrosurgical operations are discussed later.

Spontaneous recanalizations within 1 week may almost always occur irregardless of the method applied. More than one conception during the first menstrual cycle following the sterilization have been reported. Lesions of the colon caused by insufficiently cooled tubes have previously been discussed. When instructing patients on the failure rate, any procedure bearing the risk of one pregnancy per 1000 sterilizations should be pointed out. The recanalization ability of the tubes is stronger than the power of destruction exercised by the operator.

Complications of Micro-invasive Surgery

Data on clinical long-term experiences regarding complications arising from the new micro-invasive operation techniques, e.g., laparoscopically assisted vaginal extirpations of the uterus, extirpations of the uterus according to Semm, adnexal extirpations, lymphangiectomies, urological operations such as the modified "Burch" procedure, etc. Frequent cystoureteric lesions, bladder perforations, etc. are considered to be initial difficulties of the new procedures comparable to those experienced upon the introduction of laparoscopy.

The long duration of many operations generates different kinds of anaesthesia problems (see chapter on anaesthesia). The use of more than one trocar, if necessary of a larger size, may easily induce abdominal bleeding; nevertheless, their application is often indispensable. During the postoperative phase cardiorespiratory disturbances may be initiated by the transfer of the patient from the operation table onto the bed. After electrosurgical operations the patient may complain of indistinct and almost indefinable inferior abdominal pain. During the resorption phase abdominal hematoma may cause pain as well, whereas omphalic infections are rare.

Inferior to the phrenic dome unresorbed gas can be monitored by x-rays for as long as 48 h, where it appears falciform. It provokes indistinct dorsalgia due to stimulation of the phrenic nerve.

Advice to any operator: any laparotomized patient complaining of indistinct abdominal pain and unable to walk normally within 24 h after the operation should be carefully examined, either laparoscopically or by laparotomy.

If the ileum is perforated or lesioned by monopolar high-frequency current it must be resected extending far into healthy tissue. Thermic lesions reach far beyond the visible coagulation points.

Less Frequent Complications

Severe lesions of the ileum with lethal outcome in two patients were reported after electrosurgical operations in which the older generation of combined mono- and bipolar coagulation equipment together with an earthing plate placed on the femur were used. Electronic engineers of the supplier presume the following: When pushing the coagulation forceps through the metal trocar the metal end of the forceps might have come into contact with the lower part of the trocar, transforming the bipolar coagulation current into a monopolar current due to the earthing plate.

There has also been a report of an incident whereby the operator lost an eye owing to defective isolation of equipment. In another incident during an electrosurgical operation an explosion was discharged into the abdominal cavity, the reason being unknown. The patient died immediately.

It has occasionally been claimed that applying a pneumoperitoneum at excessive pressure might provoke tearings of adhesions linking the abdomen and ileum, thereby injuring the abdominal wall with ensuing peritonitis. An examination for control purposes revealed that such a perforation had been induced by thermal damage from the coagulation forceps.

Blunt separation of adhesions may damage the ileal surface. If the ileum is badly damaged, a perambulation peritonitis with all its consequences may result. Even the first incision of the scalpel into the cutis for the preparation of the entrance for the Verrres needle and laparoscope may induce vasovagal reflexes leading to cardiac arrest. Exceptional are rare infections by β-hemolytic streptococci, known as killer bacteria (necrotizing fasciitis, toxic shock syndrome), causing vast necrosis of the abdominal wall, muscles, and fascia, frequently with a lethal outcome. They are more common in surgery than in gynecology. Antibiotic therapy, difficult transplantations, and shifting of lobes seldom help to save the patient's life.

When retracting the trocar at the end of laparoscopy a fringe of the omentum might be pulled back as well. It should be pushed back into the abdominal cavity with forceps, and the incision site closed by intracutaneous suture.

In patients suffering from hypertension the introduction of the laparoscopic trocar may provoke injuries of the periumbilical artery (caput medusae). Vast abdominal hematoma, primarily encountered in patients taking marcumar, can only be stopped by operation. To avoid further hematoma additional trocars should be inserted in the area of the symphysis and transillumination and visualization of the abdominal epigastric arteris should facilitate determination of the incision sites for minimally invasive surgery. It its recommended that any local bleeding be stopped by laparotomy.

It can be argued that perforations caused by tubes introduced into the uterus for mobilization purposes should be classified as complications, but they do not require any reaction. In patients suffering from cardiac problems more intense postoperative edema of the lungs occasionally becomes manifest. The incarceration of tissue in the hernial opening is considered a relatively rare complication. During resection and coagulation of sacro-uterine ligaments in patients with chronic pelvic neuralgia, immitigable bleeding occasionally occurs; such bleeding sometimes also originates from coagulated uterine vessels. Depending on the intensity of the bleeding, laparotomy may be recommended.

During biopsies taken from fimbrial endings or the omentum, e.g., if tuberculosis or carcinoma is suspected, massive bleeding may only be stopped by laparoscopy.

Currently we cannot yet estimate to what extent minimally invasive techniques under visual guidance by laparascopy will generate new types of complications. Presentations at many international congresses do, however, include reports of complications due to, for example, laparoscopic hysterectomy, lymphadenectomy, and urological operations, such as the Burch procedure.

Summary

To summarize in brief:

1. Inexperience and insufficient knowledge of the operator are among the main reasons that give rise to complications. Operations should be taught before making use of the pelvitrainer.

2. A higher risk is involved when equipment less known to the lecturer is used during lectures. Concentration is frequently reduced by diversion owing to the demonstration.
3. Defective equipment not undergoing regular safety checks may cause complications.
4. The very complex simultaneous coincidence of various factors, e.g., insufficient preliminary examination, unsatisfactory bedding, insufficient pneumoperitoneum, and electrosurgical operations, impedes determination of the case of complications.

The operator should be well informed about unusual complications and be familiar with the symptoms. He must confess to himself that "something has happened". Immediate reaction and the availability of all necessary tools are required to possibly save the patient's life. Specialists must also be consulted. Exceptionally careful controls are imperative. Detailed, thorough, and comprehensive documentation is essential in case of legal proceedings. In a number of European countries the fact-finding boards of the Medical Chambers first become involed. They authorize a competent expert to give his opinion on the incidence and decide whether a medical technical error has happened or not. It is, however, still possible to apply to the court. Experience has shown that in 99% of all cases the opinion of the fact-finding board and its award does not differ from the judgement pronounced by the court. Long-term consequences resulting from complications are equally serious and depressing for patient and operator.

Despite possible complications the diagnostic and therapeutic value of laparoscopy is superior to that of other tools and operations. In my opinion microinvasive procedures will become directional markers in future. They must not be rejected, as is presently done in many respects.

References *

1. Beck L (1978) Intra- und postoperative Komplikationen. Thieme, Stuttgart
2. Borten M (1986) In: Friedman EA (ed) Laparoscopic complications: prevention and management. Decker, Toronto
3. Chamberlain, G.V. et al (1978) Gynecological laparoscopy: the report of the working party of the confidential enquiry into gynaecological laparoscopy. Br J Obstet Gynaecol (Suppl) 86:6
4. Cognat G, Vignaud A (1976) Le risque d'arřet cardiaque au cours de la coelioscopie. Etude à partie de 50 000 coelioscopies et d'une experimentation animale. J Gynecol Obstet Biol Reprod (Paris) 5:925–940
5. Frangenheim H (1965) Technische Fehler bei der Boelioskopie. Geburtsh Frauenheilk 25:22
6. Frangenheim H (1977) Hysteroskopie. In: Lindemann (ed) Die Laparoskopie in der Gynäkologie, Chirurige und Paediatrie. Thieme, Stuttgart
7. Frangeheim H (1975) Komplikationen bei der Laparoskopie und Vorschläge zu ihrer Verhütung. In: Obolensky W, Käser O (eds) Ovulation und Ovulationsauslösung, perioperative Probleme. Huber, Bern

* The almost impenetrable mass of literature on complications of laparoscopy restricts citations to essential references available to anybody.

8. Frangenheim H (1978) Die Komplikationen bei der gynäkologischen Laparoskopie. Ihre Ursachen, Folgen und Vorschläge zu ihrer Verhütung. In: Becke K (eds) Intra- und postoperative Komplikationen. Thieme, Stuttgart
9. Mintz M (1976) Le risque et al prophylaxie des accidents en coelioscopie gynecologique. Enquete portant sur 100 000 cas. J Gynacol Obstet Biol Reprod (Paris) 5:681
10. Palmer R (1974) Safety in laparoscopy. J Reprod Med 13:1
11. Palmer R (1974) Security in laparoscopy. In: Philips JM (ed) Gynecologic laparoscopy: principles and techniques, Stratton, New York, pp 227–241
12. Phillips Jm, Keith D, Keith L et al (1985) Survey of gynecologic laparoscopy for 1974. J Reprod Med 15:45
13. Phillips JM, Hulka JF, Hulka B (1979) American Association of Gynecologic Laparoscopists 1977 membership survey. J Reprod Med 23:76
14. Phillips JM, Hulka B et al (1978) American Association of Gynecologic Laparoscopists 1976 membership survey. J Reprod Med 21:3
15. Riedel HH, Lehmann-Willenbrock E, Mecke H, Semm K (1989) The frequency distribution of various pelviscopic (laparoscopic) operations including complications rates-statistics of the Federal Republic of Germany in the years 1983–1985. Zentbl Gynäkol 111:78–91
16. Semm K (1979) Statistischer Überblick über die Bauchspiegelung in der Frauenheilkunde bis 1977 in der Bundesrepublik Deutschland. Geburtsh Frauenheilk 39:537–544
17. Stark G (1976) Zwischenfälle und Komplikationen bei Laparoskopie, Culdoskopie und Hysteroskopie (Moderatorenbericht). Arch Gynäkol 224:272

Therapeutic Insemination

K.H. Broer and I. Turanli

One approach to the treatment of abnormal spermatozoal transport through the cervix of the uterus may be homologous insemination. This method may be in both male and female infertility (Fig. 1).

Causes of male infertility include:

1. Oligoteratoasthenospermia
2. Hypospermia
3. Fructose deficiency
4. Hyperviscosity
5. Hypo- and epispady
6. Penial induration
7. Inability to have intercourse due to disturbances of erection originating from organic or psychogenic diseases
8. Ejaculatory dysfunction caused by malformations
9. Precocious and retrograde ejaculation
10. Spermatozoal antibodies.

Homologous insemination should be considered in cases of:

1. Cervical sterility
2. Disturbed cervical mucus interaction
3. Immunological infertility
4. Inability to have intercourse
5. Morphological alterations of the cervix.

As listed earlier the most common indication for insemination is male infertility. In particular, intrauterine insemination after swim-up treatment of the ejaculate has become increasingly important during the past few years.

Success rates mainly depend on the quality of the spermatozoal parameters, i.e., the number of spermatozoa (sperm count) and their motility, i.e., their ability to move spontaneously. Therefore, male fertility diagnosis should include examination of the ejaculate with a check for bacteria and sperm penetration tests in vivo and in vitro. In female infertility treatment the success of homologous insemination varies between 10% and 20%, whereas the success rates in male infertility are significantly lower, reaching no more than approximately 10% with a reduced spermcount under the most favorable conditions. If the spermcount and motility lie below a critical level, there is little chance for a

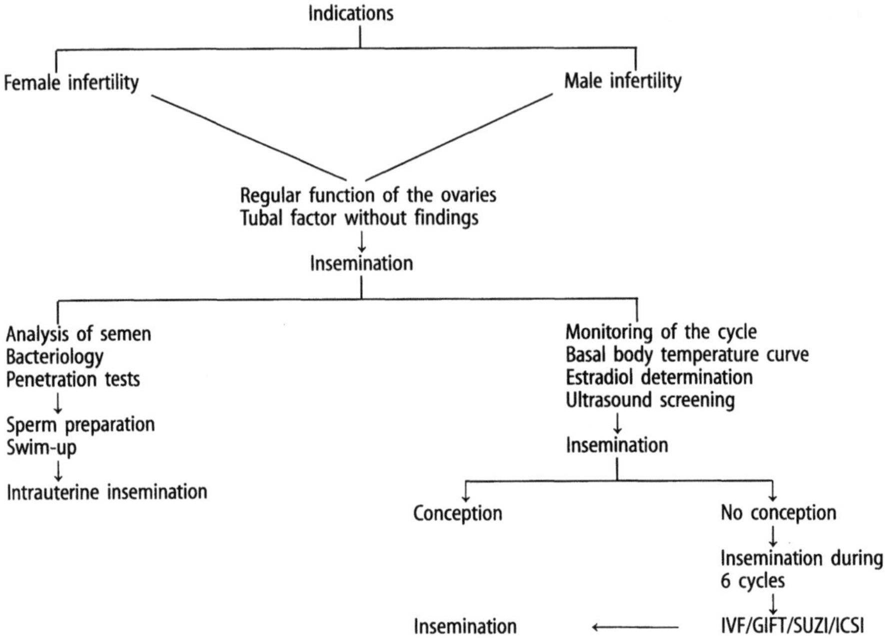

Fig. 1. Therapeutic insemination techniques. *IVF*, in vitro fertilization; *GIFT*, gamete intrafallopian transfer; *SUZI*, subzonal oocyte insemination

successful insemination. Consequently, further therapeutic techniques of assisted reproduction such as in vitro fertilization, gamete intrafallopian transfer, or subzonal oocyte insemination should be employed.

All data on success rates are difficult to compare since combined and multifactoral indications of male and female infertility very often have to be considered.

Four different techniques of homologous insemination are applied:

1. Insemination around the cervix with a cervical cap
2. Insemination into the cervix
3. Intrauterine insemination
4. Vaginal insemination.

For inseminations with cervical caps a well-fitted plastic cap is placed on the cervix with vacuum pressure. The ejaculate is then applied to the portio through a plastic tube. This insemination technique bears the advantage of optional self-injection of ejaculate by the patients who collected it at home.

For insemination into the cervix a catheter is used to introduce the ejaculate into the uterine orifice. This method is most frequently applied in hospital units performing homologous insemination. Another very common technique is so-called intrauterine insemination which is the preferred treatment in cases of disturbed spermatozoa-cervical mucus interaction. By

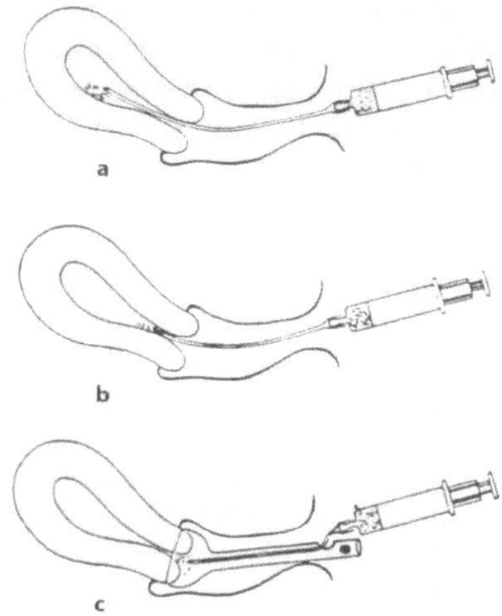

Fig. 2 a–c. Insemination techniques **a** Intrauterine and **b** intracervical insemination. **c** Portio cap. (Adapted from Whitelaw)

means of a sterile catheter the ejaculate (prepared either by the swim-up or swim-down technique) is directly inseminated into the uterus. This method is also recommended when immunological infertility – the presence of anti-sperm antibodies either on sperm cells or within the cervical mucus – has been diagnosed as it allows the sperm to cross the cervical barrier.

Vaginal insemination as a merely mechanical sperm delivery technique is no longer practiced since the success rates are significantly lower.

These insemination techniques are shown in Fig. 2.

For intrauterine insemination an appropriate sperm preparation is indispensable since cell debris, seminal plasma containing a high concentration of prostaglandins, and bacterial infections must be eliminated as far as possible. A variety of techniques for sperm preparation are suitable for intrauterine insemination of which the swim-up procedure is the most widely applied. Spermatozoa are washed in medium and recovered by centrifugation. The pellet is resuspended and the spermatozoa are allowed to swim up; in the top layer a higher concentration of morphologically motile spermatozoa can then be retrieved for insemination.

Other preparation methods are glass-wool filtration and the swim-down procedure. Special sperm-washing techniques yield a sperm concentration that provides improved sperm quality for the intrauterine insemination.

Appropriate timing is an important aspect to be considered when proceeding with insemination. The basal body temperature curve, determination of the volume of cervical secretion and estradiol level, the cervical index proposed by Insler (1972), and follicular size measured by ultrasound are crucial parameters. If no increase in the basal body temperature is measured within 48 h after insemination, a second attempt can be made if the cervical factor is diagnosed as normal.

The highest conception rates are achieved during the first four to six insemination cycles. Conceptions are seldom reported thereafter. At this point other technologies of assisted reproduction should be considered such as gamete intrafallopian transfer (GIFT), in vitro fertilization (IVF), or microinsemination.

If no conception is achieved by either IVF or GIFT treatment, a further course of insemination therapy may be initiated since conceptions are still possible; at this point, however, the success rates are clearly lower.

In conclusion, therapeutic inseminations should be applied in cases where spermatozoa are hindered from penetrating the genital tract. Causes may be disturbances in the storage of sperm, reduced quality of the ejaculate, a disturbed cervical mucus-spermatozoa interaction, or female infertility due to the cervical factor. Insemination represents a less costly and time-consuming method that hardly causes discomfort. As such it is constantly gaining importance in the treatment of female and male infertility.

References

Adoni A, Palti Z (1979) Better postcoital test for oligospermia patients using split ejaculate artifical insemination. Fertil Steril 31:587

Aparicio NJ, Schwarzstein L, Turner EA, Turner D, Mancini R, Schally AV (1976) Treatments of idiopathic normogonadotropic oligoasthenospermia synthetic luteinizing hormone-releasing hormone. Fertil Steril 27:549

Bain J, Schwarzstein L, Schill W-B (1981) Treatment of male infertility. Springer, Berlin Heidelberg New York

Bartsch G, Schreiber K (1980) Tamoxifen, ein neues Anti-Östrogen. In: Semm K, Schirren C (eds) Fortschritte der Fertilitätsforschung, vol VIII: Diagnostic und Therapie der gestörten Virilität und Fertilität. Grosse, Berlin

Bregulla K (1980) Gefrierkonservierung der menschlichen Ei- und Samenzellen. Gynaekol Prax 4:243

Comhaire F (1976) Treatment of oligospermia with tamoxifen. Int J Fertil 21:232

Eliasson R, Lindholmer C (1972) Distribution and properties of spermatozoa in different fractions of split ejaculates. Fertil Steril 23:252

Emperaire J-C, Audebert A (1978) Artifical insemination homologous and male subfertility. Proceedings of the 1st international symposium, Institut Aquitaine de Recherches sur la Reproduction Humaine, Bordeaux

Gigon U, Haldemann R (1979) Heterologe Insemination. Medizinische, genetische und juristische Probleme. Med Klin 74:1375

Haberland GL, Rohen JW, Suzuki T (1977) Kininogenases, Kallikrein 4. Schattauer, Stuttgart

Heiss H (1972) Die künstliche Insemination der Frau. Urban and Schwarzenberg, Munich

Insler V, Melmed H, Eichenbrenner I, Serr DM, Lunenfeld B (1972) The cervical score. Int J Gynaecol Obstet 10:223

Labrie F, Belanger A, Pelletier G, Seguin C, Cusan L, Kelly PA, Lemay A, Auclair C, Raynaud JP (1980) LHRH agonists: inhibition of testicular function and possible clinical applications. In: Cunningham GR, Schill WB, Hafez ESE Regulation of male fertility. Nijhoff, The Hague, p 65

Nuley WC, Kitchin JD III, Thiagarajah S (1978) Homologous insemination. Fertil Steril 30:510

Schill W-B (1972) Humane Spermakonservierung und therapeutische Ausblicke. Hautarzt 23:525

Schill W-B (1973) Probleme der homologen und heterologen Insemination aus andrologischer Sicht. In: Braun-Falco O, Petzoldt D (eds) Fortschritte der Dermatologie und Venerologie, vol VII. Springer, Berlin Heidelberg New York, p 187

Schill W-B (1976) Die Behandlung männlicher Fertilitätsstörungen mit Kallikrein. Dtsch Med Wochenschr 101:1773
Schill W-B (1978) Neuere Aspekte der Hormontherapie männlicher Fertilitätsstörungen. Ther Gegenw 117:24
Schill W-B (1979) Recent progress in pharmacological therapy of male subfertility – a review. Andrologia 11:77
Schirren C (1973) Therapieprobleme der Andrologie. Urologie [B]13:1
Schirren C (1978) Kallikrein in der Andrologie. In: Schirren C (ed) Fortschritte der Andrologie, vol VI. Grosse, Berlin
Schoysman-Deboeck A, Schoysman R, Devroey P (1980) 1000 grossesses par insemination artificielle par donneur (I.A.D.). Referat Brüssen
Sherman JK (1973) Synopsis of the use of frozen human semen since 1964: state of the art of human semen banking. Fertil Steril 24:397
Steiman RP, Taymor ML (1977) Artificial insemination homologous and its role in the management of infertility. Fertil Steril 28:146
Zander J, Mickan H (1973) Probleme der homologen und heterologen Insemination aus gynäkologischer Sicht. In: Braun-Falco O, Petzoldt D (eds) Fortschritte der praktischen Dermatologie und Venerologie, vol VII. Springer, Berlin Heidelberg New York, p 179

In Vitro Fertilization and Related Techniques

T. Rabe, Ü.B. Gör, K. Grunwald, and B. Runnebaum

Introduction

In 1978 the medical journal *Lancet* published a summary by the English gynecologist Patrick Steptoe and the physiologist Robert Edwards on the birth of the first extra corporeally fertilized child in England on 25 July 1978, a so-called test-tube baby (Steptoe and Edwards 1978).

The extracorporeal fertilization of an oocyte with sperm with subsequent transfer of the embryo into the uterus is known as in vitro fertilization (IVF). The introduction of this treatment method has, during the past few years, allowed fulfilment of the desire for a child of many couples who would not have had a child otherwise; moreover, it has been possible to scientifically answer numerous questions related to reproductive medicine and reproductive biology. An additional advantage due to the more intense research on human reproduction mechanisms has been the optimization of already existing methods [e.g., timing of an intrauterine insemination (IUI) following ultrasound biometry of the follicles].

Historical Survey

The first attempts at IVF and embryo transfer date back to the last century; as so often in medicine, the pioneering work involved experiments on animals.

Successful IVF in an animal experiment was first reported in the literature more than 100 years ago in Vienna. In 1880 Schenk succeeded in fertilizing in vitro oocytes of rabbits and guinea pigs, observing cellular mitosis (Schenk 1880). On 27 April 1890 Walter Heape carried out the first successful transfer of animal embryos (Heapa 1891, 1897). At that time he worked with rabbits, investigating whether the uterine environment influences the phenotype of an embryo. Heape's research was continued by F.H.A. Marshall and Sir J. Hammond, constituting the basis for the first book on reproductive physiology in 1910 (Marshall 1910). Between 1920 and 1930 the relation between the hypophysis and the ovaries became more evident. Decisive progress was made in the field of artificial insemination and first studies were performed on in vitro cultivation of oocytes. First examinations on human oocytes were initiated in the early 1940s. In 1944 Rock and Menkin performed in vitro inseminations on 138 human oocytes. In two of them fertilization and development to the bicellular stage were observed (Rock and Menkin 1944). In 1949 Hammond successfully cultivated mice embryos from the eight-cell stage to blastocytes in new, artificially composed culture medium (Hammond 1949). An essential improvement of the culture technique for preimplantation embryos was described by Whitten in 1956 (Whitten 1956). Extensive studies on lipid metabolism chiefly performed on extracorporeally cultivated embryos by Biggers and Brinster in the 1960s contributed greatly to the improvement of embryonic culture (Biggers and Brinster 1965). Since 1968 it has been possible to cultivate in vitro until the late blastula stage in chemically defined medium. Medium presently used for the culture of human preimplantation embryos mainly has its origin in these preliminary works.

The first pregnancy achieved in a human by extracorporeal fertilization was reported from Australia: it ended, however, in an early miscarriage (De Kretzer et al. 1973). At first Steptoe and Edwards were also denied definitive success. In one of their first attempts in 1976 the patient carried an ectopic pregnancy (Steptoe and Edwards 1976). Only in 19978 did they report the birth of the first child procreated by IVF (Steptoe and Edwards 1978).

In 1982 a study group around Craft reported on successful pregnancies in patients from whom oocytes had been retrieved 7 h before and transferred into the uterus 1 h after insemination with sperm (Craft et al. 1982). Due to its simplicity this technique attracted international interest; however its relatively low success rate compared to conventional IVF made it fall into oblivion.

In vitro fertilization and embryo transfer (IVF/ET) was originally developed for patients with pathological tubal factor. Now patients with different types of sterility also have access to IVF programs in cases where conventional treatment schemes have failed. Many of these patients have normal tubes capable of normal gamete transport and allowing adequate early embryonic development. These considerations have led to the development of the GIFT technique (gamete intra fallopian transfer) for women with normal tubes, i.e., the simultaneous introduction of oocytes and spermatozoa into the ampullary part of the tubes as an alternative to IVF (Asch 1985, 1986). In 1983 the first report on a pregnancy following gamete transfer into the tube on the occasion of a microsurgical tube operation was published (Tesarik et al. 1983). The successful outcome of experiments on animals (rhesus monkeys) was followed by a gamete transfer into properly working tubes, resulting in a pregnancy in 1984 (Asch et al. 1984, 1986).

The historical development of IVF and related techniques of human reproduction medicine is summarized in Table 1.

Table 1 Historical development of new techniques in human reproductive medicine

Year	Author	Procedure
1944	Rock and Menkin	In vitro fertilization of human oocytes
1953	Bunge and Sherman	Cryo-conservation of human semen
1973	De Kretzer	In vitro fertilization – embryo transfer: intrauterine pregnancy, but miscarriage
1976	Steptoe and Edwards	In vitro fertilization, embryo transfer but ectopic pregnancy
1978	Steptoe and Edwards	In vitro fertilization, embryo transfer and fully carried pregnancy in England
1980	Lopata et al.	In vitro fertilization, embryo transfer and fully carried pregnancy in Australia
1981	Trotnow et al.	In vitro fertilization, embryo transfer with ensuing pregnancy in Germany
1982	Craft et al.	Gamete transfer (introduction of oocyte and sperm into the uterus)
1983	Tesarik et al.	Gamete transfer into the tube during microsurgery
1983	Trounson and Mohr	Cryo-conservation of embryo, in vitro fertilization, fully carried pregnancy
1984	Asch	Gamete transfer (GIFT), fully carried pregnancy
1984	Lutjen et al.	Oocyte donation, fully carried pregnancy
1986	Chen	Cryo-conservation of human oocytes
1986	Devroy et al.	Intra-tubal zygote transfer (ZIFT)
1986	Forrler et al.	Transperitoneal insemination (TPI)
1987	Jansen and Anderson	Tubal embryo transfer (TET)
1987	Laws-King et al.	Subzonal insemination (SUZI)
1988	Balmaceda et al.	Intratubal embryo transfer (TET)
1988	Gordon et al.	"Zona triplet" from human oocytes
1988	Jansen et al.	Vaginal intratubal insemination (VITI)
1988	Ranoux et al.	Intravaginal culture (IVC)
1989	Veersma	Transcervical oocyte and sperm transfer (TOAST)
1989	Cohen et al.	Assisted hatching (AHA)
1990	Ng et al.	Intracytoplasmatic sperm injection (ICSI)
1990	Bongso et al.	Co-cultures
1990	Gordon and Gang	Blastomere biopsy

Standard Techniques

In Vitro Fertilization and Embryo Transfer (IVF-ET)

Description of Procedure. After hormonal hyperstimulation of the ovaries, oocytes are collected by vaginal ultrasonically guided aspiration (in particular cases by laparoscopic follicle aspiration). The oocytes are extracorporeally fertilized and ca. 48 h later the embryos are transvaginally transferred into the uterus. The principle and procedure of IVF are shown in Fig. 1.

Indications. Prior to an ultrasonically guided or laparoscopic aspiration of follicles for oocyte retrieval within IVF a conscientious evaluation of the indication is required, considering the risks. Alternative treatment methods

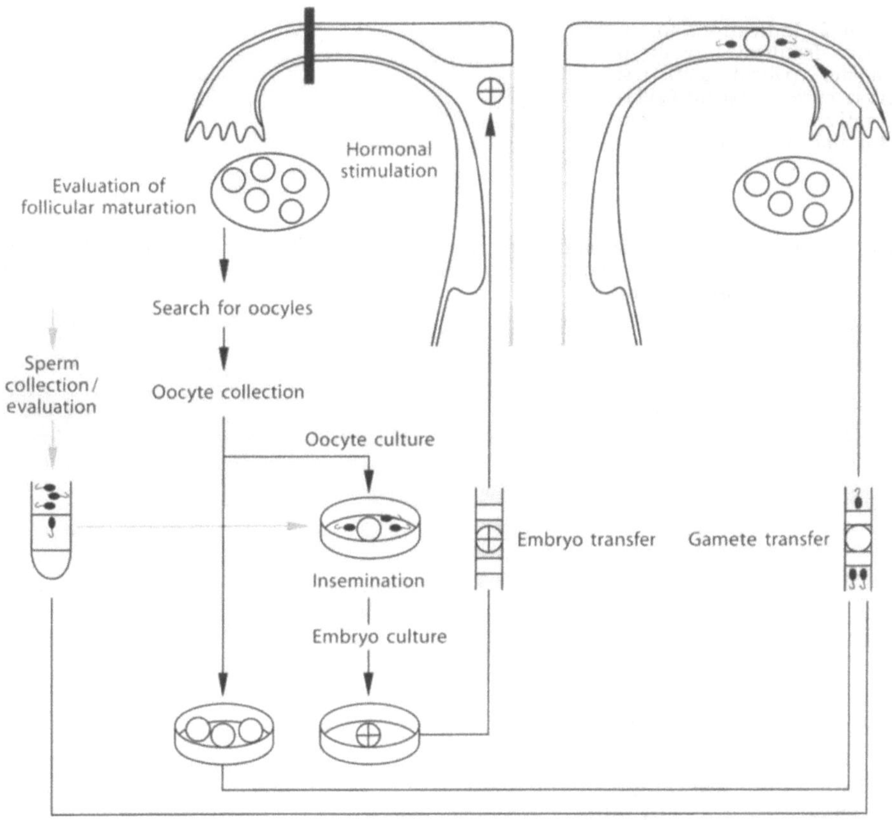

Fig. 1. In vitro fertilization and gamete transfer: schematic representation of the principle and procedure

available such as conservative treatment of infertility, e.g., insemination when tubes are not conglutinated, should be taken into consideration or even the adoption of a child or a microsurgical refertilization operation.

a) Unrestricted indications:
   Tubal ooclusion or tubal insufficiency that is not treatable (by microsurgery); bilateral tubectomy or unilateral tubectomy combined with tubal occlusion
b) Restricted indications:
   - Certain forms of male subfertility
   - Immunological infertility
   - Disturbed tubal function due to endometriosis
   - Idiopathic infertility may be considered as an indication only when all diagnostic and other methods of infertility treatment have been applied.

The international data on indications for IVF-ET in 1989–1991 are shown in Table 2.

Table 2 Indications for in vitro fertilization/embryo transfer (world statistics: 41251 cycles) (World Collaborative Report Bilan Mondial 1989/1991)

Tubal infertility	64.9%
Male subfertility	15.1%
Endometriosis	5.0%
Idiopathic infertility	10.2%
Other indications	4.8%

Table 3 Clinical pregnancy and birth rates relative to the various indications for in vitro fertilization (IVF-ET) and gamete transfer (GIFT) in the USA in 1989 (Medical Research International 1991)

	IVF			GIFT		
Diagnosis	Embryo transfers	Clinical pregnancies	Number of births	Transfer cycles	Clinical pregnancies	No. of births
Tubal factor	2348	468 (20%)	333 (14%)	335	82 (24%)	58 (17%)
Unexplained female infertility	247	58 (23%)	50 (20%)	378	126 (33%)	99 (26%)
Immunological female infertility	150	36 (24%)	21 (14%)	81	28 (35%)	19 (23%)
Endometriosis	904	180 (20%)	129 (14%)	704	229 (33%)	177 (25%)
Female factor	807	162 (20%)	121 (15%)	578	180 (31%)	146 (25%)

Contraindications:
- Pregnancy
- In possible Anesthesia
- Allergy to gonadotropin.

Success rates. Clinical pregnancy rates and take home baby rates vary from 20% to 24% and from 14% to 20% (referring to embryo transfer) respectively almost independent of the indication (Table 3). Latest results on the number of IVF cycles and pregnancy rates in various countries are summarized in Table 4.

The clinical pregnancy rate appears to be relatively low: a comparison with available alternatives, e.g., microsurgical interventions on the tubes, reveals that the efforts needed for a microsurgical operation including post-operative care are comparable to the efforts invested in two to three IVF cycles.

At Bonn University, where 2.4 follicles per patient are aspirated, a cumulative pregnancy rate of 42% was calculated. Comparison with the pregnancy rates obtained from microsurgery (salpingectomy, 30%–60%; reanastomosis, 40%–60%; adhesiolysis, 30%–40%; microsurgery in patients with bilateral occlusion or following fimbriectomy and tubectomy <10%), shows IVF to represent a viable alternative treatment (Diedrich and Krebs 1990).

Information on Risks. Since IVF is regarded as a facultative operation, detailed information on possible risks is absolutely essential:

Table 4 IVF cycles and pregnancy rates in various countries (worldwide report, 1991, presented at the 8th World Congress on In Vitro Fertilization, Kyoto, 1993)

Country/ region	Cycles	Aspirations		Transfers		Clinical pregnancy		Births	
		n	%	*n*	% of asp.	*n*	% of asp.	*n*	% of asp.
Australia	7366	6588	89.4	5457	82.8	727	11	517	7.8
Belgium	3000	2720	90.7	2220	81.6	630	23.2	484	17.8
Germany	6901	5314	77	4088	76.9	839	15.8	555	10.4
France		26951		21207	78.7	4922	18.3	3634	13.5
Greece	5090	3932	77.2	3080	78.3	597	15.2	403	10.2
UK	13156	10774	81.9	9747	90.5	2186	20.3	1604	14.9
Israel	4593	4088	89	3501	85.6	718	17.6	425	10.4
Japan	10247	9667	94.3	7610	78.7	1502	15.5	1144	11.8
Canada	3783	3048	80.6	2558	83.9	550	18	407	13.4
Latin America	2035	2036	85.7	1721	84.5	362	17.8	276	13.6
The Netherlands	3414	3173	92.9	2676	84.3	720	22.7	564	17.8
Austria	465	412	88.6	366	88.8	65	15.8	42	10.2
Scandinavia	9817	8759	89.2	7369	84.1	1857	21.2	1330	15.2
Spain	762	625	82	531	85	145	23.2	120	19.2
Taiwan	1292	1202	93	1085	90.3	254	21.1	196	16.3
Czechoslovakia	1520	1209	84.9	823	63.8	107	8.3	71	5.5
USA	24671	21083	85.5	18372	87.1	4017	19.1	3215	15.2

- Possibility of multiple pregnancy in 10%–20%. An analysis of ca. 10000 IVF pregnancies showed an outcome of 73.4% single pregnancies, 21.9% twin pregnancies, 4.3% triple pregnancies, and 0.4% quadruplet pregnancies (World Collaborative Report Bilan Mondial 1989/1991).
- Risk of vasal and intestinal lesions possibly necessitating laparotomic intervention by longitudinal section; the incidence is less than 1% of all cases; in less than 1/1000 there is a need for hysterectomy due to immitigable bleeding, resulting in lasting childlessness.
- Risk of inflammation in the small pelvis; incidence of less than 1%.
- Risk of ovarian hyperstimulation possibly necessitating hospitalization. Cases with a lethal outcome have been reported when no medical treatment was applied (e.g., thromboembolism due to hemoconcentration).

Procedure:
- Stimulation of follicle maturation (the following types of stimulation may be applied: stimulation by antiestrogens, by gonadotropins, by antiestrogens+gonadotropins, by GnRH analog+gonadotropins, by growth hormones+gonadotropins)
- Supervision of follicle/oocyte maturation:
  a) Ultrasonically guided.
  b) Hormonal supervision: the monitoring of typical response to estradiol (Jones et al. 1983) and LH (Urbancsek et al. 1991) reflected the relation to successful treatment schemes.
- Ovulation induction by HCG

- Ultrasonically guided (90%) or laparoscopic (10%) aspiration of follicles for oocyte retrieval
- Sperm collection and processing ("swim-up", Percoll gradient, glass wool, albumin column, and sedimentation methods)
- Fertilization of oocytes
- Cultivation of oocytes
- Transvaginal embryo transfer into the uterine cavity
- Supporting the luteal phase (an analysis of more than 35000 IVF cycles revealed that in 40% of all cases progesterone and in 35% of all cases HCG was chosen as medical support of the luteal phase after IVF stimulation. Thirteen percent received no medical support, and 10% received other medication (World Collaborative Report Bilan Mondial 1989/1991).

Comment. If IVF attempts fail or if male subfertility becomes manifest with markedly reduced spermiograms (e.g., OAT syndrome) one should proceed to micromanipulation techniques (intracytoplasmatic spermatozoal injection).

Gamete Intrafallopian Transfer (GIFT)

Description of Method. By means of hormonal therapy the ovaries are stimulated and when the follicles have reached maturity they are aspirated under sonographic guidance by laparoscopy to retrieve the oocytes, which shortly afterwards are laparoscopically (or transvaginally) reinjected into the ampullary part of the tubes together with processed sperm (100000 motile sperms per oocyte). The principle and implementation of gamete transfer are schematically described in Fig. 1 (Fig. 1); at least one unobstructed and well functioning fallopian tube in indispensable.

Indications:
- Endometriosis
- Immunological infertility
- Unexplained (idiopathic) infertility can only be considered an indication when all diagnostic examinations have been carried out and all therapeutic efforts have failed.
- Some kinds of male fertility disturbances that cannot be treated by other means including intrauterine insemination, but only if a high fertilization rate is proved by diagnostic IVF.

The worldwide breakdown of indications for gamete transfer in 1989 is shown in Table 5.

Contraindications:
- Absolute contraindications: all contraindications affecting pregnancy
- Restricted contraindications: in particular cases where the implementation might bear very high medical risks to the woman's life or the child's development
- Psychogenic infertility.

Table 5 Indications for GIFT, based on an analysis of 3733 cycles (World Collaborative Report Bilan Mondial 1989/1991)

Endometriosis	15.2%
Male subfertility	21.3%
Idiopathic sterility	41.8%
Mixed and other indikations	21.7%

Information on Risks:
- Risks concerning laparoscopy
- General risks (see In Vitro Fertilization)
- Possibility of ectopic pregnancies (10%–20%).

Implementation (Laparoscopic Gamete Transfer):
- Controlled hyperstimulation of the ovaries
- Ovulation induction by HCG
- Laparoscopic or ultrasonically guided aspiration of follicles
- Sperm preparation and concentration
- Aspiration of sperms and oocytes into a transfer catheter
- Introduction of transfer catheter into the ampullary part of the tube for gamete transfer.

Implementation (Transvaginal Intratubal Gamete Transfer; TV-GIFT):
- Hyperstimulation of the ovaries
- Ovulation induction by HCG
- Ultrasonically guided aspiration of follicles
- Sperm collection and preparation
- Aspiration of sperm and oocytes into a transfer catheter
- Transfer of sperm and oocytes transcervically into the tubes under sonographic control.

Success rates. Clinical pregnancy and delivery rates ("take home baby rates") vary from 24%–35% and from 20%–24% respectively almost irrespective of the indication (Tables 3, 6).

Table 6 Treatment results of IVF-EF, GIFT, and other (ZIFT, PROST, TET) methods of assisted reproduction in the USA (Medical Research International 1991) and worldwide (World Collaborative Report Bilan Mondial 1989/1991)

		Follicle aspiration	Clinical pregnancy	Miscarriage	Ectopic pregnancy	Birth
USA 1989	IVF-ET	15 392	2811 (18%)	655 (23%)	154 (5%)	2104 (14%)
	GIFT	3652	1112 (30%)	247 (22%)	43 (4%)	848 (23%)
	(ZIFT, PROST, TET)	908	190 (21%)			151 (17%)
World 1989	IVF-ET	76 030	12480 (16%)	21%	5%	8595 (12%)
	GIFT	11 141	3060 (28%)			1587 (20%)

Alternative Methods for Embryo Transfer After IVF: PROST, ZIFT, and TET

Description of Methods. These methods involve transfer of pronuclear stages or zygotes (PROST=pronuclear stage transfer, ZIFT=zygote intra fallopian transfer) or embryos (TET=tubal embryo transfer) into the tube following vaginal (Jansen et al. 1988) or transabdominal (mini-laparotomy: Balmadeca et al. 1988; laparoscopy: Hamori et al. 1988) follicle aspiration, after introduction of a transfer catheter into the tube (laparoscopic or transvaginal).

Indications:
- Tubal disturbance of oocyte deposition mechanism
- Immunological infertility
- Male subfertility
- Endometriosis.

Contraindications. Tubes not functioning.

Success rates. Success rates of 26% (Balmaceda et al. 1988) and 29% (Hamori et al. 1988) have been reported. Data for the United States (1989) are shown in Table 6.

Information on Risks. Higher risk of ectopic pregnancies.

Precondition. At least one functioning tube; intact uterus.

Implementation:
- Stimulation
- Follicle aspiration
- In vitro fertilization
- Laparoscopic or transcervical transfer of zygotes (pronuclear stages) 1 day after oocyte retrieval or transfer of embryos 48–50 h after aspiration.

Advantages. As compared to GIFT, it is possible to control fertilization and eliminate pathologically developed zygotes (triploidity).

Sperm

Sperm Collection/Sperm Processing

Microsurgical Epididymal Sperm Aspiration (MESA)

Principle. Sperm collection by microsurgical sperm aspiration from the epididymis.

Indications:
- Congenital deficiency of the vasa deferentia (20%–30% of all males with obstructed sperm release)
- Inoperable infectious obstructive azoospermia (genital tuberculosis, venereal diseases)
- Failure of anastomotic operation after vasectomy.

Procedure:
- Controlled ovarian hyperstimulation
- Microsurgical epididymal sperm aspiration. Sperm collected from the most proximal site (area nearest to the testicle) of the epididymis is most fresh, with superior motility and quality for fertilization and achieving pregnancy
- In vitro fertilization after sperm capacitation
- Transvaginal oocyte retrieval
- ZIFT or IVF-ET.

Alternative Methods. In the past a bursa was formed by surgical intervention to achieve sperm collection in a pool below the scrotal cutis appropriate for needle aspiration. This technique as well as similar devices aimed at the accumulation of sperm collected for a possible insemination of oocytes have hardly been successful.

Assessment. As a result of microsurgical epididymal sperm aspiration, fertilization rates varying from 6%–20% have been obtained in patients suffering from cystic fibrosis (Oates et al. 1992) and in cases of congenital absence of the vasa deferentia (Silber et al. 1988; Bladou et al. 1991) or obstructive azoospermia (Siddiq 1992). Ensuing embryo transfer has produced a number of pregnancies (Patrizen et al. 1988; Kodama et al. 1991; Cognat et al. 1992). It may thus be concluded that MESA in combination with the techniques of in vitro fertilization offers a promising therapeutic approach in cases of obstructive azoospermia.

Swim-up Technique

Principle. Swimming up of adequately motile sperm cells in a nutrient solution.

Indication. Selection and concentration of motile spermatozoa.

Procedure:
- Liquefaction of the sperm sample
- Dilution of the liquefied seminal plasma in a 1:2 ratio of culture medium and seminal fluid
- Centrifugation
- Removal of the fluid supernatant
- Second dilution and centrifugation, discarding the fluid supernatant
- Resuspension of Ham's-F-10 medium and human serum (0.5–1 ml)
- Incubation at 37°C (10–60 min) to allow motile sperm to migrate from the pellet into the overlay
- Careful collection of the overlay (0.2–0.5 ml) and analysis.

Evaluation. The swim-up technique represents a simple and inexpensive preparation method; it is, however, associated with a low recovery rate of sperm cells (5% according to Ng et al. 1992) of inferior quality whereas its advantage is the optimization of motile and optimally configurated spermatozoa (90%–100%).

Percoll Technique

Principle. Separation of nonvital sperm cells from morphologically intact and motile spermatozoa making use of the different density.

Indication. Selection and concentration of motile spermatozoa.

Procedure:
- Liquefaction of the sperm sample
- Placing layers of discontinuous gradients of Percoll in a sterile centrifuge tube
- Layering of liquefield semen on top of the gradient
- Centrifugation (layer of highly motile sperms with higher density at the bottom)
- Removal by pipetting and discarding of fluid supernatant by keeping the sperm pellet
- Resuspension of the remaining material in fresh culture medium (approx. 2 ml)
- Second centrifugation, removal of the supernatant layer, and resuspension of the sperm in 0.2–0.5 ml culture medium or Ham's-F-10+serum
- Analysis of motility, morphology, and amount.

Evaluation. In cases of oligo- and asthenospermia the Percoll technique may be the only means to collect viable sperm given the higher recovery rates (57%–66% according the Rhemrev et al. 1988); the motile fraction collected is very efficient yet less than when using the swim-up technique.

Spermatozoa Viability Tests

Hypo-osmotic Sperm Swell Test (HOS Test)

Principle. Swelling of spermatozoa under hypo-osmotic conditions.

Indications. Sperm viability test to control the functional integrity of the spermatozoa membrane for evaluating successful fertilization.

Procedure. Incubation of spermatozoa in a hypo-osmotic fructose and sodium citrate solution (Jeyendran et al. 1984).

Evaluation. The HOS test represents an attempt to give a prognostic estimation of in vitro fertilization behavior of spermatozoa. Jeyendran et al. (1984) found that there is a significant correlation between spermatozoa with swelling ability and spermatozoa of the same semen being able to penetrate zona-free hamster oocytes, which led to the assumption of a possible predictive value regarding the success rates of in vitro fertilization.

Van den Saffele et al. (1992) reported on a correlation between the HOS test and the results of the spermiogram. In a study examining 187 semen samples of fertile and subfertile men it became apparent that the group featuring normal spermiograms contained a greater number of HOS-reactive sperms ($P<0.001$) than the group showing pathological spermiograms while there was no significant correlation between the swelling ability of the sperm and in vitro fertilization capacity in the zona-free hamster penetration assay (Smith et al. 1992). Avery et al. (1990) did not confirm a correlation between the results of the HOS test and various causes for fertilization disturbances (oligospermia, unexplained infertility) and questioned the potential predictability for successful in vitro fertilization. At the present time it is not possible to obtain any additional information relevant to routine sperm analyses by using the HOS test (Chan et al. 1988; Van den Saffele et al. 1992).

Zona-Free Hamster Oocyte Penetration Test

Principle. Determination of penetration ability of sperm from infertile patients in zona pellucida-free hamster oocytes for the evaluation of fertilization ability.

Indication. Different causes of infertility.

Procedure. After removal of the zona pellucida from hamster oocytes, semen samples of infertile men are incubated with ensuing observation of the penetration ability.

Evaluation. The test published by Yanagimachi et al. (1976) is based on the assumption that for the prediction of fertilization ability of spermatozoa it is possible to use hamster oocytes as a replacement for human oocytes. According to Margalioth et al. (1989) the specificity and the positive predictive value are estimated to be higher than in spermiograms (77% vs 57% and 48% vs 37%). Prasad (1984) reported lower penetration rates in subfertile patients (<10%) than in fertile men (20%–100%). High penetration rates might be an indicator of an increased probability of successful in vitro fertilization whereas penetration rates of 0% by no means exclude pregnancy. The implementation of this test might be of value in cases of unexplained infertility which cannot be diagnosed by normal sperm analyses. Disadvantages of the zona-free hamster oocyte test are (a) high cost and time consuming (Chan et al. 1985, 1990; Schmidt 1988), (b) somewhat varying success rates from which it must be concluded that it is not absolutely reliable (sensitivity: 0.00–1.00, specifity: 0.51–1.00 for diagnosing male infertility; sensitivity: 0.00–0.78, specifity: 0.95–1.00 for predicting an IVF failure) (Mao u. Grimes 1988), and (c) there is no control of the sperms' ability to penetrate the zona pellucida, leading to the conclusion that a positive test result is not a guarantee for the fertilization of human oocytes (Prasad 1984).

Sperm Treatment

Sperm Processing with Pentoxifylline

Principle. The incubation of spermatozoa with pentoxifylline aims at increasing sperm motility, thus optimizing the chances for successful fertilization.

Indication. Male infertility with oligo-/asthenozoospermia and immotile sperm in combination with micromanipulation methods.

Procedure. Following sperm retrieval and pretreatment, spermatozoa are incubated with 3.5 m*M* pentoxifylline, washed again, and fertilized in vitro. Further to the treatment in vitro it is possible to apply an oral therapy with daily administration of 1200 mg pentoxifylline for a period of 3 months (Micic et al. 1988; Shen et al. 1991).

Evaluation. A study conducted by Yovich et al. (1990) revealed that sperm pretreated with pentoxifylline resulted in an increased fertilization rate in oligospermic men as compared to control groups not treated (20%, n=21/103 vs 47%, n=81/171, P<0.001). Various authors have reported on an augmentation of sperm motility following incubation with pentoxifylline in patients suffering from asthenospermia (P<0.05) (Chang et al. 1992) and when applied in cryoconserved sperms (Hammitt et al. 1989; Mbizvo et al. 1993). Yovich et al. (1988) reported on improved sperm motility (0.18±0.06 mill/ml vs 0.44±0.14 mill/ml, P<0.02) and five fully carried pregnancies in cases of oligo-/asthenozoospermia in nine couples. Sikka and Hellstrom (1991) observed 2–3 times increased motility depending on the pentoxifylline doses administered. Comparative studies between treated and untreated sperm revealed another aspect, i.e., a prolongation of sperm activity (Melo-Abreu 1992; Aparicio et al. 1980). Gavella et al. (1991) state that spermatozoa incubated with pentoxifylline release less (P<0.001) oxygen radicals than untreated controls. This inhibitory effect might be a major factor contributing to improved sperm quality, with a simultaneous increase in the chance of achieving fertilization. During oral administration of pentoxifylline for a period of 3 months an augmentation in sperm motility was observed in oligo-/asthenospermic patients (23%±9% prior to therapy vs 31%±11% after therapy, P<0.01) (Micic et al. 1988). Shen et al. (1991) also registered an increase of sperm motility from 24%–57% (P<0.05). An influence on sperm concentration was not observed (Wang et al. 1983; Shen et al. 1991). Further to an augmentation of spermatozoa motility it is being discussed whether pentoxifylline supports the acrosome reaction (Yovich et al. 1993); pentoxifylline should, however, be washed out after incubation to exclude any hindrance to oocyte maturation. According to these results, pentoxifylline pretreatment might increase the chances for conception where indicated.

Sperm Pretreatment with 2-Deoxyadenosine (2-DXA)

Principle. Increase in spermatozoa motility by incubation with 2-DXA.

Indications:
- Asthenospermia
- Reduced sperm motility.

Procedure:
- Sperm retrieval
- Sperm preparation
- Incubation with 2-DXA
- Washing of sperm
- In vitro fertilization.

Evaluation. In patients having undergone previous ineffective conventional IVF trials the application of this method produced a higher number of motile sperm (71%±31% vs 52%±26%, $P<0.025$) as compared to untreated control groups as well as an increased fertilization rate (46/107, 43% vs 13/94, 14%; $P<0.00025$) Imoedemhe et al. (1992a) reported three normally carried pregnancies following sperm pretreatment with 2-DXA.

Hammitt et al. (1989) achieved an augmentation in motility in cryoconserved sperm by 48.7% ($P<0.05$). Due to the low number of clinical applications only a restrictive prognosis as to the possible future value of this method can be given.

Oocyte

Oocyte-Sperm Interaction

Hemizona Assay (HZA)

Principle. Determination of the number of sperm bound to a zona pellucida divided into two equally sized parts in subfertile and definitely fertile men.

Indications. Prognostic evaluation of behaviour during in vitro fertilization relevant to fertilizing ability of sperm.

Procedure:
- Division of the zona pellucida of an oocyte into two equal parts
- Placement of a semen specimen from the subfertile patient into one part and a specimen from the definitely fertile donor into the other part
- Counting of the sperm bound in each part 4–5 h later.

Evaluation. Various studies confirm that sperm originating from fertile men have a higher binding capacity than those of infertile men (38±8.1 vs 5.9±2.3; $P<0.01$) (Burkmann et al. 1988). In patients with successful IVF trials a greater number of bound sperm were observed than in patients achieving no successful IVF trials (36.1±7 vs 10.4±4; $P<0.05$) (Franken et al. 1989). Also in men with antisperm antibodies a reduction in the number of bound sperm as compared to control groups is described (19.5±8 vs 77.1±49; $P<0.01$) Franken et al. 1991). In this respect HZA represents an appropriate method for

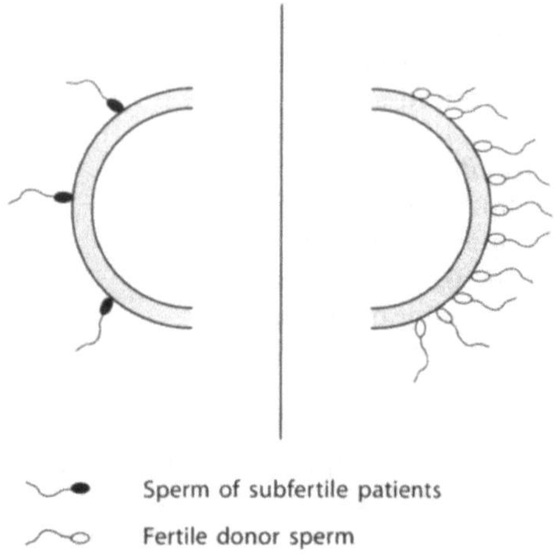

Fig. 2. Principle of the HZA

predicting fertilization ability of sperm, contributing simultaneously to the identification of patients bearing an increased risk of fertilization failure. The principle of HZA is shown in Fig. 2.

Oocyte or Embryo Treatment

Assisted Hatching (AHA)

Principle. By creating gaps in the zona pellucida by means of micromanipulation methods [mechanically, by localized application of a zona solvent (tyrode solution), or by laser] the "dis-invagination" of the embryo after transfer is facilitated, thus improving the chance of implantation.

Indications:
- Hardening of the zona with reduced embryo ability to penetrate the zona pellucida
- Density of zona pellucida>15 μm
- Failure of embryo transfer in conventional IVF trials.

Procedure. After fixation of the oocyte using a blunt suction capillary holes are drilled in the zona pellucida either mechanically by a pointed glass capillary or by a zona solvent (e.g., acid Tyrode solvent) or by applying an erbium-YAG laser.

Evaluation. Observations by Cohen et al. (1989) and Wright et al. (1990) pointed to the fact that embryos, with a lower zona pellucida density reveal improved implantation rates. Ensuing studies confirmed that AHA is most successful in embryos with a dense zona pellucida (>15 μm). Implantation rates were higher than in untreated control embryos (25% vs 18%; $P<0.05$)

(Cohen et al. 1992). Reports on implantation rates in literature vary from 9% (Tucker et al. 1991) to 36% (Strohmer and Feichtinger 1992b). The application of an erbium-YAG laser represents an alternative to the mechanical procedure of AHA, offering the advantage of precise handling. By implementing the mechanical method (Cohen et al. 1990) as well as with the use of laser (Strohmer and Feichtinger 1992a,b, Feichtinger 1992), several pregnancies were achieved in patients having had at least one ineffective IVF trial. As compared to untreated embryos, higher implantation rates were obtained (Liu et al. 1993; Gordon and Dapunt 1993). The application of AHA represents an efficient support for the normal "hatching" process. Continued clinical applications of AHA in the treatment of infertility will give final proof of its efficiency.

Biopsy of Blastomeres

Principle. Microbioptic aspiration of blastomeres followed by in vitro culturing (Nijs et al. 1988).

Indication. Chromosomal analysis for detecting genetic defects prior to embryo transfer.

Procedure:
- Mechanical or chemical opening of the zona pellucida
- Removal of blastomeres by aspiration or mechanical separation
- In vitro culture
- Chromosomal analysis.

Evaluation. Studies carried through with mice embryos reveal no negative effects on the embryonal development after the transfer (Gordon and Gang 1990; Kola and Wilton 1991; Takeuchi et al. 1992). Embryos who underwent biopsy in the four-cell stage feature implantation rates of 60% compared to 64% in control embryos (Wilton et al. 1989). Rodebush et al. (1990) achieved better results by mechanical separation than by aspiration (survival rate of mice embryos in the four-cell stage: 22.3% vs 58.9%, $P<0.001$; survival rate in the eight-cell stage 33.3% vs 66.7%, $P<0.003$). One blastomere may be retrieved from embryos in the four-cell stage and three blastomeres from the eight-cell stage without causing disturbances in embryonal development (Liu et al. 1993). Van Blerk et al. (1991) report on successful pregnancies after transfer of mice embryos that underwent biopsy, though a smaller number than with control embryos (25%–33% vs 60%; $P<0.01$). Biopsy of blastomeres with ensuing chromosomal analysis seems to be a promising future diagnostic tool in cases of specifically hereditary diseases (Morsy et al. 1992).

Co-cultures

Principle. Cultivation of embryos in cells obtained from the human tubes up to blastocyte stage with ensuing transfer.

Indication. Improvement of pregnancy rates in IVF cycles.

Procedure:
- In vitro fertilization
- Embedding of embryos in cultures of tubal cells (collected from the tubes of premenopausal hysterectomized women)
- Embryo development up to the 5th day
- Transfer of embryos into the uterus.

Evaluation. This method aims at improved and possibly faster development of the embryos in a "natural" environment. It is intended to achieve more efficient implantation results by growing embryos capable of development (Bongso et al. 1990). In a series of experiments carried out by Bongso with 50 women (68% out of whom had at least two unsuccessful IVF trials) an outcome of 22 pregnancies was reported (success rate: 44%). Other research teams have also confirmed positive effects on embryonal development in vitro using co-cultures (Yeung et al. 1992). Due to the low number of clinical applications only a qualified conclusion as to the possible future value of this method can be given at present. The implementation of co-cultures is presently in the developmental phase and may ultimately increase the stagnating success rates of IVF.

Oocyte and Embryo Donation

Principle. Oocyte donation comprises retrieval of oocytes from the ovary of a donor woman following stimulation of the ovaries and transfer of the oocytes or the embryo to a second patient called the receiver. The transfer may be effected together with the husband's sperm into the receiver's tubes (GIFT), or the oocytes may be fertilized in vitro with transfer of the resulting embryos into the uterus (IVF-ET) or the fallopian tubes (PROST, ZIFT, or TET) (Devroey et al. 1989).

Indications:
- Premature exhaustion of the ovaries
- Gonadal dysgenesis syndrome
- Iatrogenic loss of gonadal function (due to surgery, radiation, chemotherapy)
- Ovaries inaccessible for oocyte retrieval
- Persons carrying undesired genetic deseases (x-chromosomally connected or autosomally dominant)
- Repeated failure of in vitro fertilization
- Repeated unexplained abortion.

Procedure (see principle). Potential donors are GIFT or IVF patients having produced a great number of follicles who are questioned for their willingness to give away surplus oocytes. With the possibility of cryoconservation of surplus oocytes in the pronucleus stage many patients prefer, however, the freezing of additional fertilized oocytes for possible future trials. Alternatively there is the chance of finding a donor in the person of a near friend or relative who would have to undergo ovarian stimulation and oocyte collection. The major problem of oocyte donation is the discrepancy in the monthly cycles of the donor and receiver, which are difficult to synchronize. A solution to this problem is the cryoconservation of the donor embryo or cycle synchronization administering GnRH analogs.

Prognosis for success. In 1984 the first IVF-ET from a donated oocyte with ensuing pregnancy was described in a 25-year-old woman suffering from premature ovarian exhaustion (Lutjen et al. 1984). In 1988 eight patients in whom premature ovarian exhaustion was diagnosed received treatment with GIFT and oocyte donation. Six out of these eight patients became pregnant and gave birth to healthy children.

Evaluation. It is estimated that approximately 140000 women in the United States suffer from a disturbance of the ovarian function requiring oocyte donation to possibly achieve a pregnancy.

Comment. This treatment method is not allowed in the Federal Republic of Germany whereas it may be applied in Hungary, France, Greece, USA and other countries.

Surrogate Motherhood

Principle. A surrogate mother carries a pregnancy whereby the gamete originates from another couple. The patient lacking uterine function is stimulated for oocyte maturation simultaneously with the normal ovulatory cycle of the surrogate mother. After oocyte collection from the infertile women, artificial in vitro fertilization by adding the husband's sperm takes place. Shortly afterwards the zygote or embryo is directly transfered into the tubes or the uterus or else stored by cryoconservation. To women having no or a pathological uterus but intact ovaries, a surrogate motherhood offers the chance to produce children that are genetically their own.

Indikations:
- Uterine aplasia, status after hysterectomy, or pathological uterus precluding pregnancy (e.g., Asherman syndrome) in the presence of intact ovaries.

Procedure. See above.

References

Alikani M, Cohen J (1992) Advances in clinical micromanipulation of gametes and embryos: assisted fertilization and hatching. Arch Pathol Lab Med 116:373–378
Antinori S, Versaci C, Pepe G, Panci P, Fuhrberg P (1992) Erbium laser ablation of the human oocyte zona pellucida in the treatment of male factor infertility in IVF cy-

cles. XIV. World Congress on Fertility and Sterility, 22–27 Nov. 1992, Caracas (abstract 260)
Aparicio NJ, De-Turner EA, Schwarzstein L, Turner D (1980) Effect of the phosphodiesterase inhibitor pentoxyfylline on human sperm motility. Andrologia 12:49–54
Asch RH, Ellsworth LR, Balmaceda JP, Wong PC (1984) Pregnancy after translaparoscopic gamete intrafallopian transfer. Lancet II:1034
Asch RH, Ellsworth LR, Balmaceda JP, Wong PC (1985) Gamete intrafallopian transfer (GIFT): a new treatment for infertility. Int J Fertil Menopausal Stud 30:41–46
Asch RH, Balmaceda JP, Ellsworth LR, Wong PC (1986) Preliminary experiences with gamete intrafallopian transfer. Fertil Steril 45:366–371
Ausmanas M, Tureck RW, Blasco L (1985) The zona-free hamster egg penetration assay as a prognostic indicator in a human in vitro fertilization program. Fertil Steril 43:433–437
Avery S, Bolton VN, Mason BA (1990) An evaluation of the hypo-osmotic sperm swelling test as a predictor of fertilizing capacity in vitro. Int J Andrology 13:93–99
Melo-Abreu S, Bond J, Alvarez JG, Blasco L, Garside W, Mastroianni L, Storey BT, Heyner S (1992) Pentoxifylline (PX) affects sperm motility in normal and male factor samples. XIV. World Congress on Fertility and Sterility, 22–27 Nov. 1992, Caracas (abstract 57)
Balmaceda JP, Gastaldi C, Remohi J, Borrero C, Ord T, Asch RH (1988) Tubal embryo transfer as a treatment for infertility due to male factor. Fertil Steril 3:476–479
Barton M, Walker K, Weiser BP (1946) Artificial insemination. Br Med J 1:40
Biggers JD, Brinster RL (1965) Biochemical problems in the early mammalian embryos in vitro. J Exp Zool 158:39–48
Bladou F, Grillo JM, Rossi D, Noizet A, Gamerre M, Erny R, Luciani JM, Serment G (1991) Epididymal sperm aspiration in conjunction with in-vitro fertilization and embryo transfer in cases of obstructive azoospermia. Hum Reprod 6:1284–1287
Bongso TA, Sathananthan AH, Wong PC, Ratnam SS, Ng SC, Anandakumar C, Ganatra S (1989) Human fertilization by microinjection of immotile spermatozoa. Hum Reprod 4:175–179
Bongso A, Ng SC, Ratnam S (1990) Co-cultures: their relevance to assisted reproduction. Hum Reprod 5:893–900
Bongso A, Ng SC, Fong CY, Anandakumar C, Marshall B, Edirisinghe R, Ratnam S (1992) Improved pregnancy rate after transfer of embryos grown in human fallopian tubal cell coculture. Fertil Steril 58:569–574
Brandriff BF, Gordon LA, Haendel S, Singer S, Moore DH, Gledhill BL (1986) Sex chromosome ratios determined by karyotypic analysis in albumin-isolated human sperm. Fertil Steril 46:678–685
Bunge RG, Sherman JK (1953) Fertilizing capacity of frozen human spermatozoa. Nature 172:767
Burkman LJ, Coddington CC, Franken DR, Kruger TF, Rosenwaks Z, Hodgen GD (1988) The hemizona assay (HZA): development of a diagnostic test for the binding of human spermatozoa to the human hemizona pellucida to predict fertilization potential. Fertil Steril 49:688–697
Cecos, Le Lanou F, Lansac J (1989) Artificial procreation with frozen donor semen: experience of French federation: CECOS. Hum Reprod 4:757–761
Chan SYW, Fox EJ, Tang LCH (1985) The relationship between the human spermatozoa hypo-osmotic swelling test and the human spermatozoa zona-free hamster ova penetration bioassay. IRCS Med Sci 13:437–438
Chan SYW, Wang C, Ng M, So WWK, Ho PC (1988) Multivariate discriminant analysis of the relationship between the hypo-osmotic swelling test and the in vitro fertilization capacity of human sperm. Int J Andrology 11:369–378
Chang PH, Tsai EM, Shen MR, Chang JC, Linc YC, Huang CH, Chiang CP (1992) Effects of pentoxifylline in the hamster zona-free oocyte spermatozoa penetration assay and on spermatozoa transmembrane migration motility. Eur Urol 21:151–154
Chang JC, Chen LF, Lin YC, Soong YK (1992) Effect of the phosphodiesterase inhibitor pentoxifylline on human spermatozoa motility. XIV. World Congress on Fertility and Sterility, 22–27 Nov. 1992, Caracas (abstract 166)
Chen C (1986) Pregnancy after human oocyte cryopreservation. Lancet I:884–886
Coddington CC, Franken DR, Burkman LJ, Oosthuizen WT, Kruger T, Hogden GD (1991) Functional aspects of human sperm binding to the zona pellucida using the hemizona assay. J Androl 12:1–8

Cognat M, Zaroukian A, Czyba JC, Guerin JF, Pinatel C, Pinatel L (1992) Pregnancies with IVF using epididymal spermatozoa. XIV. World Congress on Fertility and Sterility, 22–27 Nov. 1992, Caracas (abstract 110)

Cohen J, De Vane GW, Elsner CW, Fehilly CB, Kort HI, Massey JB, Turner TG (1988) Cryopreservation of zygotes and early cleaved human embryos. Fertil Steril 49:283–289

Cohen J, Inge KL, Suzman M, Wiker SR, Wright G (1989a) Videochromatography of fresh and cryopreserved embryos: a retrospective analysis of embryonic morphology and implantation. Fertil Steril 51:820–827

Cohen J, Malter H, Wright G, Kort H, Massey J, Mitchel D (1989b) Partial zona dissection of oocytes when failure of zona pellucida penetration is anticipated. Hum Reprod 4:435–442

Cohen J, Elsner CW, Kort HI, Malter H, Massey JB, Mayer MP, Wiemer K (1990) Impairment of the hatching process following IVF in the human and improvement of implantation by assisting hatching using micromanipulation. Hum Reprod 5:7–13

Cohen J, Alikani M, Malter H, Adler A, Talansky BE, Rosenwaks Z (1991) Partial zona dissection or subzonal sperm insertion: microsurgical fertilization alternatives based on evaluation of sperm and embryo morphology. Fertil Steril 56:696–706

Cohen J, Alikani M, Trowbridge J, Rosenwaks Z (1992) Implantation enhancement by selective assisted hatching using zona drilling of human embryos with poor prognosis. Hum Reprod 7:685–691

Confino E, Friberg J, Dudkiewicz AB, Gleicher N (1986) Intrauterine inseminations with washed human spermatozoa. Fertil Steril 46:55–60

Corson SL, Batzer FR, Alexander NJ (1984) Sex selection by sperm separation and insemination. Fertil Steril 42:756–760

Craft I, Djahanbakch O, McLeod F (1982) Human pregnancy following oocyte and sperm transfer to the uterus. Lancet I:1031–1033

Cruz RI, Kemmanna E, Brandeis VT, Becker KA, Beck M, Beardsley Y, Sheldon R (1986) A prospective study of intrauterine insemination of processed sperm from men with oligoasthenospermia in superovulated women. Fertil Steril 46:673–677

De Kretzer D, Dennis P, Hudson B (1973) Transfer of a human zygote. Lancet II:729

Deutsch E (1987) Rechtliche Gesichtspunkte der künstlichen Insemination und extrakorporale Befruchtung. In: Dietrich-Reichart E (ed) Insemination. In-vitro-Fertilisation 251–288

Devroey P, Braeckmans P, Smitz J, van Waesberghe L, Wisanto A, Van Steirtegheim A, Heytens L, Camu F (1986) Pregnancy after translaparoscopic zygote intrafallopian transfer in a patient with sperm antibodies. Lancet:1329

Devroey P, Camus M, Van den Abbeel E, Van Waesberghe L, Wisanto A, Van Steirteghem AC (1989) Establishment of twenty-two pregnancies after oocyte and embryo donation. Br J Obstet Gynaecol 96:900–901

Diedrich K, Krebs D (1990) Indikation und Ergebnisse zur in-vitro-Fertilisation, intratubarem Gameten (GIFT) und Embryotransfer (EIFT). TW Gynäkologe 23:186–195

Edirisinghe WR, Wales RG, Chapman HM, Yovich JL (1991) Assisted fertilization of mouse oocytes and preliminary results from human oocytes using zona drilling. J Vitro Fertil Embryo Transfer 8:48–55

Feichtinger W (1992) New transfer techniques. XIV. World Congress on Fertility and Sterility, 22–27 Nov. 1992, Caracas (abstract PS9)

Feichtinger W, Strohmer H, Radner KM (1992) Erbium YAG laser for micromanipulation of oocytes and spermatozoa. Lancet II:115–116

Fishel S, Antinori S, Jackson P, Johnson J, Rinaldi L (1991) Presentation of six pregnancies established by sub-zonal insemination (SUZI). Hum Reprod 6:124–130

Focus on Reproduction (1992) Survey on assisted fertilization. Focus on Reproduction 11:II-4

Forrler A, Badoc E, Moreau L, Dellenbach P (1986) Direct intraperitoneal insemination: first results confined. Lancet II:1468

Franken DR, Oehninger S, Johnson-Burkman L, Coddington C, Kruger T (1989) The hemizona assay (HZA): a predictor of human sperm fertilizing potential in in vitro fertilization (IVF). J Vitro Fert Embryo Transfer 6:44–50

Franken D, Windt ML, Oosthuizen T, Kruger T, Menkveld R, Coddington C, Hodgen GD (1991) Assisted reproductive technologies may obviate apparent immunologic infertility. Andrologia 23:291–295

Friedler S, Giudice LC, Lamb EJ (1988) Cryopreservation of embryos and ova. Fertil Steril 49:743–764

Fugger EF, Bustillo M, Katz LP, Dorfmann AD, Bender SD, Schulman JD (1988) Embryonic development and pregnancy from fresh and cryopreserved sibling pronucleate human zygotes. Fertil Steril 50:273–278
Fukui Y, McGowan LT, James RW, Pugh PA, Tervit HR (1991) Factors affecting the in-vitro development to blastocysts of bovine oocytes matured and fertilized in vitro. J Reprod Fertil 92:125–131
Garrisi GJ, Talansky BE, Grunfeld L, Sapira V, Navot D, Gordon JW (1990) Clinical evaluation of three approaches to micromanipulation-assisted fertilization. Fertil Steril 54:671–677
Gavella M, Lipovac V, Marotti T (1991) Effect of pentoxifylline on superoxide anion production by human sperm. Int J Andrology 14:320–327
Gordon J, Gang I (1990) Use of zona drilling for safe and effective biopsy of murine oocytes and embryos. Biol Reprod 42:869–876
Gordon J, Grunfeld L, Garrisi G, Talansky B, Richards C, Laufer N (1988) Fertilization of human oocytes by sperm from infertile males after zona pellucida drilling. Fertil Steril 50:68–73
Gordts S, Garcia G, Swinnen K, Vercruyssen M, Roziers P, Campo R (1992) A prospective randomized study of SUZI in cases of male subfertility. 8th Annual Meeting of the ESHRE, The Hague, 1992 (abstract 140)
Hammond J (1949) Recovery and culture of tubal mouse ova. Nature 163:28–29
Hammit DG, Bedia E, Rogers PR, Syrop CH, Donovan JF, Williamson RA (1989) Comparison of motility stimulants for cryopreserved human semen. Fertil Steril 52:495–502
Hámori M, Stuckensen JA, Rumpf D, Kniewald T, Kniewald A, Marquez MA (1988) Zygote intrafallopian transfer (ZIFT): evaluation of 42 cases. Fertil Steril 50:519–521
Hard AD (1909) Artificial insemination. Med World 27:253
Heape W (1891) Preliminary note on the transplantation and growth of mammalian ova within an uterine forster-mother. Proc R Soc:457–458
Heape W (1897) Further note on the transplantation and growth of mammalian ova within an uterine forster-mother. Proc R Soc:178–183
Heiss H (1972) Die künstliche Insemination der Frau. Urban und Schwarzenberg, Munich, pp 7–8
Hensleigh HC, Hunter AG (1985) In vitro maturation of bovine cumulus enclosed primary oocytes and their subsequent in vitro fertilization and cleavage. J Dairy Sci 68:1456–1562
Hill DL, Adler D, Rothman C, Surrey M, Danzer H, Friedman S (1991) Micromanipulation in a center for reproductive medicine. Fertil Steril 56:36–38
Imoedemhe DAG, Sigue AB, Pacpaco EA, Olazo AB (1992a) Successfully use of the sperm motility enhancer 2-deoxyadenosine in previously failed human in vitro fertilization. J Assisted Reprod Genet 9:53–56
Imoedemhe DAG, Sigue AB, Pacpaco E, Luciano (1992b) Successful use of microinseminated oocyte fallopian transfer (MISOFT) in male factor infertility XIV. World Congress on Fertility and Sterility, 22–27 Nov. 1992, Caracas (abstract 462)
Jansen RPS, Anderson J (1987) Catheterisation of the fallopian tubes from the vagina. Lancet I:309–310
Jansen RP, Anderson JC, Radonic I, Smith J, Sutherland PD (1988) Pregnancies after ultrasound-guided fallopian insemination with cryostored donor semen. Fertil Steril 49:920–922
Jean M, Barriere P, Sagot P, L'Hermite A, Lopes P (1992) Utility of zona pellucida drilling in cases of severe semen alterations in man. Fertil Steril 57:591–596
Jeyendran RS, Van der Ven HH, Perez-Pelaez M, Crabo BG, Zaneveld LJD (1984) Development of an assay to assass the functional integrity of the human sperm membrane and its relationship to other semen characteristics. J Reprod Fertil 70:219–228
Jones HW, Acosta A, Andrews MC, Garcia JE, Jones GS, Manztawinos T, McDowell J, Sandow B, Veeck L, Whibley T (1983) The importance of follicular phased to success and failure in in vitro fertilization. Fertil Steril 40:317–321
Junca AM, Mandelbaum J, Plachot M (1984) Human sperm penetration test: value, limits and perspectives. Contracept Fertil Sex 12:491–494
Kasai M, Iritani A, Chang MC (1979) Fertilization in vitro of rat ovarian oocytes after freezing and thawing. Biol Reprod 21:839–844
Kerin JFP, Peek J, Warnes GM, Kirby C, Jeffrey R, Matthew CD, Cox LW (1984) Improved conception rate after intrauterine insemination of washed spermatozoa from men with poor quality semen. Lancet 1:533–535

Kodama H, Kigure T, Harada T, Kato M, Matsui T, Takeda S, Sekine K, Maki M (1991) In vitro fertilization using epididymal spermatozoa for the patients with obstructive azoospermia. Acta Obst Gynaec Jpn 43:1267–1269
Kola I, Lacham O, Jansen RPS, Turner M, Trounson A (1990) Chromosomal analysis of human oocytes fertilized by microinjection of spermatozoa into the perivitelline space. Hum Reprod 5:575–577
Kola I, Wilton L (1991) Preimplantation embryo biopsy: detection of trisomy in a single cell biopsied from a four-cell mouse embryo. Mol Reprod Dev 29:16–21
Lanzendorf S, Maloney M, Veck L, Slusser J, Hodgen GD, Rosenwaks Z (1988) A preclinical evaluation of pronuclear formation by microinjection of human spermatozoa into human oocytes. Fertil Steril 49:835–842
Laws-King A, Trounson A, Sathananthan AH, Kola I (1987) Fertilization of human oocytes by micro-injection of a single spermatozoa under the zone pellucida. Fertil Steril 48:637–642
Lehmann F, Haeske-Seeberg H, Seeberg B (1991) Aktueller Stand der IVF- and GIFT-Therapie in der Bundesrepublik Deutschland. Fertilität 7:150–155
Lopata A, Johnston IWH, Hoult IJ, Speirs AI (1980) Pregnancy following intrauterine implantation of an embryo obtained by in vitro fertilization of a preovulatory egg. Fertil Steril 33:117–120
Lucena E, Ruiz JA, Mendoza JC, Ortiz JA, Lucena C, Gomez M, Arango A (1989) Vaginal intratubal insemination (VITI) and vaginal GIFT, endosonographic technique: early experience. Hum Reprod 4:658–662
Lutjen P, Trounson A, Leeton J, Findlay J, Wood C, Renou P (1984) The establishment and maintenance of pregnancy using in vitro fertilization and embryo donation in a patient with primary ovarian failure. Nature 307:174–175
Maaßen B, Stauber M (1988) Die Gebrüder Hunter und die erste künstliche Befruchtung beim Menschen. In: Der andere Weg zum eigenen Kind. De Gruyter, Berlin, pp 16–18
Malter HE, Cohen J (1989) Partial zona dissection of the human oocyte: a nontraumatic method using micromanipulation to assist zona pellucida penetration. Fertil Steril 51:139–148
Malter HE, Talansky B, Gordon J, Cohen J (1989) Monospermy and polyspermy after partial zona dissection of reinseminated homan oocytes. Gamete Research 23:377–386
Mao C, Grimes DA (1988) The sperm penetration assay: can it discriminate between fertile and infertile men? Am J Obstet Gynecol 159:279–286
Margalioth EJ, Feinmesser M, Navot D, Mordel N, Broson RA (1989) The long term predictive value of the zona-free hamster ova sperm penetration assay. Fertil Steril 52:490–494
Marshall FHA (1910) The physiology of reproduction, 1st edn. Longmans, London
Medical Research International, Society for Assisted Reproductive Technology, The American Fertility-Society (1991) In vitro fertilization-embryo transfer (IVF-ET) in the United States: 1989 results from the IVF-ET registry. Fertil Steril 55:14–23
Meier U, Hienert G (1990) Tamoxifen and kallikrein in therapy of oligoasthenospermia: results of a randomized study. Eur Urol 17:223–225
Melo-Abreu S, Bond JG, Alvarez JG, Blasco L, Garside W, Mastroianni L, Storey BT, Heyner S (1992) Pentoxifylline (PX) affects spem motility in normal and male factor samples. XIV. World Congress on Fertility and Sterility, 22–27 Nov. 1992, Caracas (abstract 57)
Micic S, Hadzi-Djokic J, Dotlic R, Tulic C (1988) Pentoxifylline treatment of oligoasthenospermic men. Acte Eur Fertil 19:135–137
Morsy M, Takeuchi K, Kaufmann R, Veeck L, Hodgen GD, Beebe SJ (1992) Preclinical models for human pre-embryo biopsy and genetic diagnosis II. Fertil Steril 57:431–438
Muggleton-Harris AL, Findlay I (1991) In-vitro studies on "spare" human preimplantation embryos in culture. Hum Reprod 6:85–92
Ng SC, Bongso TA, Ratnam SS, Sathananthan HM, Chan CLK, Wong PC, Hagglund L, Anandakumar C, Wong YC, Goh VHH (1988) Pregnancy after transfer of multiple sperm under the zona. Lancet II:790
Ng SC, Bongso A, Chang S, Sathananthan H, Ratnam SS (1989) Transfer of human sperm into the perivitelline space of human oocytes after zona-drilling or zona puncture. Fertil Steril 52:73–78

Ng SC, Bongso A, Ratnam SS (1991) Microinjection of human oocytes: a technique for severe oligoasthenoteratozoospermia. Fertil Steril 56:1117–1123
Ng FLH, Liu DY, Gordon-Baker HW (1992) Comparison of Percoll, mini-Percoll and swim-up methods for sperm preparation from abnormal semen samples. Hum Reprod 7:261–266
Oates RD, Honig S, Berger MJ, Harris D (1992) Microscopic epididymal sperm aspiration (MESA): a new option for treatment of the obstructive azoospermia associated with cystic fibrosis. J Assisted Reprod Genet 9:36–40
Olar TT, La Nasa J, Dickley RP, Taylor SN, Curole DN (1990) Fertilization of human oocytes by microinjection of human sperm aspirated from the caput epididymidis on an individual with obstructive azoospermia. J Vitro Fertil Embryo Transfer 7:160–164
Palermo G, Joris H, Devroey P, Van Steirteghem AC (1992a) Induction of acrosome reaction in human spermatozoa used for subzonal insemination. Hum Reprod 7:248–254
Palermo G, Joris H, Camus M, Devroey P, Van Steirteghem AC (1992b) Assisted fertilization by direct intracytoplasmatic sperm injection to treat severe male factor infertility. 8th Annual Meeting of the ESHRE, The Hague (abstract 142)
Parker AS (1958) Factors affecting the viability of frozen ovarian tissue. J Endocrinol 17:337–343
Patrizen P, Silber S, Ord T, Balmaceda JP, Asch RH (1988) Two births after microsurgical sperm aspiration in congenital absence of vas deferens. Lancet:1364
Payne D, McLaughlin KJ, Depypere HT, Kirby CA, Warnes GM, Matthews CD (1991) Experience with zona pellucida drilling and zona cutting to improve fertilization rates of human oocytes in vitro. Hum Reprod 6:423–431
Prasad MRN (1984) The in vitro sperm penetration test: a review. Int J Andrology 7:5–22
Prins GS, Wagner C, Weidel L, Gianfortoni J, Marut EL, Scommegna A (1987) Gonadotropins augment maturation and fertilization of human immature oocytes cultured in vitro. Fertil Steril 47:1035–1037
Ranoux C, Aubriot FX, Dubuisson JB, Cardone V, Foulout H, Poirot C, Chevallier O (1988) A new in vitro fertilization technique: intravaginal culture. Fertil Steril 49:654–657
Rhemrev JPT, Jejendran RS, Vermeiden JPW, Zaneveld LJD (1988) Sperm selection by glass-wool filtration and a simple discontinuous Percoll gradient centrifugation technique. Hum Reprod 3:93
Riedel HH, Hubner F, Ensslen SC, Bieniek KW, Grillo M (1989) Minimal andrological requirements for in-vitro fertilization. Hum Reprod 4:73–77
Rock J, Menkin MF (1944) In vitro fertilization and cleavage of human ovarian eggs. Science 100:105–107
Rodebush WE, Kim JG, Minhas BS, Dodson MG (1990) Survival and cell acquisition rates after preimplantation embryo biopsy: use of two mechanical techniques and two mouse strains. Am J Obstet Gynecol 162:1084–1090
Sathananthan AH, Ng SC, Trounson A, Bongso A, Laws-King A, Ratnam SS (1989) Human micro-insemination by injection of single or multiple sperm: ultrastructure. Hum Reprod 4:574–583
Shettles LB (1978) Sex selection. Infertility 1:127–135
Schenk S (1880) Das Säugetierei künstlich befruchtet außerhalb des Muttertieres. Mitt Embr Inst KK Univ Wien 1:107
Serhal PF, Katz M (1987) Intrauterine insemination. Lancet I:52–53
Shen MR, Chiang PH, Yang RC, Hong CY, Chen SS (1991) Pentoxifylline stimulates human sperm motility both in vitro and after oral therapy. Br J Clin Pharmacol 31:711–714
Siddiq S (1992) MISA experience in Pakistan. XIV. World Congress on Fertility and Sterility, 22–27 Nov. 1992, Caracas (abstractr 111)
Siebzehnrübl ER (1989) Cryopreservation of gametes and clevage stage embryos. Hum Reprod 4 (Suppl):105–110
Sikka SC, Hellstrom WJG (1991) The application of pentoxifylline in the stimulation of sperm motion in men undergoing electroejaculation. J Androl 12:165–170
Silber SJ, Balmaceda JP, Ord T, Borrero C, Ord T, Asch R (1988) Pregnancy with sperm aspiration from the proximal head of the epididymidis: a new treatment for congenital absence of the vas deferens. Fertil Steril 50:525–528

Simon A, Younis A, Lewin A, Bartov B, Schenker JG, Laufer N (1991) The correlation between sperm cell morphology and fertilization after zona pellucida slitting in subfertile males. Fertil Steril 56:325–331
Smith AU, Polge C (1950) Survival of spermatozoa at low temperatures. Nature 166:668–669
Smith R, Madariaga M, Bustos-Obregon E (1992) Reappraisal of the hypo-osmotic swelling test to improve assessment of seminal fertility status. Int J Andrology 15:5–13
Soong YK, Lai YM, Chang SY, Chang MJ, Wang ML (1992) Subzonal sperm injection (SZI) as a treatment of patients with severe fertilization failure in IVF. XIV. World Congress on Fertility and Sterility, 22–27 Nov. 1992, Caracas (abstract 78)
Steptoe PC, Edwards RG (1976) Reimplantation of a human embryo with subsequent tubal pregnancy. Lancet I:880–882
Steptoe PC, Edwards RG (1978) Birth after the reimplantation of a human embryo. Lancet 2:8079–8092
Sterzik K, Rosenbusch B, Sasse V, Terinde R, Wolf A, Beier HM, Lauritzen C (1988) Erfahrungen und Erfolge mit der intravaginalen Fertilisation und Kultur von menschlichen Eizellen. Geburtsh Frauenheilk 48:850–853
Sterzik K, Rosenbusch B, Danasouri I, Lauritzen C (1992) Etablierung einer Schwangerschaft nach partieller Zona dissection (PZD) der Eizelle im Rahmen der In-vitro-Fertilisation (IVF). Geburtsh Frauenheilk 52:340–342
Strohmer H, Feichtinger W (1992a) Successful clinical application of laser for micromanipulation in an in vitro fertilization program. Fertil Steril 58:212–214
Strohmer H, Feichtinger W (1992b) Assisted hatching in cases of previously failed IVF-attempts. XIV. World Congress on Fertility and Sterility, 22–27 Nov. 1992, Caracas (abstract 92)
Strohmer H, Antinori S, Feichtinger W (1992) Human pregnancies after partial opening of the zona pellucida by erbium-YAG-laser. 8th Annual Meeting of the ESHRE, The Hague (abstract 139)
Sunde A, Kahn J, Molne K (1988) Intrauterine insemination. Human Reprod 3:97–99
Takeuchi K, Sandow BA, Morsy M, Kaufmann R, Beebe SJ, Hodgen GD (1992) Preclinical models for human pre-embryo biopsy and genetic diagnosis. I. Fertil Steril 57:425–430
Tesarik J, Pilka L, Dvorak M, Travnick P (1983) Oocyte recovery, in-vitro insemination, and transfer into the oviduct after its microsurgical repair at a single laparotomy. Fertil Steril 39:472–475
Trotnow S, Kniewald T, Al-Hasani S, Becker H (1981) Follikelpunktion, In-vitro-Fertilisierung, Embryotransfer und eingetretene Schwangerschaften in Dyneric/HCG-stimulierten Zyklen. Geburtsh Frauenheilk 41:835–836
Trounson A, Mohr L (1983) Human pregnancy following cryopreservation, thawing and transfer of an eight cell embryo. Nature 305:707–709
Tucker MJ, Cohen J, Massey JB, Mayer MP, Wiker SR, Wright G (1991) Partial zona dissection of the zona pellucida of frozen-thawed human embryos may enhance blastocyst hatching, implantation, and pregnancy rates. Am J Obstet Gynecol 165/2:341–345
Urbancsek J (1989) Prinzip der In-vitro-Fertilisierung mit anschließendem Embryotransfer und des Gametentransfers. In: Serum LH und seine Bedeutung bei Gonadotropinstimulationen mit und ohne GnRH-Analogon im Rahmen des In-vitro-Fertilisierungs- und Gametentransferprogrammes der Universitäts-Frauenklinik Heidelberg. Dissertation, pp 7–8
Urbancsek J, Rabe T, Grunwald K, Cumpelik S, Kiesel L (1991) Prediction of specific LH patterns before and after ovulation induction with HCG in an IVF-ET/GIFT program. In: Boutaleb Y, Gzouli A (eds) Recent developments in fertility and sterility series, vol. 5: Assisted reproduction, pp 99–114
Van den Saffele J, Vermeulen L, Schoonjans F, Comhaire FH (1992) Evaluation of the hypo-osmotic swelling test in relation with advanced methods of semen analysis. Andrologia 24:213–217
Vanderzwalmen P, Barlow P, Nijs M, Bertin G, Leroy F, Schoysman R (1992) Usefulness of partial zona dissection of the zona pellucida in a human in-vitro fertilization program. Human Reprod 7:537–544
Van Blerk B, Nijs M, Van Steirteghem AC (1991) Decompaction and biopsy of late mouse morulae: assessment of in-vitro and in-vivo development potential. Hum Reprod 6:1298–1304

Veersma S, Bernardus RE, Veersma D, Vermeiden JPW, Schoemaker J (1989) Pregnancy following transcervical transfer of oocyte and sperm. N Engl J Med 320:149
Wang C, Chan CW, Wong KK, Yeung KK (1983) Comparison of the effectiveness of placebo, clomiphene citrate, mesterolone, pentoxifylline, and testosterone rebound therapy for the treatment of idiopathic oligospermia. Fertil Steril 40:358–365
Wilmut J (1972) The effect of cooling rate, warming rate, cryoprotective agent and stage of development on survival of mouse embryos during freezing and thawing. Life Sci 11:1071–1079
Wilmut J, Rowson LEA (1973) Experiments on the low temperature preservation of cow embryos. Vet Rec 92:686–690
Wilton LJ, Shaw JM, Trounson AO (1989) Successful single-cell biopsy and cryopreservation of preimplantation mouse embryos. Fertil Steril 51:513–517
Whitten WK (1956) Culture of tubal mouse ova. Nature 177:96
Whittingham DG, Leibo SP, Mazur P (1972) Survival of mouse embryos frozen to −196°C and −269°C. Science 178:411–414
Wittemer C, Moreau L, Dellenbach P, Gerlinger P, Le Meur M-A, Chambon P (1991) A case of human pregnancy after microinjection of capacitated sperm into the pervitelline space. J Vitro Fert Embryo Transfer 8:222–224
World Collaborative Report Bilan Mondial 1989 (1991) Edited for the 7th World Congress on In Vitro Fertilization and Assisted Procreation, Paris, June 30–July 3, 1991
Wright G, Wiker S, Elsner C, Kort H, Massey J, Mitchell D, Toledo A, Cohen J (1990) Observations on the morphology of pronuclei and in human zygotes and implications for cryopreservation. Hum Reprod 5:109–115
Yanagimachi R, Yanagimachi H, Rogers BJ (1976) The use of zona-free animal ova as a test-system for the assessment of the fertilizing capacity of human spermatozoa. Biol Reprod 15:471–476
Yeung WSB, Ho PC, Lau EYL, Chan STH (1992) Improved development of human embryos in-vitro by a human oviductal cell co-culture system. Hum Reprod 7:1144–1149
Yovich YM, Edirisinghe WR, Cummins JM, Yovich JL (1990) Influence of pentoxifylline in severe male factor infertility. Fertil Steril 53:715–722
Yovich YM, Edirisinghe WR, Cummins JM, Yovich JL (1988) Preliminary results using pentoxifylline in a pronuclear stage tubal transfer (PROST) program for severe male factor infertility. Fertil Steril 50:179–181
Zaninovic N, Lucena C, Arango A, Lucena E (1992) Micromanipulation program in "CECOLFES" Colombia SA: preliminary results. XIV. World Congress on Fertility and Sterility, 22–27 Nov. 1992, Caracas (abstract 160)
Zarutzkie PW, Muller CH, Magone M, Soules MR (1989) The clinical relevance of sex selection techniques. Fertil Steril 52:891–905

Treatment of Male Factor Infertility by In Vitro Fertilization and Microinsemination

I. Psalti

Introduction

Infertility is generally considerd to be a "woman's problem". There is a tendency for men to think of fertility and virility as synonymous, a myth that needs to be dispelled (Cooke 1993).

In a series of 1242 in vitro fertilizations (IVFs) the pure male factor and mixed male factor indications represented respectively 17% and 32.5% of all indications (Psalti et al. 1992; Bouckaert et al. 1994). While the fertilization rate of tubal factor was 60%, it was only 24% in male factor (Psalit et al. 1992). So, the stage of fertilization becomes a problem when in the infertility the male partner is affected.

Referring to our own and the literature results, I will discuss the role of the IVF and the microinsemination in the treatment of male factor infertility.

Physiology of Fertilization

Fertilization in mammals is a highly regulated process that is dependent on the transport of physiologically competent spermatozoa to the upper oviduct near the time of ovulation (Overstreet 1983). The spermatozoa in vivo must penetrate and traverse the cervical mucus, ascend the female reproductive tract, undergo capacitation and acrosome reaction (AR), generate the fusogenic equatorial segment, penetrate the zona pellucida (ZP) and then undergo nuclear decondensation (Richardson and Aitken 1993).

Capacitation In Vivo and In Vitro

The physiological changes in sperm cells that are required for sperm migration to the oviduct and for fertilization are collectively termed capacitation. The term capacitation was originally proposed to refer to physiological changes in spermatozoa that render the spermatozoa capable of fertilizing the eggs (Austin 1952). Capacitation is a series of changes (see review of Yanagimachi 1988) that makes the spermatozoa capable of undergoing the acrosome reaction. It normally takes place in the genital tract of the female. It may start while the spermatozoa are passing through the cervix or cervical mucus. In vitro sperm capacitation and fertilization are certainly possible without any contributions from the female genital tract.

Because the plasma membrane of spermatozoa is directly exposed to the capacitating environment, it is not surprising that very prominent changes take place in this membrane during capacitation. The removal or alteration of coating materials from the sperm surface constitutes an important part of capacitation (Weinman and Williams 1964). Some proteins or glycoproteins are released and/or added to sperm surfaces during capacitation. There have been several articles reporting that hte phospholipid composition of sperm membrane changes. Spermatozoa exhibit increased metabolism like glycolytic activity and oxygen consumption (Boell 1985). During capacitation an increase in intracellular Ca^{2+} concentration occurs which may stimulate sperm adenylate cyclase, allowing the expression of cAMP-dependent events that are prerequisite for fertilization (Yanagimachi 1988). Capacitated sperm in vivo and in vitro undergo changes in their movement characteristics from linear, forwardly progressive motion to less linear, vigorous, hyperactivated motility. Hyperactivation is considered to be an important marker of capacitation, and may be necessary to produce the forces required for sperm migration and fertilization (Katz et al. 1989).

Acrosome Reaction

The eggs of many animals are surrounded by glycoprotein coats through which spermatozoa must pass before reaching the egg plasma membrane. All mammalian eggs are surrounded by a thick glycoprotein coat, the ZP. In most species, the ZP is further surrounded by the cumulus oophorus, which consists of cumulus cells and their matrix. The main component of the cumulus matrix is hyaluronic acid. It has been generally believed that hyaluronidase released from acrosome-reacting spermatozoa digests the cumulus matrix and that acrosin carried on the surface of acrosome-reacted spermatozoa aids in the passage of spermatozoa through the zona.

The AR has at least two functions: it renders spermatozoa capable of penetrating through the ZP and fusing with the egg plasma membrane (Yanagimachi 1988). Most probably, spermatozoa use both mechanical and enzymatical means in passing through the ZP (Yanagimachi 1988). Obviously, spermatozoa could never penetrate thick ZP if they were immotile or weakly motile. Spermatozoa must possess strong thrusting power to successfully pass through the ZP. However, strong motility alone is apparently not enough for successful sperm passage through the ZP. Acrosomal materials (including enzymes) seem to pave the way for sperm passage. Some of the acrosomal materials released may alter ZP molecules (soften the ZP) prior to sperm penetration.

Egg-Sperm Fusion

Upon passing through the ZP, the sperm head crosses the perivitelline space, becomes attached to the vitellus, and is gradually incorporated into it. Then the plasma membrane above the equatorial segment fuses first with the egg plasma membrane (Bedford et al. 1979). It is important to note that the plasma membrane above the equatorial segment becomes capable of fusing with the egg plasma membrane only after the spermatozoa has undergone its AR.

The acrosome-intact spermatozoa, regardless of whether it is capacitated or not, is unable to fuse with the egg, even if it is brought directly to the egg surface, by passing the ZP. An important physiological change must take place in the plasma membrane over the equatorial segment concurrent with (or as the result of) the AR (Yanagimachi 1988). What is exactly happening in this membrane is not yet clear.

In Vitro Fertilization

General Results

To illustrate the incidence of absence of fertilization in an IVF programme, our sample includes the 591 patients who were treated by IVF. In this series 1399 ovarian stimulation cycles, 1242 retrievals, 968 transfers, 234 pregnancies with 140 live deliveries were previously reported (Psalti et al. 1992; Bouckaert et al. 1994). Details about the procedures used for ovarian stimulation, egg retrieval, fertilization and transfer have been given in other papers (Psalti et al. 1988; De Cooman et al. 1988; Loumaye et al. 1988; Psalti et al. 1989; Loumaye et al. 1989).

Failure of Fertilization

In our sample, 591 patients were treated. This means that there were 591 first attempts at IVF. Among these, 133 (22.5%) failures of fertilization occurred. Of these patients, 59 repeated at least a second IVF subsequently. In the second attempt, the fertilization rate increased to 15% (Table 1). All parameters studied between first and second attempts at IVF were equivalent. In these 59 cases, the male factor (pure and mixed) represented 73% of indications. Without changing the ovarian stimulation protocol and sperm preparation in a subsequent IVF procedure, 15% fertilization was obtained. In 29 patients, failure of fertilization persisted. In the other 30 patients, a mean of 30% oocytes were fertilized. This means that, without any changing in IVF protocol, fertilization was achieved in 50% of patients in whom, in a previous IVF, failure of fertilization occurred. However, the fertilization rate was low. During the second attempt, 46% of patients had $<10\times10^6$ motile spermatozoa/ml in fresh semen) had a fertilization rate of 19.1% (40/209). The minimum motile

Table 1 Fertilization rate in 59 IVF patients in the first (with failure of fertilization) and second IVF attempts. The mean numbers of oocytes, of motile spermatozoa (spz) in fresh semen (FS), or normal morphology spermatozoa, and of motile spermatozoa in washed semen (WS) by the swim-up method were studied

	1st attempt	3nd attempt
Fertilization rate (%)	0	15
Embryo/oocyte	0/453	73/486
Mean oocyte per retrieaval	7.7±5.4	8.2±4.6
Motile spz in FS (M/ml)	15.7±16.2	18.3±19.9
Normal morphology in FS (%)	22.9±13.1	22.2±12.1
Motile spz in WS (M/ml)	2.3±2.2	2.6±2.2

spermatozoa in fresh semen with fertilization was 0.8×10^6/ml, the fertilization rate being 6%.

For sperm intended for IVF good progressive motility, a high percentage of normal form, a suitable linear velocity (more than 15 µm/s, De Cooman et al. 1991) and a low acrosome-reacted proportion of semen are required. It is possible to improve sperm parameters with different washing procedures. The self-migration method complies better with these criteria (Psalti et al. 1993). However, in cases of repeated failure of IVF or for men with very poor sperm, we suggest microinsemination techniques to the patient.

Fertilization with Micromanipulation Techniques

There are several instances where micromanipulation procedures might provide clinical benefit: (1) One area would be in the treatment of male infertility. Several micromanipulation techniques could be used to achieve fertilization with severely compromised males (see below). (2) Micromanipulation also aims at enhancing embryonic hatching (Cohen et al. 1990). (3) Another potential benefit of this technique would be to correct gross fertilization errors with enucleation of tripronuclear zygote (Rawlins et al. 1988). (4) The most intriguing potential use of pre-embryo micromanipulation would be in the area of early embryonic genetic diagnosis (Handyside et al. 1990).

When using micromanipulation techniques our purpose is to enhance the fertilization rate in cases of male infertility. The ZP is considered to be the main block to sperm penetration in mammalian eggs. Hence in possible situations of reduced ability of sperm to penetrate the ZP, such as oligozoospermia, zonal procedures to assist the sperm to pass through the ZP may be of assistance. Complete removal of the ZP will result in polyspermy and reduced developmental ability, because the preimplantation embryo is protected by this investment during early development (Ng et al. 1990).

Many micromanipulation techniques have been proposed in these problem cases. One consists of creating one or more holes in the ZP, either chemically with Tyrode's acid solution in the zona drilling method (Gordon et al. 1988) or mechanically with a needle in the technique of partial zona dissection (Cohen et al. 1988). The other consists of injecting one or more spermatozoa under the ZP in the subzonal insemination method (Laws-King et al. 1987) or directly into the ooplasm in intracytoplasmic sperm injection (Lanzendorf et al. 1988). Zona drilling with acid Tyrode's solution led to highest rates of oocyte damage and that embryonic development is compromised (Garrisi et al. 1990). Thus, this method is abandoned now.

Partial Zona Dissection (PZD)

PZD uses mechanical force to create an opening in the ZP to facilitate sperm penetration. In PZD the operator does not select the spermatozoa. PZD allows natural sperm selection to occur so that spermatozoa of highest motility will be able to reach the ZP incisions and enter the perivitelline space to fertilize the eggs. Moreover, the size of opening is important for the outcome of PZD. Creating small openings leads to a lower fertilization rate (Levron 1990).

The putative beneficial effect of PZD on oocyte fertilization was evaluated in 40 couples for whom no fertilization was obtained in previous IVF attempts (Psalti et al 1990). Half of the oocytes of each patient were randomly selected for micromanipulation, while the others were used as a control group to compare fertilization rate. Fertilization rate was 9.5% (16/168) and 15% (25/167) respectively for control and PZD-treated oocytes (NS). After washing, and with a sperm density $>10^6$/ml, the fertilization rate was 18.3% (11/60) and 26.7% (20/75) for control and PZD oocytes respectively (NS). In this series, replacement of 20 PZD and 16 control embryos in 15 patients resulted in two clinical pregnancies (pregnancy rate per transfer: 13.3%) (Psalti et al. 1990). The baseline semen parameters used by some authors in PZD are $10–20\times10^6$ spz/ml, motility >20% and normal morphology >40% (Sakkas et al. 1993). The procedure appeared most efficient in patients with a total motile sperm count after washing of $>5\times10^6$/ml (Simon et al. 1991). Generally, the fertilization rate with PZD is around 15% (Terriou et al. 1993). Moreover, in a review of PZD results, the mean clinical pregnancy rate per embryo transfer was as low as 11% (Laufer et al. 1991).

PZD has been associated with increased rates of polysperma (Psalti et al. 1990), abnormal cleavage and impaired compaction of the human morula, herniation of the blastocyst through the opened ZP and even expulsion of the embryo through the opened ZP during embryo transfer (Garrisi et al. 1990).

Subzonal Insemination (SUZI)

The technique of microinjection of sperm into the perivitelline space of the mature human oocyte was developed to try to improve the occurrence of fertilization in couples with severe male factor infertility in whom conventional IVF techniques have been unsuccessful. This procedure relies on the increased probability that spermatozoa capable of fertilization will come into direct contact with the oolemma of the oocyte by avoiding the necessity of making their way through the ZP. In appears useful to apply SUZI to the more extreme forms (<50 000 motile spermatozoa recoverable after semen preparation) of male factor infertility (Lippi et al. 1993), whereas PZD is more beneficial in cases of moderately abnormal semen profiles (Cohen et al. 1991). However, SUZI appears to have fewer complications than PZD (Lippi et al. 1993). Moreover, SUZI is advisable in cases of severe asthenozoospermia since Bongso et al. (1989) demonstrated that human oocytes could be fertilized with immotile spermatozoa via SUZI and that in the human, as in other species, sperm motility may not be essential for sperm-egg fusion.

Fusion of the sperm with the oocyte requires the sperm to be acrosome reacted first. Human sperm with intact acrosomes transferred into the perivitelline space do not fuse with the egg. Therefore, for single sperm transfer to be efficient, the proportion of acrosome-reacted sperm needs to be high (Ng et al. 1990). The overall fertilization rate reported with SUZI is around 12%–15% (Fishel et al. 1991; Sakkas et al. 1992; Lippi et al. 1993) or 30% (Cohen et al. 1991). When the spermatozoa were treated with follicular fluid or with electroporation to enhance AR, a fertilization rate up to 31% was obtained (Palermo et al. 1992a).

In a review of microinsemination methods, the mean clinical pregnancy rate per embryo transfer in SUZI (16.5%) appeared to be more than in the PZD (11%) method (Laufer et al. 1991).

Intracytoplasmic Sperm Injection (ICSI)

ICSI has recently been described as beneficial in alleviating infertility in couples who could not be helped by standard IVF treatment or SUZI of the oocytes (Palermo et al. 1992b; Van Steirteghem et al. 1993a, b). For ICSI, the oocyte is held by the holding pipette, the injecting micropipette is pushed through the ZP and into the ooplasm, a single spermatozoon is injected into the ooplasm, the injection pipette is withdrawn gently and the oocyte is released from the holding pipette (Palermo et al. 1992b).

The clinical results with ICSI were published recently (Van Steirteghem et al. 1993b). In this series: (1) the damage caused by the microinjection procedure concerned <10% of the injected oocytes; (2) the normal fertilization rate of the successfully injected oocytes was 65%; (3) after 24 h of further in-vitro culture >70% of the normal fertilized oocytes showed mitotic divisions; (4) 90% of patients with severe and in many cases extreme male factor infertility had embryos transferred; (5) the total and clinical pregnancy rates per started cycle were 39% and 35%, respectively.

Our preliminary data in the treatment of the severe or extreme form of male factor infertility with IVF-ICSI (with the collaboration of three clinics: Hôpital Français, Clinic Edith Cavell and Clinic Van Helmont) confirmed the results of previous authors. In our first 125 cases, overall rates of 46.6% fertilization and 23.4% clinical pregnancy were obtained.

Conclusion

In IVF, when a failure of fertilization occurs, 50% of patients have a chance to have an embryo in a subsequent attempt. However, in the cases of the severe form of male factor infertility ($<2\times10^6$ motile spermatozoa/ml in fresh semen) the fertilization process is very compromised. Previously, in these cases donor insemination was suitable for patients, but now, micromanipulation procedures are proposed.

A rather moderate success in terms of fertilization, embryo cleavage and pregnancy has been achieved by PZD and SUZI. The normal fertilization rate has never exceeded 20%–25% of the injected oocytes and the implantation and take-home baby rates have remained low. The first clinical application of ICSI seemed to be more promising in terms of fertilization and clinical pregnancy rates (Van Steirteghem et al. 1993a, b). However, the more appropriate comparison, in terms of judging the microinsemination techniques, is with IVF results in the same population of patients prior to microfertilization (Lippi et al. 1993). Such a comparison clearly demonstrates that microfertilization results in dramatically higher fertilization and embryo transfer rates and permits the establishment of pregnancies in patients who would otherwise have little chance of achieving this goal.

Some concerns have been expressed that the cumulus oophorus and the ZP are barriers that prevent abnormal spermatozoa from fertilizing oocytes, and that in bypassing them, genetically unfit spermatozoa will be allowed to fertilize and so produce defective embryos. However, there is little evidence for an association between human sperm function and their genome (Martin and Rademaker 1988). Early concerns over the risk of inducing abnormalities in embryos as a direct result of mechanically assisted fertilization procedures are now diminishing as a result of the increasing number of clinical series being published.

In male factor infertility, which treatment is beneficial to the patient? It depends on the semen quality. I believe that for PZD, a minimum of 0.5×10^6 motile spermatozoa/ml and for SUZI, $0.15–0.20 \times 10^6$ motile spermatozoa/ml are required in fresh semen to obtain fertilization. For ICSI, however, only a few spermatozoa appeared to be sufficient. Obviously, donor insemination remains the only chance of pregnancy in very extreme forms of male factor infertility and in the case of azoospermia.

References

Austin CR (1952) The "capacitation" of mammalian sperm. Nature 170:326

Bedford JM, Moore HD, Franklin LE (1979) Significance of the equatorial segment of the acrosome of the spermatozoa in eutherian mammals. Exp Cell Res 119:119

Boell EJ (1985) Oxygen consumption of mouse sperm and its relationship to capacitation. J Exp Zool 234:105

Bongso TA, Sathananthan H, Wong PC, Ratnam SS, Ng SC, Anandakumar C, Ganatra S (1989) Human fertilization by microinjection of immotile spermatozoa. Hum Reprod 4:175

Bouckaert A, Psalti I, Loumaye E, De Cooman S, Thomas K (1994) The probability of a successful treatment of infertility by in-vitro fertilization. Hum Reprod 9:448

Cohen J, Malter H, Wrigth G, Elsner C, Kort H, Massey J (1988) Implantation of embryos after partial opening of oocyte zona pellucida to facilitate sperm penetration. Lancet ii:162

Cohen J, Elsner G, Kort H, Malter H, Massey J, Meyer MP, Wiemer (1990) Impairment of the hatching process following IVF in the human and improvement of implantation by hatching using micromanipulation. Hum Reprod 5:7

Cohen J, Alikani M, Malter HE, Adler A, Talansky BE, Rosenwaks Z (1991) Partial zona dissection or subzonal sperm insertion: microsurgical fertilization alternatives based on evaluation of sperm and embryo morphology. Fertil Steril 56:696

Cooke S (1993) Counselling in donor insemination. In: Barratt CLR, Cooke ID (eds) Donor insemination. Cambridge University Press, Cambridge, pp 12–33

De Cooman S, Psalti I, Sirjacobs Y, Thomas K, Loumaye E (1988) Intérêts de la fécondation in vitro dans le traitement de la stérilité masculine. Louvain Med 107:407

De Cooman S, Psalti I, Polet W, Bianchini W, Thomas K (1991) An objective semen analysis with Autosperm® in selected IVF patients. Hum Reprod 6:(Suppl 1) 297

Fishel S, Antinori S, Jackson P, Johnson J, Rinaldi L (1991) Presentation of six pregancies established by sub-zonal insemination (SUZI). Hum Reprod 6:124

Garrisi GJ, Talansky BE, Grunfeld L, Sapira V, Navot D, Gordon JW (1990) Clinical evaluation of three approaches to micromanipulation-assisted fertilization. Fertil Steril 54:671

Gordon JW, Grunfeld L, Garrisi GL, Talansky BE, Richards C, Laufer N (1988) Fertilization of human oocytes by sperm from infertile males after the zona pellucida drilling. Fertil Steril 50:68

Handyside AH, Kentogianni EH, Hardy K, Winston RML (1990) Pregnancies from biopsied human preimplantation embryos sexed by Y-specific DNA amplification. Nature 344:768
Katz DF, Drobnis EZ, Overstreet JW (1989) Factors regulating mammalian sperm migration through the female reproductive tract and oocyte vestments. Gamete Res 22:443
Laws-King A, Trounson A, Sathananthan H, Kola I (1987) Fertilization of human oocytes by microinjection of single spermatozoon under the zona pellucida. Fertil Steril 48:637
Lanzendorf SE, Maloney MK, Veeck LL. Slusser J, Hodgen CD, Rosenwaks Z (1988) A preclinical evaluation of pronuclear formation by microinjection of human spermatozoa into human oocytes. Fertil Steril 49:835
Laufer N, Abrams T, Simon A (1991) Treatment of male infertility by gamete micromanipulation. Focus Reprod 1(5):5
Levron J, Manor D, Brander JM, Itskovitz J (1990) Human sperm and hamster oocyte interaction: a model system to assess sperm entry into the oocyte after partial zona dissection. Fertil Steril 54:342
Lippi J, Mortimer D, Jansen RPS (1993) Sub-zonal insemination for extreme male factor infertility. Hum Reprod 8:908
Loumaye E, De Cooman S, Anoma M, Psalti I, Depreester S, Schmit M, Thomas K (1988) Short term utilization of a gonadotropin releasing hormone agonist (Buserelin) for induction of ovulation in an in-vitro fertilization program. Ann NY Acad Sci 541:96
Loumaye E, Vankrieken L, Depreester S, Psalti I, De Cooman S, Thomas K (1989) Hormonal changes induced by short-term administration of a gonadotropin releasing hormone agonist during ovarian hyperstimulation for in vitro fertilization and their consequences for embryo development. Fertil Steril 51:105
Martin RH, Rademaker A (1988) The relationship between sperm chromosomal abnormalities and sperm morphology in humans. Mutat Res 207:159
Ng SC, Bongso A, Sathananthan H, Ratnam SS (1990) Micromanipulation: its relevance to human in vitro fertilization. Fertil Steril 53:203
Overstreet JW (1983) Transport of gametes in the reproductive tract of the female mammal. In: Hartmann JF (ed) Mechanism and control of animal fertilization. Academic, New York, pp 499–543
Palermo G, Joris H, Devroey P, Van Steirteghem AC (1992a) Induction of acrosome reaction in human spermatozoa used for subzonal insemination. Hum Reprod 7.248
Palermo G, Joris H, Devroey P, Van Steirteghem AC (1992b) Pregnancies after intracytoplasmic injection of single spermatozoon into an oocyte. Lancet 340:17
Psalti I, Loumaye E, De Cooman S, Thomas K (1988) Les contrôles de qualité de fécondation extracorporelle d'ovocytes humains et de transfert d'embryon. Louvain Med 107:399
Psalti I, Loumaye E, Pensis M, Depreester S, Thomas K (1989) Evaluation of a synthetic serum substitute to replace fetal cord serum for human oocyte fertilization and embryo growth in vitro. Fertil Steril 52:807
Psalti I, Loumaye E, Pensis M, Depreester S, Claudot A, Thomas K (1990) Partial zona dissection in couples without fertilization in previous attempts. 2nd Joint Meeting of ESHRE-ESCO, Milan, p 62
Psalti I, Bouckaert A, Loumaye E, De Cooman S, Thomas K (1992) Bilan de la fécondation in vitro aux Cliniques Universitaires Saint-Luc à Bruxelles (Résultats d'octobre 1986 à décembre 1989). Contracept Fertil Sex 20:1127
Psalti I, Thomas K, De Cooman S (1993) Effects of hyaluronate, strontium and prolonged incubation on different sperm parameters. Gynecol Obstet Invest 36:47
Rawlins RG, Binor Z, Radwanska E, Dmowski WP (1988) Microsurgical enucleation of tripronuclear human zygotes. Fertil Steril 50:266
Richardson DW, Aitken RJ (1993) Techniques for examining the fertilizing capacity of semen. In: Barratt CLR, Cooke ID (eds) Donor insemination. Cambridge University Press, Cambridge, pp 50–71
Sakkas D, Lacham O, Gianaroli L, Trounson A (1992) Subzonal sperm microinjection in cases of severe male factor infertility and repeated in vitro fertilization failure. Fertil Steril 57:1279
Sakkas D, Gianoroli L, Diotallevi L, Wagner I, Ferrareti AP, Campana A (1993) IVF treatment of moderate male factor infertility: a comparison of mini-Percoll, partial zona dissection and subzonal sperm insertion techniques. Hum Reprod 8:587

Simon A, Younis J, Lewin A, Bartoov B, Schenker JG, Laufer N (1991) The correlation between sperm cell morphology and fertilization after zona pellucida slitting in subfertile males. Fertil Steril 56:325

Terriou P, Giorgetti C, Hans E, Spach JL, Roulier R (1993) Partial zona dissection enhances the fertilization rate in cases of sperm defect only when total failure has occured in previous in-vitro fertilization attempts. Hum Reprod 8:722

Van Steirteghem AC, Liu J, Joris H, Nagy Z, Janssenswillen C, Tournaye H, Derde MP, Van Assche E, Devroey P (1993a) Higher success rate by intracytoplamic sperm injection than by subzonal insemination. Hum Reprod 8:1055. Report of a second series of 300 consecutive treatment cycles

Van Steirteghem AC, Nagy Z, Joris J, Liu J, Staessen C, Smitz J, Wisanto A, Devroey P (1993b) High fertilization and implantation rates after intracytoplamic sperm injection. Hum Reprod 8:1061

Weinman DE, Williams WL (1964) Mechanism of capacitation of rabbit spermatozoa. Nature 203:423

Yanagimachi R (1988) Mammalian fertilization. In: Knobil E, Neill et al (eds) The physiology of reproduction. Raven, New York, pp 135–185

Oocyte Storage

S. Al-Hasani, K. Diedrich, and M. Ludwig

Introduction

After the birth of Louise Brown in 1978, in vitro fertilization (IVF) heralded a new era in the understanding and management of human infertility and is now an integral and important part of gynaecology. Since transfer for more than one cleaved embryo increases the likelihood of achieving pregnancy, it is necessary to obtain a large number of oocytes to generate embryos for replacement. Unfortunately such procedures lead to the problem of excess oocytes and consequently a high number of embryos which ,if all were to be replaced, would increase the risk of high order multiple pregnancy. To minimize this risk most centres have adopted the approach of replacing three or fewer embryos. In Germany, as in other countries, the law requires that not more than three fertilized oocytes or embroys are transferred. Such a policy obviously creates the issue of excess oocytes and embryos. The surplus embryos thus created raise complex ethical, social, legal, moral and religious issues concerning their future use or disposal. A practical solution to this dilemma is to consider cryopreservation of the embryos. Unfortunately this may serve only to postpone confrontation of these problems. Many religious groups are opposed to embryo cryopreservation because of their belief that the embryo is the beginning of human life. An alternative approach to the problem of spare or excess embryos is to inseminate only the required number of oocytes and to store the surplus oocytes by cryopreservation for later use. With the current controversy surrounding embyro cryopreservation there is clearly a need to investigate the possibility of freezing human oocytes as an alternative. Of equal importance is the need for research into cryopreservation of the human oocyte. Little is known about the effects of deep freezing on the oocyte, its survival after thawing and its subsequent performance and development following exposure to sperm in the in vitro system. The potential significance and practical application of this research is clearly far-reaching.

History of Oocyte Cryopreservation

Attempts have been made in the past to preserve mammalian oocytes at very low temperatures. Early work in the 1950s provided evidence of this research, although little success was achieved (Sherman and Lin 1958a, 1958b, 1959; Parkes 1958).

A temporary lull ensued until the 1970s, when interest was revived again. Leibo (1977), in a study of mouse ova and embryos, obtained a higher proportion of ova surviving after deep freezing to -196°C. Survival was found to bear an inverse relationship to cooling rates and the formation of intracellular ice. These observations were fundamental to an understanding of cryobiological processes involving cells held at very low temperatures. In another important study, Whittingham (1977), using dimethyl sulphoxide (DMSO) as cryoprotectant, succeeded not only in cooling unfertilized ovulated mouse oocytes to a temperature of -196°C, permitting storage from between 24 h and 3 months, but also in obtaining 70% survival among those oocytes, thus clearly demonstrating the feasibility of oocyte cryopreservation. Fertilization rates in vitro of the frozen-thawed oocytes was significantly lower than those of freshly collected control oocytes. However, living healthy normal fetuses were obtained after transfer of the oocytes into the oviducts of recipient females when mated with fertile males. Successful, oocyte cryopreservation was achieved by Kasai et al. (1979) in the rat. The oocytes were frozen at -196°C using DMSO, with 60% surviving after thawing and 47% showing fertilization in vitro.

Parkening and Chang (1977) stored hamster oocytes at -75°C, whilst Quinn et al. (1982) obtained an 80% survival rate of oocytes after slow cooling to -80°C prior to storage at -196°C. In rabbits most of the cryopresevation experiments were done with either fertilized or cleaved oocytes (Smith 1952; Chang 1953). Until 1977 there was no interest in cryopreservation of rabbit oocytes. In this year Ogawa and Tomada claimed to be able to fertilize successfully rabbit oocytes after freezing them, but their method could not be reproduced. The first successful cryopreservation of rabbit oocytes leading to the production of living, healthy normal offspring was published by our group (Al-Hasani et al. 1989).

In a study by De Mayo et al. (1985), an attempt was made to freeze monkey oocytes as a forerunner to similar procedures with human oocytes. The monkey oocytes were collected by laparoscopy after appropriate ovarian hyperstimulation, and then frozen in DMSO before storage at -196°C. Ova were stored for 1–12 weeks in liquid nitrogen. The stored ova were thawed either slowly or rapidly and then subjected to xenogenous fertilization in the rabbit oviduct. Survival after the freezing-thawing procedure varied between 20% and 40%, with xenogenous fertilization rates of about 30%. Whilst animal studies clearly showed that the mammalian oocyte could be frozen and stored successfully, there was little evidence to indicate that this was possible in humans. Indeed, some IVF researchers thought cryopreservation of human oocytes to be extremely difficult or even technically impossible because of the potentional instability of the oocyte chromosome spindle when subjected to freezing and thawing. In one study, however, ten human ova were exposed to 35% glycerol and then frozen in liquid nitrogen (Burks et al. 1965). Nine retained their morphological integrity after thawing. In another study. Trounson (1984) obtained more than 80 oocytes from ovarian wedge samples and cultured them for 48 h in vitro prior to freezing. Only four oocytes survived both freezing and subsequent thawing. In a preliminary experiment done in our centre (Tolksdorf et al. 1985), five human oocytes were cryopreserved to -196°C and DMSO was used as cryoprotectant. Two oocytes survived after thawing. After in vitro fertilization one of these two oocytes showed two visible pronuclei 24 h after insemination. In the same year, Bernard et al. (1985), using glycerol as cryoprotectant, found that none of their oocytes were fertilizable after a cryopreservation-thawing procedure. In this study they also used 1,2-propanediol instead of glycerol; fertilization and cleavage to the eight-cell stage occurred in one ovum before termination of the experiment. Later more publications appeared concerning the cryopreservation of human oocytes with successful results.

Advantages of Cryopreservation of Human Oocytes and Its Practical Application

In view of the risk of hyperstimulation syndrome in women undergoing IVF, it is advantageous to freeze the supernumerary oocytes to attempt conception at a later date. This also has the advantages of reducing the risk of multiple pregnancies as well as the number of operative interventions. Moreover it offers a greater chance of success from embryo implants in a natural cycle and a significant reduction in costs to the patient.

Oocyte cryopreservation is also expected to increase the results of IVF by increasing the number of pregnancies from several eggs obtained in a single IVF treatment cycle. It may provide an alternative to embryo freezing, especially in countries in which freezing of embryos is not acceptable for ethical, moral and legal reasons. It also creates possibilities for patients with cancer to become pregnant after chemo- and radiotherapy which has rendered them sterile. Another possibility is the establishment of oocyte banking. Thus patients who suffer from diseases that endanger the function of the ovaries (such as cancer, endometriosis, recurrent cysts and infections) may wish to store oocytes for future use. Should their ovaries require removal to cure their disease, they could still become pregnant through IVF, using their stored oocytes.

Oocyte cryopreservation may provide a means for family planning. Thus women who defer childbearing because of the pursuit of a career, the unavailability of a marriage partner or illness may at a young age opt to have their oocytes stored for later use. The storage of the oocytes at the time of sterilization may also be important for those women who later regret the operation and desire a family, especially if a reversal operation is not possible. Stored oocytes may find a use in oocyte donation programmes to provide embryos for women with congenital or surgical absence of the ovaries, the presence of hypoplastic ovaries, the failure to produce ovulation from stimulation regimens, premature menopause, genetic diseases and ovaries which are inaccesssible to both laparoscopic and ultrasonic collection of oocytes.

Consideration should also be given to disadvantages that can arise through oocyte cryopreservation. These include problems of the prolonged storage of the oocytes, as well as patient-related matters, such as difficulties with the fees for the storage, or failing marital partnerships.

The Human Oocyte

During embryological development oocytes enter the prophase of the first meiotic division and then become arrested in the dicktyate stage. This stage extends through infancy until just prior to the onset of puberty and ends with the menopause (Chandly 1971; Baker 1976; Ohno et al. 1962; Zamboni 1970). With the onset of reproductive life, the meiotic process is resumed and the first meiotic division is then completed. The second meiotic division occurs and the oocyte is ovulated at the metaphase II stage, with the first polar body extruded and the chromosomes arranged on spindle at the second meiotic metaphase. Meiotic division then arrests again at the second phase. During this stage the oocyte may be regarded as relatively unstable. It is the view of cryobiologists that the oocyte is best cryopreserved at the ovulated phase (Polge 1977; Al-Hasani et al. 1986b). Following fertilization, resumption of meiotic maturation occurs, the second polar body is extruded and shortly after that the third polar body appears for a short while.

The oocyte at the time of ovulation is generally the largest cell found in most mammals, being a sphere varying in diameter from about 70–80 μm in the mouse, rat and hamster to about 130 μm in the rabbit, bovine and human. The oocyte is surrounded by a transparent non-cellular membrane, the zona pellucida, and a layer of follicular cells, the corona radiata and cumulus cells.

Cryobiology of Oocyte Freezing

Action of Cryoprotectants

Before starting any work on oocyte and embryo cryopreservation a general understanding of cryobiological concepts in cell freezing is essential. Successful cryopreservation is due to the application of theoretical considerations and empirical observations derived from studies in different species and cellular systems. There are two factors of utmost importance in cryopreservation work: the presence of a molar concentration of a protective solute or cryoprotectant and appropriate rates of cooling and thawing. Cryoprotective agents which are of low molecular weight are thought to prevent the potentially deleterious exposure of cells to elevated concentrations of electrolytes by their colligative action in reducing the quantity of ice formed intracellulary at any sub-zero temperature. Also precise control of the cooling and warming rate determines the ultimate fate of water that is present intracellulary during the cryopreservation process. If the cooling rate during freezing is sufficiently slow, cytoplasmic water will flow out of the cell and will freeze extracellularly, resulting in a gradual dehydration of the cell. However, damage to the cell at slow rates of cooling may be caused by solution effects which again can be reduced by the use of cyroprotectant media. On the other hand if cooling is too rapid the cytoplasm will not have sufficient time for dehydration so it will supercool and eventually freeze. The formation of intracellular ice is a lethal factor and leads to cell damage and death. Generally for different cells there is an optimal cooling rate that varies according to the cell size and type (Chen 1990).

Cellular Events During Cryopreservation

If a cell suspended in physiological medium like saline solution is cooled progressively to temperatures slightly below 0°C, ice forms first in the extracellular solution. Consequently, the dissolved solutes become more concentrated as water is removed in the form of ice. The lower the temperature decreases, the higher becomes the concentration of the solvent and the lower is the chemical potential of water. The cell responds osmotically to equalize the chemical potentials of water across its membranes; hence during freezing, it loses water extracellularly. If a cell is cooled at high enough rates, there will be insufficient time for the cell to remain in osmotic equilibrium and as the temperature falls the cell content will become increasingly supercooled, until suddenly the cell water freezes within the cell itself, resulting in cell death. Seeding or the induction of ice formation in the medium overcomes this problem of supercooling and the deleterious effect of thermal changes following the release of the latent heat of fusion.

As cooling proceeds further and the temperature reaches -40°C, 74% of the solution becomes crystallized and the solute concentration in the remaining liquid increases to 47% weight% (Rall et al. 1984). Many small ice crystals form and surround the cell, thereby obscuring it from view on cryomicroscopy. The next phase is a critical one when cell death can happen. As the temperature falls further, the intracellular contents freeze and the cell suddenly reappears. This is caused by the diffraction of light by the ice crystals formed intracellularly – a phenomenon termed "blackening out" or "flashing". If the cells is now cooled rapidly by plunging it into liquid nitrogen at -196°C, there is no additional crystallization, that is, a "glass" forms and the residual liquid "vitrifies". Cooling to -196°C results in an arrest of biological time for the cell that can then be stored virtually indefinitely. During thawing the physical events depend on whether warming is slow or rapid. Slow warming is accompanied by a complex series of changes: a "flashing" of the cytoplasm at -90°C ("first flash"), the gradual growth of a dark crystalline material extracellularly between -90°C and -70°C, gradual disappearance of the dark material between -70°C and -42°C, and a "second flash" at -55°C. With rapid warming, that is rates in excess of 100°C/min, the extracellular ice merely melts when the temperature increases above -40°C. There is insufficient time for the formation of ice nuclei or "detrification" and the glassy solid therefore "liquifies". The final step is a critical one of diluting out the cryptrotectant and a return to physiological conditions. Most cryodamage occurs to the biological material during this final step.

The role of the cryoprotectant is to protect the cell during freezing; in addition, the avoidance of supercooling by seeding, careful control of the cooling rate, the prevention of significant intracellular ice formation, the establishment of osmotic and thermal equilibrium during freezing and the control of warming rates are of importance. Both the understanding of these concepts and meticulous attention to and control of these factors during freezing and thawing are influential in successful outcome of the cryopreservation process (Chen 1990).

Factors Influencing Successful Cryopreservation

Various factors are thought to affect the outcome of rabbit and human oocyte freezing and thawing. They include oocyte selection, its size, time exposure to cryoprotectant, seeding and assessment of survival.

Oocyte Selection

We faced a problem in selecting mature oocytes for cryopreservation in our IVF centre because the oocytes of good quality mostly were taken for the conventional in vitro fertilization procedure, while the surplus oocytes were of either intermediate or immature quality. To compensate for this problem the oocytes were first cultured for about 24 h and then cryopreserved. A very small number of mature oocytes could be obtained for freezing. It is important to mention that only oocytes that appeared morphologically normal under the dissecting microscope were considered to be suitable for cryopreservation.

Size

The oocyte volume in the freezing process plays an important role. In freezing most investigators have tried to reduce the size of the oocyte-cumulus complex by removing the cumulus complex either mechanically or chemically to increase the success of survival after freezing and thawing. Polge (1977) found that the size can adversely affect the survival rate after freezing. In mouse the size of the oocyte is about half of the size of a human egg; therefore the success is twice as high as in human and rabbit (Whittingham 1977; Al-Hasani 1986a, 1989). Fuller and Bernard (1984) used the microscope to observe the time required by mouse egg to reach an appropriate volume after the addition of glycerol. They concluded that the unfertilized mouse oocytes would need at least 1 h to allow sufficient glycerol to permeate the cells. Another example of the importance of cell size is the freezing of semen. The survival rate in this case is much higher than oocyte freezing, presumably because the size of sperm is about 1/180 of the size of the oocyte in both the human and rabbit. The larger the size of the oocyte, the longer the necessary exposure to cryoprotectants.

Duration of Exposure to Cryoprotectant

The duration of exposure to cryoprotectant is again of importance and the shorter the exposure to the cryoprotectant, the better is the survival rate after freezing and thawing. If the duration of exposure is too long it can alter the intracellular pH as well as the developmental potential, as seen in mouse zygotes by Damien et al. (1990). Recently Pickering et al. (1991) found that inappropriate exposure of human oocytes to DMSO reduces the fertilization rate. In our freezing procedure the duration of exposure to propanediol was 20 min, which may be long for human oocytes. We believe that shortening this time to half might improve the survival rate.

Seeding

Controlling the seeding process by the naked eye is an important procedure, especially in the case of automatic seeding because then some of the materials will not be seeded and supercooling may occur in the straws, a lethal process for the oocytes. Seeding can be induced at −7°C. A period of 15 min for equilibration till the crystals' form in the whole straw is seen to be a favourable interval before starting with further cooling.

Assessment of Survival

Survival assessment after cryopreservation is also of importance, the oocytes being observed immediately after dilution of the cryoprotectant and again shortly before the insemination in vitro. In the case of cryopreservation of rabbit oocytes five assays are used to identify the surviving oocytes after thawing whereas with human oocytes only one assessment is undertaken, namely the morphological examination under the dissecting microscope. This examination is found to be enough for distinguishing the surviving from the non-surviving oocytes. The intact oocyte appears shiny without discolouration of the ooplasm, cell disruption or pyknosis. The cytoplasm adheres to the zona pellucida without any zona fracture whereas the damaged oocyte has a dark ooplasm and the cytoplasm is contracted and pyknotic. Sometimes the zona is also fractured. The best test of survival in cryopreservation is the subsequent performance of the intact oocyte, namely fertilization and cleavage of the embryo.

Possible Cryodamage

The Spindle Apparatus

The mature oocyte shortly before and at ovulation is in the metaphase II of the second meiotic division. At this stage the chromosomes are arranged on a spindle which is an unstable phase. The microtubuli of this stage can be affected by changing the temperature (Sathanathan et al. 1987). This change in temperature or the addition of cryoprotectant will cause the chromosomes not to arrange themselves and to be scattered in the cytoplasm, leading to their dislocation and aberration and an increasing rate of abnormality or malformation.

The depolymerization of the microtubuli of mouse eggs is mainly caused by the addition of cryoprotectant (Vincent 1988) and is reversible after its removal and after a short period of culture (Magistrini and Szollosi 1980; Pickering et al. 1987). Recently Aigner et al. (1991) observed that a high number of frozen-thawed mouse oocytes showed a normal spindle apparatus using either slow freezing or ultrarapid freezing.

The Cortical Granules

The oocytes surviving after thawing show a high percentage of polyploidy in in vitro fertilization. This phenomenon is observed in mouse (Wood 1986; Glenister et al. 1987) and in human (Al-Hasani et al. 1989; Mandelbaum et al. 1986). Normally the cortical granules are diffused under the oolemma in mature oocytes. The zona reaction in the human oocyte occurs after the movement of these granules to the periphery of the cytoplasm and this reaction is responsible for hindering the penetration of more than one spermatozoon (polysperma block). An electron microscopic examination is done on the frozen-thawed and on the freshly collected oocytes from rabbit and human. In rabbit the number of cortical granules is seen to be reduced and the margin is not sharp; some show signs of disappearance or lysis. This observation may explain the high incidence of polyploidy in frozen-thawed and in vitro fertilized oocytes. Conversely, the findings may explain how the freezing process can damage and reduce the number of cortical granules, thus leading to a high frequency of polyploidy. Similiar findings are observed in humans. Johnson et al. (1988) found that the fertilization rate was reduced in mouse oocytes after thawing, suggesting that the rapid cooling to 4°C may promote release of cortical granules and a premature zona reaction.

Freezing of Rabbit Oocytes

We have used a rabbit model to develop the technique of freezing and thawing in humans (Al-Hasani et al. 1984, 1986a). Our microscopic observations of frozen-thawed oocytes after different times of collection and culture in both DMSO and propanediol experiments are summarized in Table 1. The highest survival rates of 28.8% in the case of DMSO and 32% in the case of

Table 1 Results of morphological examination of frozen-thawed rabbit oocytes collected at different times after the injection of LH

Type of cryoprotectant	Time of collection after LH (h)	Period of culture after thawing (h)	Number of frozen/thawed oocytes	Number and (%) of oocytes morphologically intact after culture
DMSO	6	14	405	22 (5.4)
DMSO	9	7	315	63 (20)
DMSO	12	4	320	92 (28.8)
Propanediol	13	1/2	774	246 (32)

Table 2 Results of FDA examination of morphologically intact oocytes after freezing/thawing

Time of collection after LH (h)	Number of oocytes examined	FDA test	
		Positive	Negative
6	11	11	–
9	18	18	–
12	23	23	–

Table 3 Results of chromosomal analyses of frozen/thawed oocytes collected at different times after the injection of LH

Time of collection after LH (h)	Period of culture after thawing (h)	Number of fixed oocytes	Number of oocytes with visiible chromosomes	Stage of maturation
6	14	14	2	2×metaphase II
9	7	46	19	9×metaphase I 10×metaphase II
12	4	71	23	1×telophase 22×metaphase II

Table 4 Results of frozen/thawed oocytes fertilized in vitro and cultured for a further 6 days

Type of cryoprotectant	No. of oocytes inseminated	No. (%) of oocytes fertilized	No. (%) of blastocysts
DMSO	30	18(60)	1(5.5)
PROH	246	161(61)	No culture

Table 5 Transfer results of cryopreserved and in vitro fertilized rabbit oocytes cultured for 24–26 h using propanediol

	No. of recipient	No. of embryos transferred	Implantations at day 15		Fetuses		Resorptions		No. of young born
			No.	%	No.	%	No.	%	
a	2	17	3	18	2	12	1	6	2
b	2	18	–	–	–	–	–	–	–
c	2	18	2	11	2	11	–	–	2
total	6	53	5	9.4	4	7.5	1	1.9	4

Recipients were given HCG 30,24 and 18 h before embryo transfer
a: –6 h asynchronous; b: –12 h asynchronous; c: –18 h asynchronous

propanediol were obtained in the group of ovulated oocytes 2-3 h after ovulation. A total of 52 oocytes that were considered viable after freezing and thawing were incubated for 2 min in Ham's F-10 medium containing fluorescein diacetate (FDA) (Table 2). All examined oocytes were fluorescent. No oocyte that was considered to be degenerated showed fluorescence. The results of chromosomal analysis demonstrated the highest amount of metaphase II oocytes after thawing when they were collected 12 h after LH injection (Table 3). Collecting after 6 and 9 h was less effective. Morphologically intact oocytes are capable of being fertilized in vitro (Table 4). In DMSO and propanediol experiments, respectively. 18 of 30 (60%) and 161 of 246 (61%) oocytes which were incubated with capacitated spermatozoa for 6 h could be fertilized and cleaved to the two- and four-cell stages. The overall implantation rate (9.4%) and pregnancy outcome are summarized in Table 5.

Freezing of Human Oocytes

The two different freezing methods developed using rabbits have been used for freezing human oocytes.

Oocytes and Oocyte Retrieval

Oocytes were collected by either laparoscopy or by transvaginal puncture after ovarian stimulation with HMG/HCG or GnRH agonist/HMG/HCG.

The oocytes in excess of the four to six committed for IVF were used for cryopreservation. After retrieval excess oocytes were incubated for about 24 h to let them reach maturity since many oocytes used for cryopreservation were immature or at intermediate stages of maturity at the time of recovery. Furthermore, before cryopreservation of excess oocytes, it was useful to observe two pronuclei in the inseminated oocytes, indicating that fertilization had occurred.

The freezing and thawing process, similar to that used in rabbit, has been described in detail elsewhere (Al-Hasani et al. 1986 a).

Results

Two hundred and seventeen excess oocytes from 39 cycles were frozen slowly to −33°C using 1.5 *M* DMSO. Of 144 oocytes that have been thawed, 40 oocytes seemed to be morphologically intact (28%); only 20 oocytes could be fertilized in vitro, the polyploidy rate being 20% (Fig. 1).

Figure 2 summarizes observations on freezing of human oocytes by the method described previously by Lassalle et al. (1985). Sixty-six excess oocytes from nine cycles were frozen. Twelve of 38 oocytes thawed were morphologically intact and nine could be fertilized in vitro, the polyploidy rate being 44%.

The importance of oocyte quality for the success of cryopreservation is shown in Table 6, the maturational stage of oocytes before freezing playing an important role in the success of cryopreservation and the subsequent IVF procedures.

Oocyte maturation at the time of oocyte retrieval is also important. The embryos from the only two pregnancies which have been achieved originated from mature oocytes.

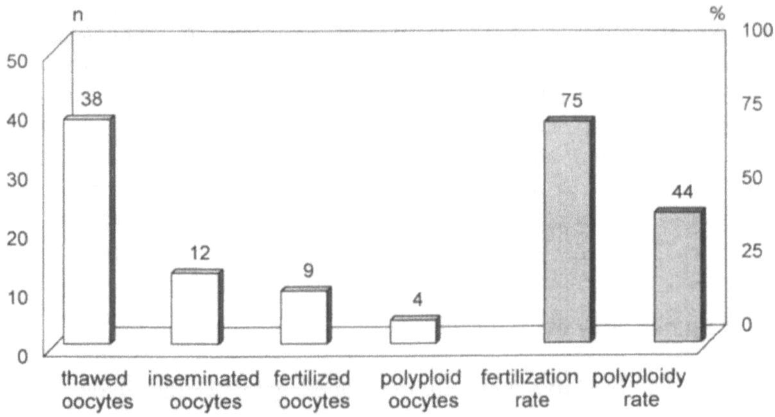

Fig. 1. In vitro fertilization results with frozen/thawed human oocytes (frozen with DMSO). No. of cycles = 39

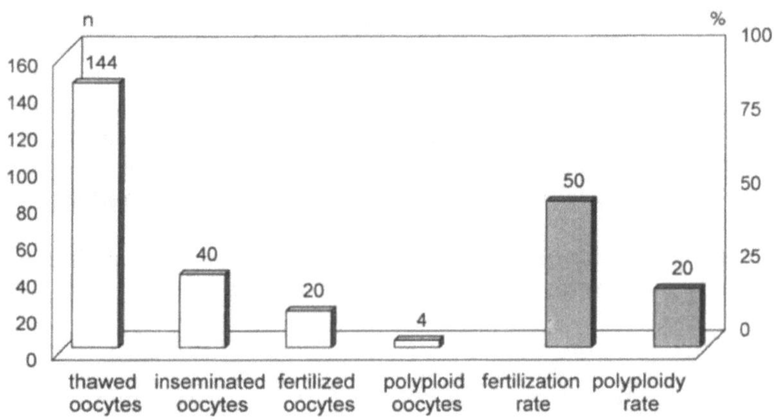

Fig. 2. In vitro fertilization results with frozen/thawed human oocytes (frozen with propanediol). No of cycles = 9

Table 6 In vitro fertilization results of frozen/thawed human oocytes (in relation to the oocyte quality)

No. of patients	No. and quality[a] of frozen oocytes			No. of thawed oocytes	No. of oocytes found after thawing	No. of oocytes inseminated (intact)			No. of fertilized oocytes (%)			No. of pregnancies
	+	++	+++			+	++	+++	+	++	+++	
48	141	101	29	182	159	10	29	16	3(30)	16(57)	19(69)	2
		283					54			30		

[a] Oocyte maturity was estimated morphologically at the time of oocytes retrieval: +, immature; ++ intermediate; +++, mature

Table 7 Word-wide reported pregnancies resulting from freezing human oocytes

Reference	Year	Pregnancies
Chen (Adelaide, Australia)	1986 1987	Twins (m+f), delivered Single (f), delivered
van Uem et al. (Erlangen, Germany)	1987	Single (f) delivered
Diedrich Bonn (Germany)	1987	Miscarriages (2)
Kolodziej et al. (Essen Germanny)	1991 1991	Single (f), delivered Miscarriage (1)

m, Male; f, female

Results Concerning Pregnancies World-wide After Human Oocyte Cryopreservation

To date, a total of seven pregnancies derived from frozen human oocytes have been reported (Table 7). All the pregnancies were achieved using a slow-freeze and fast-thaw technique, with DMSO as cryoprotectant. Four of the pregnancies have delivered and all of the infants, a male and four females, are healthy and normal. The remaining three pregnancies resulted in first trimester miscarriages.

Perspective

The human preovulatory oocyte can be successfully frozen and stored. Mouse oocytes had already been successfully cryopreserved by Whittingham (1977), who reported that oocytes could survive deep freezing at –196°C with a survival rate of about 70%. These thawed mouse oocytes were capable of fertilization in vitro although with lower rates than control unfrozen oocytes and, on transfer to recipient females, normal live offspring were produced. However, the technique may not be applicable to the human oocyte because of species differences, as there are structural differences between the chromosomes of mouse and man (Chen 1990).

Pathenogenetic activation of frozen-thawed oocytes has not been seen with either rabbit nor human oocytes. With the human oocytes there is clear morphological evidence of the appearance of both male and female pronuclei with subsequent syngamy and cell cleavage. The only and most practical means of assessing the survival and subsequent performance of the fertilized frozen-thawed human oocytes is by its morphological appearance on light microscopy. Polyploidy rates are higher after cryopreservation of human oocytes regardless of which cryoprotectant is used. Reducing the number of inseminating spermatozoa may reduce the polyploidy rate. The risk of fetal malformation resulting from freezing-thawing of the human oocytes is not known as only five normal children have been born without malformation after cryopreservation of oocytes. Presumably only the most robust normal cells survive.

Since cryopreservation of oocytes in the pronuclear stage and cleaved embryos is widely performed with better results with regard to survival rate and pregnancy outcome, cryopreservation of oocytes today is just practiced for certain indications, e.g. oocyte banking for patients with diseases endangering ovarian function.

References

Aigner S, Siebzehnruebl E, Van der Elst J, Spitzer M, Van Steirtghem AC, Lang L (1991) Veränderungen des meiotischen Spindelapparates von Mäuseeizellen nach verschiedenen Einfrierverfahren. Dreiländertagung Fertilität und Sterilität Goslar, pp 267–268

Al-Hasani S, Hahn J, Dankowski K, Schneider U (1984) In-vitro fertilization and embryo transfer of rabbit oocytes collected at different times after P-LH injection. Eur J Obstet Gynecol Reprod Biol 17:417–423

Al-Hasani S, Tolksdorf A, Diedrich K, van der Ven H, Krebs D (1986a) Successful in-vitro fertilization of frozen-thawed rabbit oocytes. Hum Reprod 1:309–312

Al-Hasani S, van der Ven H, Diedrich K, Krebs D (1986b) Successfull in-vitro fertilization of frozen-thawed human oocytes. Workshop on embryos and oocytes freezing (Reports). Collection Fondation Marcel Merieux, Annecy, pp 25-39

Al-Hasani S, Diedrich K, van der Ven H, Reinecke A, Hartje M, Krebs D (1987) Cryopreservation of human oocytes. Hum Reprod 2:695–700

Al-Hasani S, Kirsch J, Diedrich K, Blanke S, van der Ven H, Krebs D (1989) Successful embryo transfer of cryopreserved and in vitro fertilized oocytes. Hum Reprod 4:77–79

Baker TG (1976) Oogenesis and ovulation. In: Austin CR, Short RV (eds) Fortpflanzungsbiologie der Säugetiere, vol 1, Keimzelle und Befruchtung, Parey, Berlin, pp 19–42

Burks JL, Davies ME, Bakken AH, Tomasovic JJ (1965) Morphologic evaluation of frozen rabbit and human ova. Fertil Steril 16:638–664

Bernard A, Imoedemhe DA, Shaw RW, Fuller B (1985) Effects of cryoprotectants of human oocyte. Lancet 1:632–633

Chandly AC (1971) Culture of mammalian oocytes. J Reprod Fertil (Suppl) 14:1–6

Chang MC (1953) Storage of unfertilized rabbit ova: subsequent fertilization and the probability of normal development. Nature 172:353

Chen C (1986) Pregnancy after human oocyte cryopreservation. Lancet 1:884–886

Chen C (1987) Pregnancies after human oocyte cryopreservation. Fifth world congress on in-vitro-fertilization and embryo transfer. Norfolk, USA, 5–10 April 51:19 (Abstract)

Chen C (1990) Oocyte freezing. In: Wood C, Trounson A (eds) Clinical in vitro fertilization, 2nd edn. Springer, Berlin Heidelberg New York, pp 113–126

Damien M, Luciano AA, Peluso JJ (1990) Propanediol alters intracellular pH and developmental potential of mouse zygotes independently of volume change. Hum Reprod 5:212–216

De Mayo FJ, Rawlins RG, Dukelow WR (1985) Xenogenous and in vitro fertilization of frozen-thawed primate oocytes and blastomere separation of embryos. Fertil Steril 43:295–300

Diedrich K (1987) Cryopreservation of rabbit and human oocytes. Fifth, world congress on in vitro fertilization and embryo transfer. Norfolk, 5–10 April (Abstract)

Fuller BJ, Bernard A (1984) Successful in-vitro fertilization of mouse oocytes after cryopreservation using glycerol. Cryo Letters 5:307–312

Glenister PH, Wood MJ, Kirby C, Whittingham DG (1987) Incidence of chromosome anomalies in first cleavage mouse embryos obtained from frozen-thawed oocytes fertilized in vitro. Gamete Res 16:205–216

Johnson MH, Pickering SJ, George MA (1988) The influence of cooling on the properties of the zona pellucida of the mouse oocyte. Human Reproduction 3:383-387

Kasai M, Iritani A, Chang MC (1979) Fertilization in vitro of rat ovarian oocytes after freezing and thawing. Biol Reprod 21:839-844

Lassalle B, Testort J, Renard JP (1985) Human embryo features that influence the success of cryopreservation with the use of 1,2-propanediol. Fert Steril 44:645–651
Leibo SP (1977) Fundamental cryobiology of mouse ova and embryos. In: Elliot K, Whelan J (eds) The freezing of mammalian embryos. Elsevier Excerpta Medica. Amsterdam, pp 69-96 (Ciba Foundation 52 (new series))
Magistrini M, Szollosi D (1980) Effects of cold and isopropyl-*N*-phenylcarbamate on the second meiotic spindle of mouse oocytes. Eur J Cell Biol 22:699-707
Mandelbaum J, Junca A, Plachot M, Alnot MO, Tibi C, Cohen C, Salat-Baroux J (1986) Cryopreservation of human oocytes and embryos using 1–2 propanediol with or without sucrose as cryoprotective agents. Workshop on Embryos and Oocytes Freezing. Collection Fondation Marcel Merieux, Annecy (Reports) pp 95–122
Ohno S, Klinger HD, Atkin NB (1962) Human oogenesis Cytogenetics 1:42–51
Parkening TA, Chang MC (1977) Effects of cooling rate and maturity of the animal on the recovery and fertilization of frozen-thawed rodent eggs. Biol Reprod 17:527–531
Parkes AS (1958) Factors of the viability of frozen ovarian tissue. J Endocrinol 17:337–343
Pickering SJ, Johnson MH (1987) The influence of cooling on the organization of the meiotic spindle of the mouse oocyte. Hum Reprod 2:207–216
Pickering SJ, Braude PR, Johnson MH (1991) Cryopreservation of human oocytes: inappropriate exposure to DMSO reduces fertilization rates. Hum Reprod 6:142–143
Polge C (1977) The freezing of mammalian embryos: perspectives and possibilities. In: Elliott K, Whelan J (eds) The freezing of mammalian embryos. Elsevier Excerpta Medica Amsterdam pp 3–18 (Ciba Foundation 52 (new series))
Quinn P, Barros C, Whittingham DG (1982) Preservation of hamster oocytes to assay the fertilizing capacity of human spermatozoa. J Reprod Fert 66:161–168
Sathanathan AH, Trounson A, Freeman L (1987) Morphology and fertilization of frozen human oocytes. Gamete Res 16:343–354
Sherman JK, Lin TP (1958 a) Survival of unfertilized mouse eggs during freezing and thawing. Proc Soc Biol Med 98:902–905
Sherman JK, Lin TP (1958 b) Effect of glycerol and low temperature on survival of unfertilized mouse eggs. Nature 181:785–786
Sherman JK, Lin TP (1959) Temperature shock and cold storage of unfertilized mouse egg. Fertil Steril 10:384–396
Smith AU (1952) Behaviour of fertilized rabbit eggs exposed to glycerol and to low temperatues. Nature 170:374–375
Tolksdorf A, Al-Hasani S, Diedrich K, van der Ven H, Krebs D (1985) An attempt to freeze rabbit follicular oocytes. Hum Reprod Bonn, FRG 23–26 June 1985; 93:33 (Abstract)
Trounson A (1984) In vitro fertilization and embryo preservation. In: Trounson A, Wood C (eds) In vitro fertilization and embryo transfer. Chuchill, Edinburgh, pp 111-130
Vincent C, Heymann Y, Garnier V, Renard JP (1988) Cryopreservation of ovulated rabbit oocytes: cryoprotectant effect in microfilament and microtubule organisation. In vivo survival after freezing. 25th Annual Meeting of Cryobiology Society. Aachen abstr 157
Whittingham DG (1977) Fertilization in vitro and development to term of unfertilized mouse oocytes previously stored at –196°C. J Reprod Fert 49:89–94
Wood MJ (1986) An increased incidence of polyploidy in embryos derived from frozen oocytes. Workshop on Embryos and Oocytes Freezing (Reports). Collection Fondation Marcel Merieux. Annecy. pp 41–51
Zamboni L (1970) Ultrastructure of mammalian oocytes and ova. Biol Reprod (Suppl) 2:44–63

The Role of Doppler-Ultrasonography in Reproductive Medicine

S. KUPESIC, A. KURJAK, A.K. ERTAN, M.M. BABIC, and W. SCHMIDT

Introduction

The newly developed color Doppler modality and pulsed-wave Doppler provide a unique noninvasive method for evaluating normal and abnormal conditions in the female pelvis (Kurjak et al. 1995). This method acts as a logical extension of digital examination, but it is also a method of choice for follicular monitoring and has rapidly replaced laparoscopy for follicle aspiration in in vitro fertilization programs. Transvaginal color flow has superior accuracy, reproducibility, and enables the visualization of small vessels under physiologic conditions, such as follicular vascularity and corpus luteum blood flow. The role of this new modality in the field of human reproduction is to evaluate intraovarian and uterine perfusion. It may also help to predict ovulation and detect certain ovulatory disorders and the luteal phase defect. Doppler investigation of ovarian blood flow may improve the early diagnosis of ovarian hyperstimulation syndrome in patients with ovulation induction. Initial impressions concerning the usefulness of blood flow studies in the infertile patient have been confirmed by numerous studies during last 3 years. However, it is still not clear whether blood flow changes play a role in infertility, or whether a failure of adequate perfusion could result in early pregnancy loss. It is hoped that this simplified examination technique will be used as a clinical therapeutic aid and exciting future developments are anticipated.

Transvaginal Color Flow Doppler in the Assessment of Uterine and Ovarian Blood Flow

Transvaginal color flow Doppler ultrasound is a powerful tool for the investigator studying and observing the female reproductive system and vascular changes within the pelvis. The follicle and corpus luteum of the ovary and endometrium are the only areas in the normal adult body where angiogenesis occurs (Kurjak et al. 1991; Findlay 1986). Blood flow in the main pelvic vessels can easily be visualized and recognized (Gratton et al. 1990). Iliac vessels can be seen on the side wall of the pelvis, often lying deep and close to the ovary. The color Doppler signal of the main uterine vessels may be seen in all patients laterally to the cervix. Waveform analysis shows high to moderate flow velocity. The resistance index depends on age, phase of the menstrual cycle, and special conditions (such as pregnancy, uterine tumors, etc.).

Transvaginal color Doppler can be used to obtain flow velocity waveforms from the uterine arteries at any time during the menstrual cycle (Kurjak et al. 1991). It is apparent that there is a complex relationship between the concentration of ovarian hormons in peripheral venous plasma and uterine artery blood flow parameters (Goswamy and Steptoe 1989; Goswamy et al. 1988; Bourne et al. 1991). In most women, there is a small amount of end-diastolic flow in the uterine arteries in the proliferative phase. Goswamy and Steptoe (1989) found an increasing resistance index and systolic/diastolic ratio during the postovulatory drop in the serum estradiol concentration.

During the normal menstrual cycle there is a sharp increase in end-diastolic velocities between the proliferative and secretory phase of the menstrual cycle. It is particularly interesting that the lowest blood flow impedance occurs during the time of peak luteal function, during which implantation is most likely to occur. It is logical that blood supply to the uterus should be high in the late luteal phase as reported by Kurjak et al. (1991). Goswamy and Steptoe (1989), Battaglia et al. (1990), and Steer et al. (1991). In anovulatory cycles these changes are not present, and a continuous increase in the resistance index is seen. In some infertile patients the end-diastolic flow is not present.

In experimental studies, an increase of the ovarian blood flow was found during cycle stimulation. Deutinger et al. (1989) performed transvaginal pulsed-wave Doppler measurements of the ovarian arteries in stimulated cycles before and after follicle puncture. Four days before follicle puncture, high flow velocities in systole were found compared with diastole. Toward the day of embryo transfer, a marked increase of the diastolic blood flow velocity was observed. In patients with high endocrine response, the pulsatility index was significantly lower compared with that of patients with low endocrine response.

Ovarian steroids alter the function of periarterial sympathetic nerves through changes in α-1-adrenergic receptor numbers and lead to marked changes in the blood flow.

Scholtes et al. (1989) used a combined transvaginal two-dimensional (2-D) real-time and pulsed-wave Doppler method for recording flow velocity waveforms in the uterine and ovarian arteries from 16 healthy women during the follicular and luteal phase of the normal menstrual cycle. In contrast to earlier reports , their study revealed forward end-diastolic velocities in at least 70% of the ovarian artery flow velocity waveforms and in nearly all uterine flow velocity waveforms. When end-diastolic velocities were absent, this was always during the early follicular stage (day 7) of the menstrual cycle.

The observation that left-right differences in pulsatility index were not related to the site of ovulation suggests that there is no essential difference in blood supply to the left and right ovarian artery. Serial assessment of the flow velocity waveforms reveals a decrease in pulsatility index from the ovarian arteries supplying the ovary carrying the dominant follicle and subsequent corpus luteum, which is only statistically significant on day 21, whereas the pulsatility index from the contralateral ovarian artery depicts an increase that is only statistically significant on day 16. The significant correlation between the pulsatility index from the ovarian artery and the uterine artery on the side of the corpus luteum, as opposed to the contralateral side during the menstrual cycle – despite a marked reduction in pulsatility index from this artery on the side of the ovary carrying the corpus luteum – was only documented on day 21. A comparison with the pulsatility index on the side of the ovary bearing the developing corpus luteum suggested reduced down stream impedance or increased blood flow. The highest pulsatility index (PI) value was recorded in the uterine arteries on day 16 (Table 1).

Sterzik et al. (1989) investigated uterine and ovarian blood flow by vaginal Doppler ultrasonography in 45 women from an in vitro fertilization program. All of the subjects had normal menstrual cycles and in all cases the tubal factor was felt to be responsible for sterility. This group of investigators also used a resistance index (RI) to evaluate the blood pattern. They compared the patients who became pregnant after embryo transfer (group 1) with those who did not conceive (group 2). In group 1 RI values of uterine arteries on the day of follicular aspiration were 0.78±0.06. In group 2, RI values were 0.84±0.08. It was evident that in group 1 the vascular resistance of the uterine arteries was significantly lower on the day of follicular aspiration When the flow parameters for patients in whom pregnancy occurred are compared with the values of women who did not become pregnant, no difference can be detected for ovarian blood flow (Table 1).

Thaler et al. (1990) performed flow measurements of the uterine and ovarian arteries from 10 in vitro fertilization/embryo transfer (IVF/ET) protocol patients who were treated with gonadotropins. The Doppler studies were performed every 2 days, starting from the 3rd day of the cycle, prior to treatment. The day of human chorionic gonadotropin (hCG) administration was marked as day 0 and all measurements were expressed in relation to this time point. Daily measurements of serum estradiol (E_2), progesterone, and follicular growth were obtained in each patient.

Thaler et al. measured the changes in the resistance index throughout the treatment cycle in both uterine arteries. There was no difference between sides. The values obtained initially before treatment were relatively low and demonstrated a gradual increase until the day of follicular aspiration. A rapid decline occurred thereafter throughout the luteal phase. Blood flow in the uterine arteries decreased gradually, reaching the lowest levels at about day 0. Within 24 h after the administration of hCG, there was a steep increase in flow rates in this vessel throughout the luteal phase. The periovulatory increase in RI and the decrease in volume flow rates coincided with the decrease in E_2 levels at midcycle. The subsequent increase in flow rates and the rapid decline in RI were associated with the exponential increase in progesterone levels in the luteal phase.

In spontaneous ovarian cycles, the resistance index in the uterine artery fell with a rise in the estrogen level during the early follicular phase and increased in the periovulatory phase along with the drop in this hormone. A

Table 1 Uterine artery perfusion in infertile patients

Authors (year)			
		PI	
Scholtes et al. (1989	Day 13	Day 16	Day 21
Nondominant artery	0.05±0.15	0.33±0.22	0.12±0.13
Dominant artery	0.07±0.17	0.29±0.14	0.12±0.14
		RI	
Sterzik et al. (1989)	Day of follicular aspiration		
Pregnant		0.78±0.06	
Nonpregnant		0.84±0.08	
		PI	
de Ziegler et al. (1991)		5.2±0.4	
Before treatment			
(exogenous E_2)	Days 13 to 14		Days 26 to 27
	1.5±0.2		1.7±0.3
		RI	
Kurjak et al. (1991)	Proliferative phase		Day 18 (nadir)
	0.88±0.04		0.84±0.04
	PI		Pregnancy rate
Steer et al. (1992)			
Low-PI group	1.00–1.99		0.41
Medium-PI group	2.00–2.99		0.47
High-PI group	>3		0
		PI	
Kupesic and Kurjak (1993)	2 days before ovulation		Day before ovulation
Spontaneous cycles	3.16		2.22
		Periovulatory period	
Stimulated cycles		3.06	
Steer et al. (1995)	Day 7	Day 14	Day 21
Pregnant	3.8 (1.5–5.3)	2.65 (1.3–3.4)	2.55 (1.3–4.4)
Nonpregnant	3.3 (1.3–3.6)	3.85 (1.8–6.8)	2.83 (1.3–5.0)

PI, pulsatitily index; RI, resistance index; E_2 estradiol

decrease in uterine impedance was noted in the luteal phase along with rising progesterone levels.

As with the uterine artery, the changes in vessel resistance and flow volume throughout the treatment cycle demonstrate an association with estrogen and particularly with progesterone levels.

To clarify the effect of physiological levels of ovarian hormones on vascular resistance of uterine arteries, de Ziegler et al. (1991) conducted a study in young women deprived of ovarian function who received physiological E_2

and progesterone (P) replacement. Their results indicated that in the absence of ovarian hormone, uterine arteries showed a high degree of vascular resistance. A profound modification of the Doppler flow pattern suggesting a marked decrease in vascular resistance was seen, however, after the elevation of plasma E_2 to menstrual cycle levels.

The results of de Ziegler et al. showed that in the absence of estrogen production by the ovary, uterine arteries have a high degree of vascular resistance expressed by narrow systolic Doppler flow waves and high PI values. This observation differed from the findings obtained during the early follicular phase of the menstrual cycle, which showed a persistence of blood flow during at least part of the diastolic interval in several women.

According to their findings, transdermal administration of E_2 in quantities ranging from 0.1 to 0.4 mg/day which duplicates the ovarian production of E_2 seen during the menstrual cycle, decreased the uterine vascular resistance.

That P administration from days 15 to 28 induced a minor change of uterine artery Doppler flow waves in only two of the six women studied appears to indicate that P does not interfere markedly with the vasodilative effect of E_2 on uterine arteries. From their results, de Ziegler et al. anticipate that transvaginal Doppler studies of uterine arteries will prove to be a valuable indicator of the biological efficacy of various estrogenic treatments (Table 1).

Kurjak et al. (1991) performed serial measurements of the flow velocity of the uterine and ovarian arteries throughout the menstrual cycle in women attending an infertility clinic and compared them with those in volunteers coming for annual examinations. Uterine flow velocity had a resistance index of 0.88±0.04 (2 SE) in the proliferative phase and started to decrease the day before ovulation. A nadir of 0.84±0.04 was reached on day 18 and remained at that level for the rest of the cycle. In anovulatory cycles, these changes did not occur. A subgroup of 12 women who lacked end-diastolic flow in the uterine arteries during the secretory phase as identified. Of the 11 of these women who were infertile, 8 had primary infertility. Ovarian artery flow velocity was usually detected when the dominant follicle reached 12–15 mm. The resistance index was 0.54±0.04 and also declined the day before ovulation. A nadir of 0.44±0.04 was reached 4±5 days later and the RI slowly rose to 0.05±0.04 before menstruation (Table 1).

Steer et al. (1992) tried to assess whether a measure of uterine blood flow impedance (the pulsatility index, PI), as determined by transvaginal ultrasonography with color blood flow imaging, may be used to assess endometrial receptivity immediately before the time of embryo transfer (ET) after assisted conception. Their study had demonstrated that transvaginal blood flow imaging and use of the PI could have an important role in medically assisted conception and might theoretically improve pregnancy rates to almost 50% per ET.

Kupesic and Kurjak (1993) measured the flow velocity of the uterine, radial, spiral, and ovarian arteries during the periovulatory period in spontaneous (Table 2) and induced ovarian cycles with confirmed ovulation. They performed daily measurements during the periovulatory period in 78 patients attending an infertility clinic for reasons involving the male factor in

Table 2 Uterine, radial, and spiral artery blood flow during the periovulatory period assessed by transvaginal color Doppler

Day from ovulation	Peak systolic blood flow velocity (cm/s)	Resistance index	Pulsatility index
Uterine artery flow velocity			
−3	33.02±10.2	0.88±0.09	2.91±0.82
−2	33.20±8.7	0.90±0.08	3.10±0.90
−1	35.24±7.2	0.86±0.03	2.05±0.72
0	36.02±7.5	0.62±0.08	2.90±0.68
+1	36.12±8.2	0.87±0.03	2.88±0.45
Radial artery flow velocity			
−3	11.35±4.21	0.72±0.70	1.79±0.65
−2	10.34±4.21	0.72±0.70	1.79±0.65
−1	13.87±2.25	0.66±0.05	1.19±0.32
0	12.18±2.12	0.76±0.08	2.02±0.92
+1	13.95±2.85	0.68±0.03	1.54±0.96
Spiral artery velocity			
−3	6.21±0.04	0.55±0.02	0.86±0.05
−2	6.02±0.09	0.54±0.03	0.85±0.09
−1	6.32±0.12	0.48±0.04	0.83±0.12
0	6.68±0.68	0.48±0.06	0.84±0.14
+1	7.46±1.31	0.49±0.05	0.72±0.12

Values are expressed as the mean±SD.

infertility. Two days before ovulation uterine flow in spontaneous cycles had a pulsatility index of 3.16, and it started to decrease the day before ovulation (PI=2.22). In stimulated cycles these changes did not occur, and the mean PI of 3.06 remained at that level during the periovulatory period. Clear flow velocity waveforms were obtained from the endometrium and myometrium around the time of ovulation. Data obtained from the radial arteries suggest better myometrial perfusion in patients with natural cycles compared with induced ovarian cycles. Spiral artery flow velocity in spontaneous cycles had a PI of 1.13 the day before ovulation, and a nadir of 0.72 was reached the day after ovulation. In contrast the mean PI of the spiral artery blood flow in the group with ovulation induction rose during the day before ovulation (PI=2.32) and reached a nadir of 1.09 the day after ovulation. These data suggest better uterine receptivity during the periovulatory phase of natural cycles compared with induced ovarian cycles (Table 1).

Weiner et al. (1993) studied the changes that occur in vascular resistance to blood flow in the uteroovarian circulation and correlated them with the number of follicles and steroid hormone levels in 11 patients undergoing ovarian stimulation with gonadotropin. They concluded that induced cycles are associated with decreased impedance to blood flow in the uteroovarian circulation. Intraovarian PI correlates negatively at each stage of the cycle with the eventual numbers of preovulatory follicles. Little or no changes are observed when the response to ovarian stimulation is poor.

Coulam et al. (1994) tried to assess the utility of endometrial thickness, echogenic pattern, and uterine artery impedance (measured as the pulsatility index) in predicting implantation.

When conception and nonconception cycles were compared, no difference in mean endometrial thickness was seen, but significant differences in the frequency of nonmultilayered pattern and pulsatility index>3.3 were observed. Forty-seven percent of nonconception and 9% of conception cycles were associated with at least one of these factors.

Sterr et al. (1994) compared the midluteal uterine artery impedance to blood flow as measured by the pulsatility index in women with various causes of infertility with that of women with normal fertility and correlated the result with endometrial thickness. All the infertile groups had significantly different median pulsatility indexes when compared with the normal group and the pulsatility indexes correlated with endometrial thickness. The impedance to uterine arterial blood flow is significantly different in women with various causes of infertility from that in women with normal fertility. Increased resistance to uterine blood flow in the midluteal phase may be an important contributing factor to some causes of infertility and the cause of some previously unexplained infertility.

Wada et al. (1994) tried to determine whether the addition of low-dose aspirin to a standard hormone replacement therapy (HRT) protocol improved uterine perfusion during assisted conception. In the first attempts, those with impaired perfusion (group 1, n=37) received low doses of aspirin starting from day 13 of HRT. Women with normal perfusion (group 2) did not receive aspirin. In subsequent attempts, those from group 1 were arbitrarily allocated to start aspirin on day 1 or day 13 of HRT, and 10 women from group 2 were arbitrarily selected to receive aspirin from day 1 of HRT. In group 1, the cancellation (46% versus 36%) and pregnancy rates (15% versus 25%) in those who received 150 or 300 mg aspirin daily were similar. In those with canceled first attempts, good perfusion was achieved in 82% versus 20% of subsequent attempts using aspirin from day 1 versus day 13 of HRT. Higher pregnancy rates (47% versus 17%) were achieved in those taking aspirin from day 1 of HRT. In group 2, pregnancy rates were not statistically different in those who did or did not receive aspirin during their subsequent attempts (10% versus 35%). The addition of low-dose aspirin to a standard HRT protocol in women with impaired uterine perfusion is associated with improved blood flow and satisfactory pregnancy rates. The initial assessment of uterine perfusion in each treatment cycle was done on day 13 of HRt. The blood flow velocity waveform of the anterior branch of the left and right uterine arteries was measured and classified according to the following criteria (Goswamy et al. 1988): (1) type 0, when there was no diastolic forward flow; (2) type A, when the diastolic flow was present but not continuous with the preceding systolic waveform; (3) type B, when the diastolic flow was continuous with the preceding systolic waveform but not extending to the next cardiac cycle; and (4) type C, when the diastolic and systolic waveforms were continuous from one cycle to the next.

The pulsatility index was defined as the peak-to-peak excursion of the waveforms divided by the mean height (Thaler et al. 1990). The results were classified as PI<3 or PI>3 (Steer et al. 1992). Uterine perfusion was considered to be impaired when there was bilateral blood flow velocity waveform type o or A and PI>3, or adequate when there was unilateral or bilateral blood flow velocity waveform type B or C and PI<3. In those with impaired perfusion, the Doppler examinations were repeated atg 2-day intervals until uterine blood flow improved; otherwise the cycle was abandoned on day 21 of HRT if poor perfusion persisted.

Failure of implantation is the major hurdle to improved success rates with IVF therapy today, and any method that allows an accurate prediction of the likelihood of implantation would be a major advance in therapy. Steer et al. (1995) investigated the correlation between uterine artery impedance with immunohistochemical, histologic, and ultrasonographic markers of uterine receptivity.

Nineteen of 76 patients who had a successful ET became pregnant. The pulsatility index on day 14 of both trial and ET cycles was significantly lower in those who achieved pregnancy compared to those who did not conceive: 2.65 (range 1.3–3.4) versus 3.85 (1.8–6.8) and 2.85 (1.4–3.6) versus 4.15 (2.1–6.8), respectively (Table 1). There were significant correlations between pulsatility index and 24-kD protein, E_2 receptor, and endometrial histology but not between PP14 and endometrial thickness. Uterine artery impedance had a significant correlation with biochemical markers of uterine receptivity and accurately predicted the probability of pregnancy in frozen embryo replacement cycles.

Tekay et al. (1995) assessed the role of transvaginal pulsed-wave Doppler ultrasound in predicting the outcome of in vitro fertilization therapy in 30 patients during stimulated cycles. The pulsatility index of the uterine arteries did not change significantly until the midluteal phase. Within 6 days after the beginning of stimulation, the maximum peak systolic velocity increased significantly from 27.6±8.9 to 36±12.8 cm/s. No difference was found in uterine PI between pregnant and nonpregnant women. The PI of intraovarian flow was also similar in both groups. These investigators found a significant increase in uterine receptivity when the PI of the uterine artery was between 2.0 and 2.99 on the day of embryo transfer.

There are no data yet as a basis for speculation on whether absent diastolic flow is associated with infertility or poor reproductive capacity. It seems that transvaginal color Doppler may be used as noninvasive assay of uterine receptivity that would enable clinicians to cryopreserve the embryos if uterine conditions are adverse, and to reduce the number of transferred embryos when conditions are optimal.

Women with poor uterine perfusion could be advised that pregnancy is not likely to occur in their current treatment cycle, and they could have their embryos cryopreserved for transfer at a later date. One of the major problems associated with current IVF practice is the necessity of using multiple embryo transfers to increase the pregnancy rate, which leads to an increased incidence of multiple-gestation pregnancies. This may contribute to an increasesd obstetric risk and a less favorable perinatal outcome compared to single-gestation pregnancies. It is well known that the probability of pregnancy is strongly related to embryo quality and uterine receptivity. Instead of endometrial biopsy, which may cause trauma and bleeding at the implantation site, color Doppler ultrasound should be used to assess uterine receptivity. This noninvasive procedure is rapid, easy to perform, and may predict the likelihood of implantation, minimizing the risk of multiple-gestation pregnancy (Kupesic et al. 1994).

Circulatory changes similar to those observed in the main uterine arteries are seen in the minute arterial vessels (radial and spiral arteries). The endometrium has an exceptional capacity to undergo changes in structure and function during the menstrual cycle. The histological changes include a striking alteration of the spiral arteries, which become more developed during the menstrual cycle. The increase in endometrial vascularity during the menstrual cycle depends on the changes in uterine, arcuate and radial artery blood flow. Flow velocity waveform changes in spiral arteries during normal ovulatory cycles can now be visualized for the first time using transvaginal color Doppler (Kupesic and Kurjak 1993).

Endometrial perfusion presents an accurate noninvasive assay of uterine receptivity that may be used to predict the implantation success rate, to reveal unexplained infertility problems, and to select patients for correction of endometrial perfusion abnormalities by appropriate treatment (Kupesic et al. 1994).

The same method allows assessment of the intraovarian blood flow during the ovarian cycle. Color Doppler facilitates the detection of small vascular areas in the ovarian stroma and follicular rim (Kurjak et al. 1991). Blood flow velocity waveforms from the follicle can be seen when the follicle reaches 10–12 mm in diameter, and they may be a hemodynamic parameter of its growth, maturation, and ovulation. The resistance index is approximately 0.54±0.04 until ovulation approaches. A decline beginning 2 days prior to ovulation reaches its nadir at ovulation (0.44±0.04). Vascular changes at the time of presumed ovulation show increased vascularity on the inner wall of the follicle and a coincident surge in blood velocity just prior to eruption. This may represent the dilatation of new vessels that have developed between the relatively vascular theca cell layer and the normally hypoxic granulosa cell layer of the follicle (Bourne et al. 1991; Collins et al. 1991). These vascular changes intensify the effects of the oxygen concentration across the follicular epithelium. Immediately after follicular rupture there is a further dramatic increase in the velocity of blood flow to the early corpus luteum. The resistance index remains at that level for 4–5 days, then gradually climbs to a level of 0.50±0.04, which is still lower than that seen in the proliferative phase. It is hoped that transvaginal color flow and pulsed-wave Doppler ultrasound can be used to optimize the time of recovery of oocytes of the highest quality. Collins et al. (1991) found that the changes in PI observed in the wall of the dominant follicle and corpus luteum were less marked than the changes in blood velocity. Merce et al. (1992) obtained Doppler shift waveforms from the parenchyma of the nondominant ovary and from the parenchyma adjacent to the dominant follicle or corpus luteum in the dominant ovary. Like Kurjak et al. (1991), they detected a lower blood flow velocity waveform index in the dominant ovary during the luteal than in the follicular phase. Increased resistance to blood flow was observed in the late luteal phase. These blood flow changes reflect changes in vascularization and function of the corpus luteum. Some experimental studies (Ratmacher and Andersson 1968;

Bassett 1943) have shown that blood flow to the dominant ovary decreased dramatically during the late luteal phase of the cycle. The nondominant ovary (Merce et al. 1992) presented a slightly higher blood flow velocity waveform index in the luteal than in the follicular phase. A higher blood flow velocity and lower impedance detected in the vessels of the dominant ovary in the late follicular and early luteal phase indicate increased blood flow to the dominant ovary. The increased blood supply to the ovary containing the dominant follicle and corpus luteum is necessary for delivery of steroid precursors to the ovary and removal of progesterone. Doppler technique and uptake of radioactive microspheres by the ovary in ewes (Niswender et al. 1975) demonstrated a three- to sevenfold increase in blood flow during the luteal phase. Therefore, in both uterine and ovarian vessels changes in flow velocity occur before ovulation, implying that these changes are complex and not purely secondary to progesterone action. Undoubtedly, many other vasoactive compounds (e.g., prostaglandins) are involved in regulation of the vasculature.

Transvaginal ultrasonography is useful not only for imaging, but also for invasive techniques and therapeutic procedures. The main advantages of such procedures are accurate needle placement, simplicity, low complication rates, low cost, avoidance of general anesthesia, reduced operating and personnel time, and overall patient acceptance. Addition of color Doppler might be quite useful in most of these procedures (Kupesic and Kurjak 1994).

The ideal method of oocyte recovery should allow easy access to the largest number of available oocytes, be simple to perform, and be associated with low morbidity and cost. Laparoscopy under general anesthesia was formerly a standard method of ova retrieval in in vitro fertilization/embryo transfer programs (Steptoe and Edwards 1970). Despite the major advantage of this method, consisting in the direct view of the pelvic organs during the procedure, it is associated with significant postoperative discomfort, some morbidity and, rarely, mortality (Gonen et al. 1990a). Several studies (Lopata et al. 1974; Lewin et al. 1986; Lavy et al. 1988) have demonstrated that both prolonged exposure to the anesthetic agents and the potential drop in follicular fluid pH caused by CO_2 pneumoperitoneum may have deleterious effects on the oocyte (Boyers et al. 1987; Mastroyanii et al. 1987). The transvaginal oocyte retrieval procedure has several outstanding advantages: avoidance of general anesthesia, lower expense, reduced operating and personnel time, less morbidity, less risk, and greater patient acceptance (Feichtinger and Kameter 1986; Russell et al. 1987). In our IVF unit, transvaginal oocyte pickup has replaced all other methods of follicular aspiration; thus, laparoscopic oocyte retrieval is reserved only for patients who need a simultaneous evaluation of the pelvic anatomy. More recently, we have been using transvaginal color Doppler for ovarian follicle aspiration. By this method it is possible to minimize the risk of perforation of the main pelvic vessels and significantly reduce bleeding from puncture sites. The needle is advanced firmly and quickly through the vaginal wall into the follicle, avoiding the intraovarian vascular network with the help of color images. The aspirate is always bloodstained, and the microcirculatory network, which is necessary for normal development of the corpus luteum, should not be damaged.

Intrauterine transfer of early embryos is the last critical step in the IVF process. Failure at this stage is attributed to poor embryo quality, poor uterine receptivity or inaccurate placement of the embryos within the uterus. This technique is useful in patients with uterine anomalies, submucosal myomas, or in cases where the catheter has coiled itself in the region of the internal cervical os (Leeton 1984; Hurley et al. 1991). Transfundal embryo transfer is an alternative to cervical transfer in patients in whom it is difficult to pass the catheter through the cervix (Lenz et al. 1987; Parsons et al. 1987). Transvaginal color flow, with its superior accuracy, reproducibility and capacity to visualize small vessels may help in analyzing endometrial function prior to embryo transfer, which depends both on hormonal and on adequate vascular support (Glissant et al. 1985; Gonen et al. 1989; Steer et al. 1992). The advantages of this technique in transfundal embryo transfer might be the shorter puncture route and the precision of needle placement, both of which reduce the risk of inadvertent injury to adjacent uterine vessels.

The introduction of powerful drugs for ovulation induction and in vitro fertilization has resulted in an increased frequency of multiple gestations, which are associated with high fetal and maternal complication rates (Stone et al. 1987). Initially, a transabdominal ultrasound-guided technique was used during the transabdominal or transcervical needle approach for selective reduction of the number of multiple gestations (Brandes et al. 1987; Berkowitz et al. 1988; Itskovitz et al. 1989). The introduction of transvaginal ultrasonography with an attached needle guide has simplified this technique. The advantages of such an approach are the shorter puncture route, clear images that reduce the risk of injury to adjacent gestational sacs and employment of a thinner-gauge needle, while the main disadvantage is that the number of the fetuses is not "settled" during early gestation (Gonen et al. 1990). There are several advantages of using color Doppler here. First, with this new modality the vascularity of maternal and fetal blood flow can be assessed for each embryo separately. Furthermore, color Doppler imaging enables the surgeon to insert the needle in the correct direction during perforation of the fetal thorax. This modality is also helpful in observing the heartbeats of targeted fetuses after the injection of 2 mEq/ml of potassium chloride in the vicinity of the heart.

In conclusion, transvaginal color Doppler imaging promises to play a major role in gynecology in the next decade. This noninvasive technique makes it possible to study the development of the follicle and the corpus luteum and to describe to blood flow velocity waveform changes in the uterine, arcuate, radial and spiral arteries during the menstrual cycle. Changes in blood flow velocity patterns of the uterine and ovarian arteries are present during the normal menstrual cycle. Because these changes in flow velocity begin prior to ovulation, we suspect that they may involve angiogenesis as well as hormonal factors. The observed changes are statistically significant and may be used as an additional diagnostic tool in the study of infertility or menstrual cycle irregularities.

References

Bassett DL (1943) The changes in the vascular pattern of the ovary of the albino rat during the estrous cycle. Am J Anat 73:251–291
Battaglia C, Larocca E, Lanzani A, Valentini M, Genazzani AR (1990) Doppler ultrasound studies of the uterine arteries in spontaneous and IVF cycles. Gynecol Endocrinol 4:245–250
Berkowitz RI, Lynch L, Chitkara V, Wilkins IA, Mehalek KE, Alvarez A (1988) Selective reduction of multifetal pregnancies in the first trimester. N Engl J Med 318:1042
Bourne T, Jurkovic D, Waterstone J, Campbell S, Collins WP (1991) Intrafollicular blood flow during human ovulation. Ultrasound Obstet Gynecol 1:53
Boyers SP, Lavy G, Russell JB, DeCherney AH (1987) A paired analysis of in vitro fertilization and cleavage rates of first versus last recovered preovulatory human oocytes exposed to varying intervals of 100% CO_2 pneumoperitoneum and general anesthesia. Fertil Steril 48:987
Brandes JM, Itskovitz J, Timor Tritsch IE, Drungan A, Frydman R (1987) Reduction of the number of embryos in multiple pregnancy. Fertil Steril 48:326
Collins W, Jurkovic D, Bourne T, Kurjak A, Campbell S (1991) Ovarian morphology, endocrine function and intra-follicular blood flow during periovulatory period. Hum Reprod 3:319–324
Coulam CB, Bustillo M, Soenksen DM, Britten S (1994) Ultrasonographic predictors of implantation after assisted reproduction. Fertil Steril 62:1004–1010
De Ziegler D, Bessis R, Frydman R (1991) Vascular resistance of uterine arteries: physiological effects of estradiol and progesterone. Fertil Steril 55:775–779
Deutinger J, Reinthaller A, Bernaschek G (1989) Transvaginal pulsed Doppler measurement of blood flow velocity in the ovarian arteries during cycle stimulation and after follicle puncture. Fertil Steril 51:466–470
Feichtinger W, Kameter P (1986) Transvaginal sector scan sonography for needle guided transvaginal follicle aspiration in gynecologic routine and research. Fertil Steril 45:722
Findlay JK (1986) Angiogenesis in reproductive tissues. J Endocrinol 111:357
Glissant A, de Mouzon J, Frydman R (1985) Ultrasound study of the endometrium during in vitro fertilization cycles. Fertil Steril 44:701
Gonen Y, Casper RF, Jacobson W, Blanker J (1989) Endometrial thickness and growth during ovarian stimulation: a possible predictor of implantation in in vitro fertilization. Fertil Steril 52:446
Gonen Y, Blanker J, Casper RF (1990a) Transvaginal ultrasonically guided aspiration: a comparative study with laparoscopically guided follicular aspiration. J Clin Ultrasound 18:257
Gonen Y, Blankier J, Casper RF (1990b) Transvaginal ultrasound in selective embryo reduction for multiple pregnancy. Obstet Gynecol 75:720
Goswamy RK, Steptoe PC (1989) Doppler Ultrasound studies of the uterine artery in spontaneous ovarian cycles. Hum Reprod 3:721
Goswamy RK, Williams G, Steptoe PC (1988) Decreased uterine perfusion a cause of infertility. Hum Reprod 3:955
Gratton RC, Lyons EA, Harrington JC, Levi CS (1990) Basic physics and instrumentation of transvaginal color imaging. In: Kurjak A (ed) Transvaginal color Doppler. Parthenon, Carnfort, pp 9–17
Hurley VA, Osborn JC, Leoni MA, Leeton J (1991) Ultrasound guided embryo transfer: a controlled trial. Fertil Steril 55:559
Itskovitz J, Boldes R, Thaler I, Bronstein M, Erlik Y, Brandes JM (1989) Transvaginal ultrasonography-guided aspiration of gestational sacs for selective abortion in multiple pregnancy. Am J Obstet Gynecol 160:215
Kupesic S, Kurjak A (1993) Uterine and ovarian perfusion during the periovulatory period assessed by transvaginal color Doppler. Fertil Steril 60:439–443
Kupesic S, Kurjak A (1994) The role of color Doppler in vaginal sonographic puncture procedures. In: Kurjak A (ed) Atlas of transvaginal color Doppler. Parthenon, London, pp 171–197
Kupesik S, Kurjak A, Stilinovic K (1994) The assessment of female infertility. In: Kurjak A (ed) Atlas of transvaginal color Doppler. Parthenon, London, pp 171–197

Kurjak A, Kupesic-Urek S, Schulman H, Zalud I (1991) Transvaginal color Doppler in the assessment of ovarian and uterine blood flow in infertile women. Fertil Steril 56:870
Kurjak A, Kupesic S, Zalud I, Predanic M (1995) Transvaginal color Doppler. In: Dodson MG (ed) Transvaginal ultrasound. Churchill Livingstone, New York, pp 325–339
Lavy G, Restrego-Candelo M, Diamond M, Shapiro B, Grunfield L, DeCherney AH (1988) Laparoscopic and transvaginal ova recovery: the effect on ova quality. Fertil Steril 49:1002–1004
Leeton J (1984) Embryo transfer. In: Trounson A, Wood C (eds) In vitro fertilization and embryo transfer. Churchill Livingstone, Edinburgh, p 197
Lenz S, Leeton J, Rogers P, Trounson A (1987) Transfundal transfer of embryos using ultrasound. J In Vitro Fertil Embryo Transf 4:13
Lewin A, Laufer N, Rabinowitz R, Margalioth BJ, Bar I, Scheneker JG (1986) Ultrasonically guided oocyte collection under local anesthesia: the first choice for in vitro fertilization – a comparative study with laparoscopy. Fertil Steril 46:257–258
Lopata A, Johnston IWH, Leeton JF (1974) Collection of human oocytes at laparoscopy and laparotomy. Fertil Steril 25:1030–1032
Mastroyanii C, Hosoi Y, Yoshimura Y, Atlas SJ, Walach EE (1987) The effect on carbon dioxide pneumoperitoneum on rabbit follicular oocytes and early embryonic development. Fertil Steril 47:1025
Merce LT, Garces D, Barco MJ, De la Fuente F (1992) Intraovarian Doppler velocimetry in olvulatory, dysovulatory and anovulatory cycles. Ultrasound Obstet Gynaecol 2:197–202
Niswender GD, Moore RT, Akbar AM, Nett TM, Diekman MA (1975) Flow of blood to the ovaries of ewes throughout the estrous cycle. Biol Reprod 13:381–388
Parsons JH, Bolton VN, Wilson L, Campbell S (1987) Pregnancies following in vitro fertilization and ultrasound directed surgical embryo transfer by periurethral and transvaginal techniques. Fertil Steril 48:691
Ratmacher RP, Andersson LL (1968) Blood flow and progesterone levels in the ovary of cycling and pregnant pigs. Am J Physiol 214:1014–1018
Russell JB, DeCherney AH, Hobbins JC (1987) A new transvaginal probe and biopsy guide for oocyte retrieval. Fertil Steril 47:350
Scholtes MC, Wladimiroff JW, van Rijen HJM, Hop WCJ (1989) Uterine and ovarian flow velocity waveforms in the normal menstrual cycle: a transvaginal Doppler study. Fertil Steril 52:981–985
Steer CV, Mills CV, Campbell S (1991) Vaginal color Doppler assessment on the day of embryo transfer (ET) accurately predicts patients in an in vitro fertilization programme with suboptimal uterine perfusion who fail to be pregnant. Ultrasound Obstet Gynecol 1 [Suppl]:79
Steer CV, Campbell S, Tan SL, Crayford T, Mills C, Mason BA, Collins WP (1992) The use of transvaginal color flow imaging after in vitro fertilization to identify optimum uterine conditions before embryo transfer. Fertil Steril 57:372–376
Steer CV, Seang Lin Tan, Mason BA, Campbell S (1994) Midluteal-phase vaginal color Doppler assessment of uterine impedance in a subfertile population. Fertil Steril 61:53–58
Steer CV, Lin Tan S, Dillon D, Mason BA, Campbell S (1995) Vaginal color Doppler assessment of uterine artery impedance correlates with immunohistochemical markers of endometrial receptivity required for the implantation of an embryo. Fertil Steril 63:101–108
Steptoe P, Edwards RG (1970) Laparoscopic recovery of preovulatory human oocytes after priming the ovaries with gonadotropin. Lancet 1:683
Sterzik K, Grab D, Sasse V, Huetter W, Rosenbusch B, Terinde R (1989) Doppler sonographic findings and their correlation with implantation in an in vitro fertilization program. Fertil Steril 52:825–828
Stone SC, Schimberni M, Schuster PA, Werlin LB, Weatherbee P (1987) Incidence of multipe gestations in the presence of two or more mature follicles in the conception cycle. Fertil Steril 48:503
Tekay A, Martikainen H, Jouppila P (1995) Blood flow changes in uterine and ovarian vasculature, and predictive value of transvaginal pulsed colour Doppler ultrasonography in an in vitro fertilization programme. Hum Reprod 10:688–693
Thaler I, Itskovitch J, Manor D, Brandes J (1990) Blood flow measurements in the uterine and ovarian arteries in patients undergoing IVF/ET and in early pregnancy,

performed with a transvaginal Doppler duplex system. In: Maschiach S et al (eds) Advances in assisted reproductive technologies. Plenum, New York, pp 545–557
Wada I, Hsu CC, Williams G, Macnamee MC, Brindsen PR (1994) The benefits of low-dose aspirin therapy in women with impaired uterine perfusion during assisted conception. Hum Reprod 9:1954–1957
Weiner Z, Thaler I, Levron J, Lewit N, Itgskovitz-Eldor J (1993) Assessment of ovarian and uterine blood flow by transvaginal color Doppler in ovarian-stimulated women: correlation with the number of follicles and steroid hormone levels. Fertil Steril 59:743–749

Andrology

New Trends in Andrology

G. Haidl

Introduction

The most recent developments in assisted reproduction [subzonal insemination (SUZI), (ICSI)] are used very successfully, especially in the therapy of male factor infertility (Van Steirteghem et al. 1993). By these new techniques, male fertility disturbances can be overcome in patients who previously had no chance of achieving pregnancy, e.g., those with globozoospermia. Moreover, dogmas have been questioned that until recently were generally accepted, e.g., the role of the epididymis in sperm maturation, given that epididymal and even testicular spermatozoa have also been used successfully in the above-mentioned methods. Alternative possiblilites of drug treatment in andrology are very limited; those which were thought to be useful in the past, e.g., kallikrein, are doubted today (Glezerman et al. 1993). Consequently, at present, there is considerable uncertainty in andrology, so that the role of traditional andrology in reproductive medicine is questioned.

The new methods of micromanipulation require a lot of technical equipment and experience and are very expensive. If they were restricted to cases in which alternative treatment is not possible, these new developments might represent a challenge for andrology, possibly leading to a greater demand for the development of new diagnostic methods and alternative treatment forms.

Nosology and Classifications of Sperm Morphology

There is general agreement that common sperm parameters – count, motility, and morphology (which is mostly confined to the counting of normal forms) – do not allow reliable prognosis of fertilization and introduction of rational therapy. Specification of andrological disturbances according to sperm parameters permits "diagnoses" such as the OAT syndrome, but correlation to basic causes and, therefore, establishment of a nosology is not possible. However, it is very important to classify fertility disorders according to causes, origin, and severity in order to undertake appropriate steps. Apart from the essential clinical examination, a possible approach is the exact analysis of sperm morphology. Counting merely the percentage of normal-shaped spermatozoa, which is suggested in most classifications of sperm morphology,

Table 1 Düsseldorf classification of sperm morphology

Normal forms
Alterations of the sperm head
Hyperelongation of the postacrosomal region (I–III°) (Fig. 1)
Acrosome defects (I–II°)
Combined acrosome-defective and hyperelongated forms (I–II°) (Amorphous heads, megalo- and microforms, twin- and multiheaded spermatozoa)
Midpiece and tail disturbances
Ia° Atypical staining behaviour (Fig. 2)
ib° Structural shaft disturbance
II° Breaking and coiling
III° Rudiments

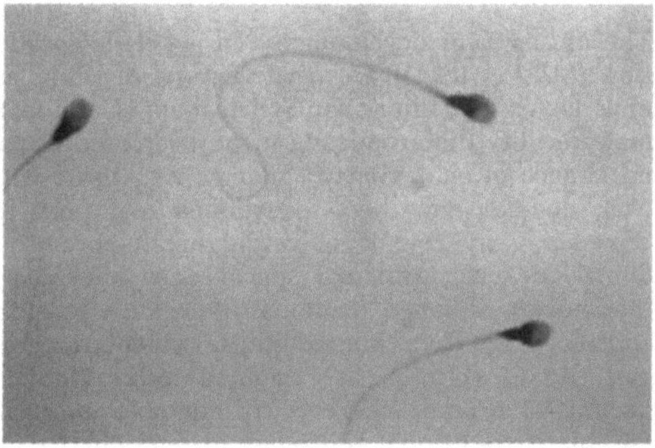

Fig. 1. Spermatozoa with hyperelongation of the postacrosomal region. Papanicolaou, ×1000

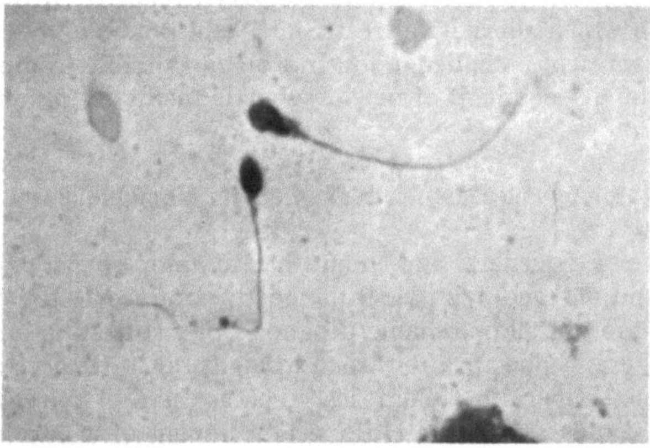

Fig. 2. Spermatozoa with normal red staining of the flagellum; acrospermatozoa of atypically bluish staining. Shorr, ×1000

will only give information on the present fertility potential of a semen sample and does not allow any conclusions about the kind, severity, and possible treatment of a disturbance. These considerations are paid due respect in the Düsseldorf classification of sperm morphology, which is based on the following observations: Although there are numerous variations of malformed spermatozoa, some characteristics can be recognized: The changes share common principles, they are frequently observed, often in defined disorders, and they show different degrees of severity. These malformations can be detected in testicular sections and, therefore, reflect disturbances of spermiogenesis. The Düsseldorf classification differentiates between hyperelongation of the postacrosomal segment, disturbed acrosomal development, the combination of both, and different alterations of midpiece and flagellum (Table 1). By means of enzyme histochemical studies on testicular tissue, hyperelongated forms could be attributed to disturbed function of Sertoli cells and myoid cells of the lamina propria. Such malformations are frequently observed in varicocele orchipathy but may have other causes, e.g., circulatory disturbances of the testes or injuries. Acrosomal defects are predominantly caused by disturbed synthesis of steroids in the Leydig cells. Normally, this block cannot be overcome by drugs. These forms are characteristic of constitutional disturbances such as cryptorchidism or toxic influences. In addition, functional histochemical enzyme defects of spermatogonia and spermatocytes may be detected. The combination of acrosomal defects and hyperelongated postacrosomal segments reflects a severe disturbance, because all testicular compartments (Leydig cells, spermatogonia, Sertoli cells) are affected (Hofmann and Haider 1985). Finally, disturbances of midpiece and flagellum are included in the Düsseldorf classification; these are testicular or epididymal origin and wil lbe discussed below.

The Tygerberg classification with strict criteria for sperm morphology, which is increasingly used as the international standard, concerns only normal-shaped spermatozoa. Using this classification, fertile samples show 14% normal forms, a figure established by means of in vitro studies (Kruger et al. 1986). Studies based on naturally occurring pregnancies, in which sperm morphology was calculated according to the Düsseldorf criteria, revealed an average of 30% normal spermatozoa in fertile men (Haidl and Schill 1993) (Table 2). This threshold is also suggested by the WHO (1992).

Table 2 Sperm parameters in 78 fertile men divided into three groups according to sperm density (from Haidl and Schill 1993)

Mean value	SEM	Range	$n=13$:		$n=32$:		$n=33$:	
			$5–19\times10^6$/ml	SEM	$20–50\times10^6$/ml	SEM	$>50\times10^6$/ml	SEM
No. of spermatozoa ($\times10^6$/ml)								
72.26	81	5.4–295.2	10.98	1.1	34.84	1.5	133.20	13.2
Progressive motility (%)								
37.99	1.5	2.0–67.0	36.58	3.9	33.60	2.4	43.09	2.0
Normal-shaped spermatozoa (%)								
29.50	1.3	5.0–50.0	22.25	2.2	27.84	2.3	37.06	1.3

Sperm Morphology and Sperm Function Tests

In contrast to strict or WHO criteria, the approach of the Düsseldorf classification allows examination of the fertilizing capacity of defined malformed spermatozoa by special studies of sperm function. This is important with regard to the new methods of micromanipulation, which also use abnormal spermatozoa. Apart from fertilization under in vitro conditions, there is no test that would be informative regarding all steps required during the fertilization process. Therefore, several sperm function tests are necessary to define whether or not fertilization might occur. In addition to determination of sperm motility and penetration into the cervical mucus, the hemizona assay (Menkveld et al. 1991), determination of acrosome reaction and acrosin activity, the HOP (hamster ovum penetration) test (Schill et al. 1994) and assessment of the chromatin condensation by means of the aniline blue staining technique (Haidl and Schill 1994a) may be applied. Evaluation of sperm motility and determination of the percentage of hyperactivated spermatozoa by CASA (computer-assisted sperm analysis) will not be discussed because CASA has been disappointing so far with regard to additional information for clinical andrology.

Correlation of the above-mentioned sperm function tests with sperm morphology according to the Düsseldorf criteria showed that exclusively normal-shaped spermatozoa and those with slightly hyperelongated postacrosomal segments bind to the zona pellucida (Menkveld et al. 1991). Studies with the HOP test revealed that spermatozoa with minor malformations are able to fuse with the zona free hamster egg and can lead to fertilization, which is not the case with spermatozoa with defective acrosomes (Heywinkel 1991). Under in vivo conditions, the latter have further handicaps with regard to their fertilizing capacity: There is no or too little acrosin to penetrate the zona pellucida. Moreover, they frequently show disturbed chromatin condensation. During spermiogenesis, the hereditary material has to be condensed in the course of the extreme morphological modification of the gamete. Particular nucleoproteins, the histones, are replaced by different proteins, the protamines. In the case of disturbed chromatin condensation, the histones persist, which is demonstrable by aniline blue staining. A highly significant correlation between regular chromatin condensation and fertilization rate in IVF has been shown (Haidl and Schill 1994a); in contrast to all other sperm functions that are not necessarily required for the ICSI procedure, regular chromatin condensation is a prerequisite for the subsequent decondensation of the paternal hereditary material in the oocyte and, therefore, most probably only spermatozoa with normal chromatin condensation can be used for ICSI. Disturbed chromatin condensation is frequently observed in acrosome-defective spermatozoa, to a lesser degree in hyperelongated forms, and in approximately 20% of normal-shaped spermatazoa (Hofmann et al. 1990). In acrosomeless round-headed spermatozoa, a genetic defect in which the acrosomal vesicle cannot attach to the nucleus because of absence of a "cementing" protein, chromatin condensation is normally not disturbed. Therefore, successful fertilization by ICSI – the only treatment option in such cases –

can be expected (Lundin et al. 1993). Apart from cases of round-headed spermatozoa, ICSI should also be successful with hyperelongated spermatozoa. ICSI is also indicated in patients with immotile spermatozoa or those with severe flagellar defects.

New perspectives may arise in epididymally caused motility disturbances. These can be recognized by atypical staining behavior of the sperm tails in Shorr or Papanicolaou staining. Normally, sperm tails stain red in these techniques; if epididymal maturation is disturbed, they appear bluish. Such spermatozoa are completely immotile without showing further structural defects. Studies on immotile spermatozoa from the epididymal head with a high percentage of atypical staining behavior revealed a significant increase in motility and progressive motility, accompanied by a reduction of atypically stained flagella, after in vitro addition of phosphatidylcholine (Fig. 3). This points to missing membrane lipids in epididymal spermatozoa, an observation that is underlined by the detection of increased membrane rigidity in immotile spermatozoa (Haidl et al. 1993). In future, this may allow a new therapeutic approach in patients in whom epididymal spermatozoa have to be used for methods of assisted reproduction. If in vitro addition of phosphatidylcholine improves the motility and fertilizing capacity, intra-uterine inseminations with stimulated spermatozoa could be performed instead of the highly expensive and difficult ICSI procedure that is used today.

Increased frequency of spermatozoa with atypically stained flagella can also be observed in chronic inflammatory processes of the epididymis that are easily overlooked because of absence of discomfort to the patient, but may be causally treated by anti-inflammatory drugs.

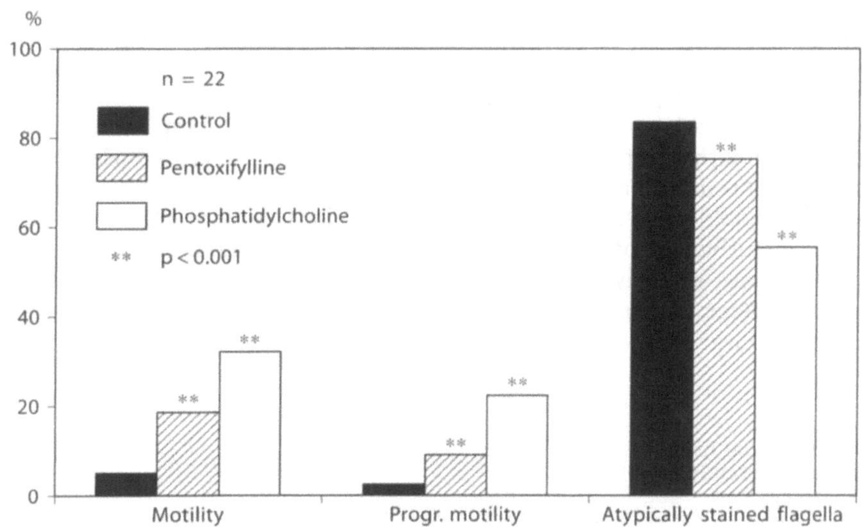

Fig. 3. Changes in motility, progressive motility, and staining of sperm tails after stimulation of epididymal spermatozoa with pentoxifylline and phosphatidylcholine

Treatment of Male Fertility Disorders

In general, there are hardly any new developments in the therapeutic sector, although regimens thought to be effective in the past are doubted today. As long as there is no reasonable nosology in andrology, studies that are based only on symptoms (for example "idiopathic OAT") must be interpreted with caution. A new hope may be the administration of pure or recombinant FSH. One study did not result in changes in the sperm parameters in patients with severe male factor infertility, but a significantly better fertilization rate in IVF was observed (Acosta et al. 1992). Anohter study particulary showed improvement of the acrosomal status of spermatozoa after treatment with FSH (Bartoov et al. 1994). However, more multicenter studies are needed to confirm these preliminary results. Also, the role of growth factors and paracrine regulation in the treatment of male fertility disturbances has to be determined (Spiteri-Grech and Nieschlag 1993). A further causal approach is the treatment with antioxidants such as vitamin C and E in the presence of reactive oxygen species. There is increasing evidence for the significance of these radicals in impaired sperm function (Aitken and Clarkson 1988). Unless new therapeutic approaches are developed, perhaps based on molecular biological studies, the only proven treatment regimens remain (a) hormonal replacement therapy in cases of hypogonadotropic hypogonadism, (b) anti-inflammatory and antibiotic treatment in cases of inflammatory diseases of the testes, epididymis and accessory glands, (c) alpha-sympathomimetic drug therapy for sperm emission failures, such as retrograde ejaculation (Schill and Haidl 1993) (Table 3).

The significance of varicocele treatment is still controversial (Glezerman 1994). Recent studies have confirmed previous reports pointing out that patients with pathological GnRH tests should be treated in any case. In addition, the most significant improvement of sperm parameters after varicocele treatment was observed in patients with increased appearance of hyperelongated spermatozoa (Haidl and Schill 1994b).

So far, there exists no treatment for genetically caused disturbances, which are thought to be responsible for a relatively high number of male fertility disorders: chromosomal causes (gonosomes and autosomes, meiotic chromosomes) are held responsible for 1%–17%, and in 30% of infertility patients genetic disturbances of spermatid differentiation are assumed (Lange et al. 1990). Despite extensive studies in patients whose spermatozoa showed a high percentage of impaired acrosomal development and chromatin condensation and in groups with severe flagellar defects, no abnormal genetic find-

Table 3 Causal drug treatment currently used in andrology

Hormonal substitution in hypogonadotrophic hypogonadism
Antibiotics
Antiphlogistics
Antioxidants
Alpha-sympathomimetics

Table 4 Genetic disturbances of spermatogenesis

Chromosomal causes (aberrations of gono- and autosomes, meiotic chromosomes)
Microdeletions of the y-chromosome
Genetic disturbance of spermatid differentiation – Globozoospermia – Immotile cilia syndrome

ings have so far been established (Hofferbert et al. 1993). Genetic disturbances of spermatid differentiation have only been demonstrated in globozoospermia (Flörke Gerloff et al. 1984) and immotile cilia syndrome, both of which are inherited as an autosomal recessive trait (Table 4). Further molecular biological projects are ongoing. Recently, microdeletions of the y-chromosome have been detected as a cause of fertility disorders in patients with severe oligozoospermia or azoospermia, which underlines the significance of the y-chromosome for spermatogenesis (Vogt et al. 1992). Perhaps this will lead to the development of molecular biological techniques of treatment for such patients. New knowledge from basic research needs to be integrated into clinical androlgoy to provide a differentiated view of andrological disturbances with exact diagnoses and rational therapeutic approaches. This should result in more exact prognoses of fertility and reduced performance of assisted reproduction procedures for andrological reasons. Moreover, prophylactic measures, such as early treatment of cryptorchidism, should be kept in mind, as well as avoidance of toxic influences. Recent reports point to increased exposure to environmental substances with estrogen-like effects. These are claimed to be responsible for the decreasing sperm quality in men over recent decades (Sharpe and Skakkebaek 1993); confirmation of this interesting theory requires further research.

Conclusion

In summary, andrological knowledge considerably lags behind knowledge at the gynecological level. Therefore, increased research efforts are necessary to make andrology an equal counterpart to gynecological reproductive medicine; then there will be no question about the significance of andrology in the future.

References

Acosta AA, Khalifa E, Oehninger S (1992) Pure human follicle stimulating hormone has a role in the treatment of severe male infertility by assisted reproduction: Norfolk's total experience. Hum Reprod 7:1067–1072

Aitken RJ, Clarkson JS (1988) Significance of reactive oxygen species and antioxidants in defining the efficacy of sperm preparation techniques. J Androl 9:367–376

Bartoov B, Eltes F, Lunenfeld E, Har-Even D, Lederman H, Lunenfeld B (1994) Sperm quality of subfertilie males before and after treatment with human follicle-stimulating hormone. Fertil Steril 61:727–734

Flörke-Gerloff S, Töpfer-Petersen E, Müller-Esterl W, Mansouri A, Schatz R, Schirren C, Schill W-B, Engel W (1984) Biochemical and genetic investigation of round-headed spermatozoa in infertile men including two brothers and their father. Andrologia 16:187–202
Glezerman M, Lunenfeld E, Potashnik G, Huleihel M, Soffer Y, Segal S (1993) Efficacy of kallikrein in the treatment of oligozoospermia and asthenozoospermia: a double-blind trial. Fertil Steril 60:1052–1056
Glezerman M (1994) Varicocele: questions and answers on etiology, pathophysiology, and management. In: Colpi GM, Balerna M (eds) Treating male infertility. Karger, Basel, pp 87–98
Haidl G, Schill W-B (1993) Sperm morphology in fertile men. Arch Androl 31:153–157
Haidl G, Schill W-B (1994a) Assessment of sperm chromatin condensation: an important test for prediction of IvF-outcome. Arch Androl 32:263–266
Haidl G, Schill W-B (1994b) When to treat varicocele. Acta Chir Acad Sci Hung (in press)
Haidl G, Badura B, Hinsch KD, Ghyczy M, Gareiß J, Schill W-B (1993) Disturbances of sperm flagella due to failure of epididymal maturation and their possible relationship to phospholipids. Hum Reprod 8:1070–1073
Heywinkel E (1991) Bedeutung der Morphologie und der Motilität der Spermatozoen für die assistierte Reproduktion. PhD Thesis, Medical Faculty, Heinrich Heine University, Düsseldorf
Hofferbert S, Burfeind P, Hoyer-Fender S, Lange R, Haidl G, Engel W (1993) A homozygous deletion of 27 basepairs in the coding region of the human outer dense fiber protein does not result in a pathologic phenotype. Hum Molec Gen 2:2167–2170
Hofmann N, Haider SG (1985) Neue Ergebnisse morphologischer Diagnostik der Spermatogenesestörungen. Gynäkologe 18:70–76
Hofmann N, Hilscher B, Bierling C (1990) Quantitative studies on the correlation between disturbances of the chromatin condensation and sperm morphology (in German). Fertilität 6:208–213
Kruger TF, Menkveld R, Stander FSH, Lombard CJ, van der Merwe JP, van Zyl JA, Smith K (1986) Sperm morphologic features as a prognostic factor in in-vitro fertilization. Fertil Steril 46:1118–1123
Lange R, Michelmann HW, Engel W (1990) Chromosomal causes of male infertility – a review (in German). Fertilität 6:17–28
Lundin K, Sjögren A, Hamberger L (1993) Fertilization of human oocytes with acrosomeless spermatozoa. J Reprod Fertil 12 (Abstr. Series):55
Menkveld R, Franken DR, Kruger TF, Oehninger S, Hodgen GD (1991) Sperm selection capacity of the human zona pellucida. Molec Develop Reprod 30:346–352
Schill W-B, Haidl G (1993) Medical treatment of male infertility. In: Insler V, Lunenfeld B (eds) Infertility – male and female, 2nd edn. Churchill, Edinburgh, pp 575–622
Schill W-B, Henkel R, Miska W (1994) Biotests of sperm function. In: Armas OR (ed) Fertility and sterility. Progress in research and practive. Parthenon, Casterton Hall
Sharpe RM, Skakkebaek NE (1993) Are oestrogenes involved in failling sperm counts and disorders of the male reproductive tract? Lancet 341:1392–1395
Spiteri-Grech J, Nieschlag E (1993) Paracrine factors relevant to the regulation of spermatogenesis – a review. J Reprod Fertil 98:1–14
Van Steirteghem AC, Liu J, Joris H, Nagy Z, Janssenswillen C, Tournaye H, Derde MP, Van Assche E, Devroey PC (1993) Higher success rate by intracytoplasmic sperm injection than by subzonal insemination: report of a second series of 300 consecutive treatment cycles. Hum Reprod 8:1055–1060
Vogt P, Chandley AC, Hargreave TB, Keil R, Ma K, Sharkey A (1992) Microdeletions in interval 6 of the Y-chromosome of males with idiopathic sterility, point to disruption of AZF, a human spermatogenesis gene. Hum Genet 89:491–496
WHO (1992) Laboratory manual for the examination of human semen and sperm-cervical mucus interaction, 3rd edn. Cambridge University Press, Cambridge

Operative Therapy for Male Infertility

J. Zumbé, M.J. Mathers, and U. Engelmann

Introduction

Approximately 15% of all marriages are involuntarily childless. In one-third of these cases a disturbance in male fertility is the sole cause. For a normal in vivo conception the ejaculate must contain millions of sperm with a normal morphology and sufficient progressive motility.

Since 1978 in vitro fertilization (IVF) with subsequent embryo transfer (ET) has been successfully performed in tubal sterility. However, pregnancy rates have not been significantly improved in cases of severe pathological seminal profiles [28, 31]. Conservative treatments of severe oligo- or azoospermia mainly pertain to the correction of hormonal dysregulation and functional disorders of ejaculation.

In recent years the technological developments in reproductive medicine and increased experience in microsurgery of the reproductive system, as well as a close cooperation with different medical subspecialties, have enhanced possible therapies for infertile marriages. Modern aspects of urological therapy of male infertility include prophylactic measures as well as correction of already existing male fertility problems (Table 1).

Table 1 Surgically correctable disturbances in male fertility

Cryptorchism
Varicocele testis
Obstructive azoospermia
Aplasia of the vas deferens
Epi-/hypospadia
Penile deviation
Peyronie's disease (induratio penis plastica)
Disorders of erection

Cryptorchism

Nowadays the surgical therapy for correcting the undescended testis is standardized. The optimal time for operative treatment is up to the age of 2 years. The sperm density during the first year of life does not differ between a descended and an undescended testis. This changes, however, during the second year of life and a significant decrease in germinal cells can be found [8].

A complete retention of one or both testes in the abdomen is a special case and usually makes it impossible to obtain sufficient cord length by surgical dissection [7]. Here the existence of a testis should be ascertained by laparoscopy and the dystopic testis microsurgically autotransplanted during the same procedure [22]. The sequence of diagnostic measures proving the existence of a testis should be as follows: sonography, computer tomography/ NMR, laparoscopy, and phlebography.

Varicocele Testis

In general a varicocele is viewed as a hemodynamic disturbance in the venous drainage system of the testis, especially in the pampiniform plexus. The significance of the interrelationship between a varicocele and male infertility has still not been clarified. Besides pathological changes of testicular tissue caused by retarded venous outflow, decreased oxygenation and therefore a disturbed hormonal metabolism and an elevated temperature of the testis have been discussed as possible mechanisms [9]. Furthermore adrenal hormones can be found in the spermatic vein, possibly caused by retrograde venous filling.

Recent studies have shown a correlation between a varicocele and secondary sterility. The extent and severity of the clinical finding of a varicocele do not necessarily correlate with the degree of infertility. However, a varicocele is still generally accepted as a possible cause of an oligo- or azoospermia. One important fact is that approximately 50% of surgically treated patients show an improved semen quality. Treatment of varicoceles in mature males is indicated when there is dysspermatogenesis or presence of symptoms from the varicocele. The severe varicocele in boys should be surgically corrected during the age of 12 through 14 years as a prophylactic measure. Mild cases in boys should be treated as soon as a size difference in the testicles occurs. Compared with the established methods of spermatic vein resections, antegrade sclerosis is nowadays the most important (Table 2). From the viewpoint of the urologist this method has a low complication rate combined with a high success rate and low cost [29]. In addition the operation can be performed as an outpatient procedure and is minimally invasive.

Table 2 Current methods of operative varicocele treatment

Suprainguinal resection of the spermatic vessels [17]
Infrainguinal resection of the spermatic vein [10]
Retrograde sclerosis of the spermatic vein [18]
Antegrade sclerosis of the spermatic vein [29]
Laparoscopic resection of the spermatic vein [5]

Operative Technique of Antegrade Sclerosis

After infiltration of the spermatic cord and the scrotal skin with an anesthetic, a transverse incision is made approximately 2 cm under the penile base. After preparation of the spermatic cord, a varicose vein of the pampiniform plexus is dissected. Distally this vein is sutured. Proximally the opened vein is canalized with a 24-G needle. Through this needle a non-ionized contrast medium is injected in order to prove the correct position of the needle in a vein leading to the spermatic vein. After injecting 1 ml of air as an "airblock", approximately 3 ml of the sclerosing medium (e.g., Varicocid) is injected.

Obstructive Azoospermia

Basically obstructive azoospermia can be differentiated according to whether there is obstruction of the duct on both sides or within the epididymis (Table 3). The microscopic correction of obstructive azoospermia is the main interest of the clinically involved andrologist surgeon. Here is the reconstruction of the semen-transporting system such as a vasovasostomy or epididymovasostomy and the microaspiration of sperm from the epididymis are the current goals.

Vasectomies for contraception are becoming more and more popular. In 1988 approximately 25000 were performed in Germany. At the same time approximately 1500 patients requested a refertilization, this is a percentage of 6%. Their main motives, were a new partnership, death of a spouse and psychosomatic adjustment problems following vasectomy. In 473 of these patients a recanalization of the duct was performed (1.9%) [6]. According to a study conducted in the United States in 1983, the potential for refertilization operations taking divorces into account would probably be ca. 10% [12].

Other reasons for bilateral ejaculatory duct obstruction should be mentioned here even though they are quite seldom:

1. Scarring after infection and after vasography
2. Resection of the vas deferens during surgery for other reasons.

Table 3 Classification of obstructive azoospermia

Obstruction of the vas deferens on both sides
Following vasectomy
Following infection
Scarring after vasography
Lesions of the duct following surgical procedures or trauma
Aplasia of the duct
Obstruction with intact vas deferens
Secondary to a granuloma or extravasation
Following epididymitis
Malformation of the epididymis
Following epididymal surgery

Vasovasostomy

Vasovasostomy is indicated and technically possible in patients with a localized blockage of the vas deferens. The main goal here is tension-free and fluid-tight anastomosis. Clinically three different surgical approaches are widely used:

1. The macroscopic method with or without a splinting of the duct
2. The one-layer suture technique with magnifying glasses
3. The two-layer microsurgical suture technique.

The macroscopic approach unfortunately does not allow an exact adaptation of the lumen and therefore often causes scarring or sperm granulomas. However, postoperatively one can often find sperm in the ejaculate. This is most probably due to spontaneous recanalization after the formation of a sperm fistula [14].

The patency rate of the one-layer technique with magnifying glasses is up to 87%. The pregnancy rate is reported to be up to 48% [12]. The one-layer surgical technique using four 8×0 resorbable sutures in each quadrant is usually used. Four to six serosa sutures (7×0) guarantee a fluid-tight closing. The anastomosis is performed with magnifying glasses with a fourfold magnification.

Of the different microscopic techniques it seems that the nonsplinted two-layer approach recommended by Silber shows the best results [23]. After atraumatically freeing the two ends of the vas using a loupe, both ends can usually be easily bridged together. Using a microscope with approximately a 16- to 20-fold magnification a tension-free anastomosis of the inner mucosa can be performed. Usually the testicular side lumen is dilated because of the chronic high pressure obstruction. The reanastomosis should only by performed if the presence of sperm can be found in the sperm fluid from the testicular side of the vas. This fluid should be examined under a conventional laboratory microscope. According to Silber the microscopic characterization of the sperm morphology in the vas fluid will allow accurate prediction of the success or failure of the vasovasostomy [25]. At this point sperm motility does not seem to play an important role. The patency of the abdominal part of the vas is proven by the injection of saline solution. Vasography performed with contrast medium is absolete. This in itself could result in an obstruction caused by scarring or fusing of the mucosal walls.

The two ends of the vas are brought into close approximation under the microscope using a vasovasostomy clamp. Five to six mucosal sutures are placed with 10×0 nylon while carefully approximating the different sized lumina (Fig. 1). The second layer is achieved by accurately suturing the muscularis with eight to ten Nylon sutures (9×0). This will ensure adequate strength to the anastomosis whereas the separate mucosal layer will allow a leak-proof connection (Fig. 2).

Similar patency rates can be achieved by using either loupes or the microscope. Therefore this issue is at present still controversial. However, pregnancy rates are higher when operating under a microscope since the exact adaptation of the mucosa prevents a sperm granuloma.

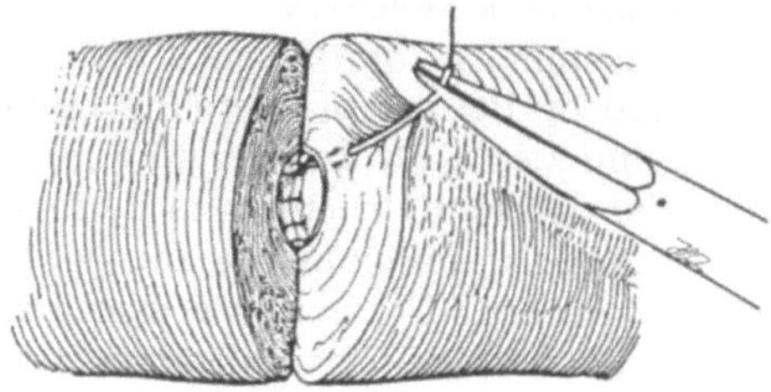

Fig. 1. Vasovasostomy in the two-layer technique with mucosa-mucosa sutures (10×0)

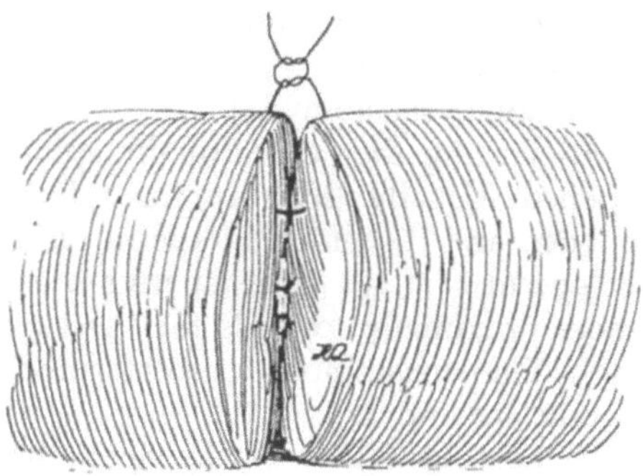

Fig. 2. Vasovasostomy in the two-year technique with muscularis-muscularis sutures (9×0)

Therapy for Obstructive Azoospermia and an Intact Duct

The reasons for obstructive azoospermia and an intact duct are usually obstructive changes in the epididymal tubuli (Table 3). Only through a direct correction of the duct to the prestenotic part of the tubuli system can patency of the ejaculatory duct be achieved.

Prerequisites for an epididymo- or tubulovasostomy are:

1. Normal spermatogenesis proven by testicular biopsy
2. Patency of the duct
3. Azoospermia in the seminal fluid after spontaneous recanalization.

Depending on the interval after vasectomy a so-called blow-out occurs in the epididymis; this is caused by increased pressure within the tubulus apparatus and a sperm granuloma is the result. For this reason one does not often find a normal spermiogram even though the vasovasostomy anastomosis is patent.

Because of the correlation between the viscosity and the operative results Silber recommends the following strategy:

1. If the fluid is clear and the interval since the vasectomy is less than two years, a vasovasostomy can be attempted.
2. If the fluid is creamy or opaque, an epididymovasostomy should be performed.
3. Regardless of the viscosity, a vasovasostomy should be tried first if the ligation of the vasectomy was high. Should this approach fail a tubulovasostomy should be attempted.

Epididymotubulovasostomy

The anastomosis of the duct to a tubule of the epididymis can only be achieved by the use of operating microscopes and sophisticated microsurgical techniques. Only an operating microscope can magnify sufficiently to enable the different structures to be seen distinctly. The lumen of the epididymal tubule is approximately 100–300 µm in diameter and has a wall thickness of 30 µm. The accurate placement of stitches for the anastomosis requires up to a 24× magnification. Obviously one has to see the structures properly. In 1978 Silber described an end-to-end epididymovasostomy which in his hands revealed a patency of 78% [24]. Because of the difficulty of recognizing the intact tubules' canal during the dissection, a modified technique was developed. For the first time in 1983 Belker illustrated the end-to-side tubulovasostomy [1].

By cutting the serosa of the epididymis tail a so-called serosa window is opened. Usually three so ten tubules are visible. One of these tubules is opened and the efflux of sperm fluid is examined for the adequate presence of sperm (Fig. 3). If no sperms are found, other serosa windows are made more proximally towards the head of the epididymis until sperms are found [19]. The anastomosis is performed at the distalmost level where normal sperm are found.

After preparation of the duct, the specific tubule which is effluxing the sperm fluid should be anastomosed tension free with the lumen of the duct in an end-to-side tubulovasostomy manner. In a first step three or four muscularis-serosa stitches are placed with 9×0 nylon. Then the mucosa-mucosa sutures are placed with 11×0 stitches to form a watertight anastomosis (Fig. 4); further muscularis-serosa sutures complete the anastomosis (Fig. 5).

In order to prevent an infection a wound drain should not be used. Perioperative use of antibiotics is not necessary. A period of sexual restriction should be maintained for about 4 weeks. The first semen analysis can be performed after approximately 6 weeks. However, a final evaluation of the operation can only be made after a year. Long-term semen analysis controls are

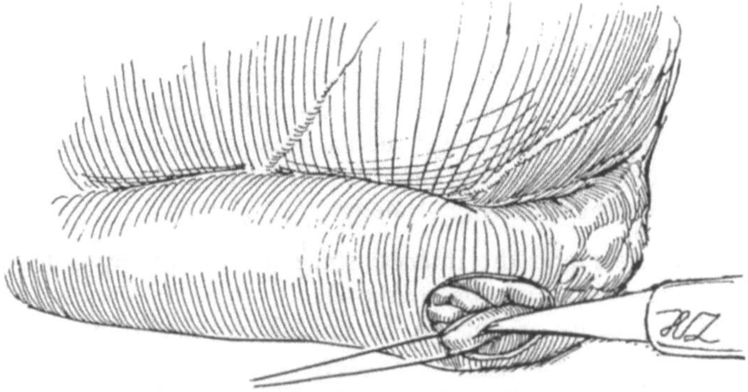

Fig. 3. Within a serosa window of the epididymis a tubule is opened. The fluid can be examined

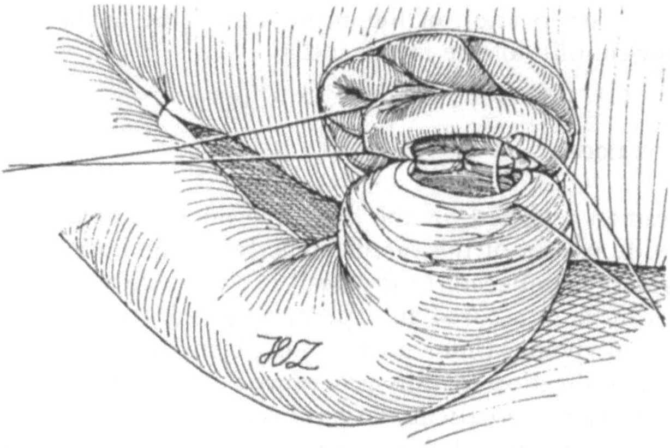

Fig. 4. Tubulovasostomy in the two-layer technique with mucosa-mucosa sutures (11×0)

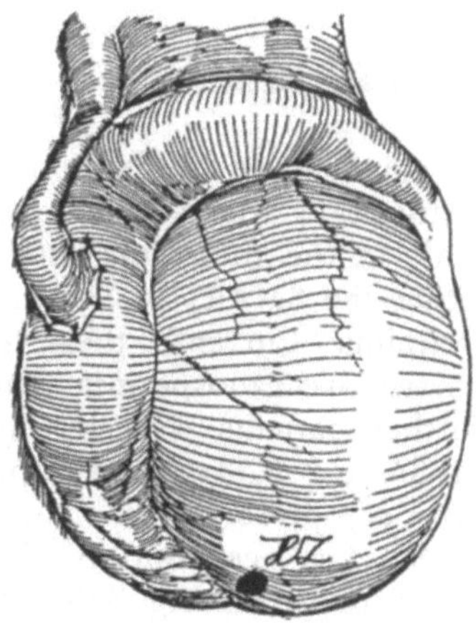

Fig. 5. Tubulovasostomy in the two-layer technique with muscularis-serosa sutures (9×0)

difficult to accomplish since patients are often non-compliant after either a pregnancy or disappountment with the results.

A direct comparison of different study groups with regard to patency and pregnancy rates after tubulovasostomy or vasovasostomy is difficult because of different methods and undefined patients. The presence of sperm can be the result of a sperm granuloma. Reasons for the azoospermia are frequently not given. The time since obstruction is repeatedly not mentioned even though this information would be important for assessing the possibility of sperm antibodies which are influential in the process of fertility. Long-term semen analysis controls are usually not done and repeatedly there is no information concerning the fertility status of the partner.

In 1989 Silber published an exemplary study of tubulovasostomies in 190 patients over a period of 4 years [26]. He concluded that the pregnancy rate depended on (a) the location of the anastomosis (the farther distal the better) and (b) the motility of the found sperm.

Alloplastic Spermatocele

In 1968 Schoysman reported for the first time on an alloplastic spermatocele in a patient with aplasia of the vas deferens [20]. The basic idea was to create a sperm reservoir adjacent to the head of the epididymis. At a later time this reservoir can be punctured and sperm obtained, which then can be used to impregnate an ovum. Unfortunately long-term results are discouraging. Nevertheless the indication for this procedure is given in patients with ejaculation difficulties as these patients do have a chance to profit from the method. An absolute prerequisite for this procedure is the presence of progressive propelling sperm. If possible this operation should be combined with the spermatozoa microaspiration retrieval technique (SMART) and subsequent IVF.

SMART and MESA

In 1985 Temple-Smith reported on the first pregnancy achieved by in vitro fertilization after surgically obtaining the spermatozoa from the epididymis [30]. In the meantime more than 200 children have been born by using either the SMART or the microscopic epididymal sperm aspiration (MESA) technique. Currently these techniques are mainly indicated in patients with obstructive azoospermia (Table 4). In the future increased experience with further patients with fertility problems will facilitate the combination of MESA and ICSI (intracytoplasmatic sperm injection) [15, 16 27]. However, until cryopreservation of minute amounts of sperm fluid, as are acquired by MESA, has been optimized, these advances in reproductive technology require correct timing: After stimulation of the follicle it is retrieved transvaginally by puncture and the quality of the egg is examined. Should the results be positive, the partner is simultaneously operated on using the following surgical procedure:

1. Microsurgically the serosa window is made as far distal as possible (Fig. 4)
2. Preparation of the epididymis, with due care in achieving hemostasis
3. Piercing of the tubule and aspiration of the sperm fluid

Table 4 Indications for MESA/SMART

Aplasia of the duct
Inoperable obstruction of the duct
Failure after refertilization
In addition to a tubulovasostomy (cryopreservation) in order to increase the chance of fertility
Disturbances of ejaculation (e.g., paraplegia, diabetes)

4. Evaluation of the sperm under a laboratory microscope [21]
5. If this examination is positive regarding the count and motility, a new exprimate should be sought
6. Incubation in Ham's F10 solution which has to be combined with serum from the partner in a 5% CO_2 atmosphere.

The separation of the spermatozoa is achieved either after several centrifugal sequences, such as by "mini-Percollcentrifugation", or through direct selection of the spermatozoa in the exprimate. Cryoconservation of abundant spermatozoa and oocytes in the "pronucleus stage" can enable further microinjections to be performed.

Prognostic Criteria

When developing the different IVF therapies it was believed that, through better technique, results would be improved. Unfortunately these hopes could not be fulfilled. Therefore it is essential to identify prognostic factors in male infertility so that the different methods of assisted reproduction can be selectively used in different situations. In 1986 Kruger proposed strict criteria regarding sperm morphology when evaluating the spermiogram. He was able to find a direct correlation between sperm morphology and the results of IVF [11]. Membrane intrinsic defects of the spermatozoa are of prognostic significance, and in some cases an electron microscope is necessary for the diagnosis.

The functional differentiation between the degrees of infertility is important. Miscellaneous functional tests such as the hamster penetration test, the hemi-zona test or the cervix mucus penetration test can be helpful in selected cases.

References

1. Belker AM, Jimenez-Cruz DJF, Kelami A, Wagenknecht LW (1986) Alloplastic spermatocele: poor sperm motility in intraoperative epididymal fluid contraindicates prosthesis implantation. J Urol 136:408
2. Brindley GS (1981) Reflex ejaculation under vibratory stimulation in paraplegic men. Paraplegia 19:299
3. Cos LR, Valvo JR, Davis RS, Cockett ATK (1983) Vasovasostomy: current state of the art. Urol 22:567
4. Denil J, Ohl DA, Menge AC, Keller LM, McCabe M (1992) Functional characteristics of sperm obtained by electroejaculation. J Urol 147:69
5. Donovan JD, Winfield HN (1992) Laparoscopic varix ligation. J Urol 147:77
6. Engelmann U, Deindl F, Hertle L, Wilbert D, Senge Th (1989) Die Refertilisierungssituation in der BRD – Ergebnisse einer Umfrage. Urologe B 29:29
7. Fowler R, Stephens FD (1959) The role of testicular vascular anatomy in the salvage of high undescended testes. Aust NZ J Surg 2992
8. Hadziselimovic F, Hecker E, Herzog B (1984) The value of testicular biopsy in cryptorchism. Urol Res 12:171
9. Hadziselimovic F, Herzog B, Liebundgut B, Jenny P, Buser M (1989) Testicular and vascular changes in children and adults with variocele. J Urol 142:583
10. Ivanissevich O (1960) Left varicocele due to reflux. J Int Coll Surg 349:742

11. Kruger TF, Acosta AA, Simmons KF et al (1987) New method of evaluating sperm morphology with predictive value for human in vitro fertilization. Urology 30:248
12. Lee HY (1986) A 20-year experience with vasovasostomy. J Urol 136:413
13. Marcourt D, Engel S, Jones RF, Zaki M (1991) Pregnancy by gamete intrafallopian transfer (GIFT) with sperm aspirated from their vaso-epididymal junction of spinal injured man. Paraplegia 29:550
14. Noldus J, Otto U, Salamon J, Schulze W, Klosterhalfen H (1992) Vasovasostomie nach Vasektomie. Operationsergebnisse 1986–1989. Urologe A31:103
15. Oates RD, Honig S, Berger MJ, Harris D (1992) Microscopic epididymal sperm aspiration (MESA): a new option for treatment of the obstructive azoospermia associated with cystic fibrosis. J Ass Reprod Gen 9:36
16. Palermo G, Joris H, Devroey P, Van Steirteghem AC (1992) Pregnancies after intracytoplasmatic injection of single spermatozoa into an oocyte. Lancet 340:17–18
17. Palomo A (1949) Radical cure of varicocele by a new technique: preliminary report. J Urol 61:604
18. Salgarello G (1990) Transvenous sclerotherapy of the gonadal veins for treatment of varicocele: long-term results. J Vasc Diseases 427
19. Schlegel PN, Goldstein M (1993) Microsurgical vasoepididymostomy: refinements and results. J Urol 150:1165
20. Schoysman R (1968) Creation of an artificial spermatocele in agenesis of the deferent duct. Bull Soc Belge Gynec Obstet 38:307
21. Sikka SC, Hellstrom WJG (1991) The application of pentoxifylline in the stimulation of sperm motion in men undergoing electroejaculation. Androl 12:165
22. Silber SJ, Keller J (1976) Successful autotransplantation of an intraabdominal testis to the scrotum by microvascular technique. J Urol 115 452–454
23. Silber SJ (1977) Perfect anatomical reconstruction of the vas deferens with a new microscopic surgical technique. Fertil Steril 28:72
24. Silber SJ (1978) Microscopic vasoepididymostomy: Specific microanastomosis to the epididymal tubule. Fertil Steril 30:565
25. Silber SJ (1988) Microsurgery for male infertility. Microsurgery 9:251
26. Silber SJ (1989) Results of microsurgical vasoepididymostomy: role of epididymis in sperm maturation. Hum Reprod 4:298
27. Van Steirteghem AC, Nagy Z, Joris H, Liu J, Staessen C, Smitz J, Wisanto A, Devroey P (1993) High fertilization rates after intracytoplasmatic sperm injection. Hum Reprod 1061–1066
28. Steptoe RC, Edwards RG (1978) Birth after reimplantation of a human embryo. Lancet II:366
29. Tauber R, Johnsen N (1994) Antegrade scrotal sclerotherapy for the treatment of varicocele: technique and late results. J Urol 151:386–390
30. Temple-Smith PD, Southwick GJ, Yates CA, Trounson AD, de Kretser DM (1985) Human pregnancy by in vitro fertilization (IVF) using sperm aspirated from the epididymis. J Vitro Fert Embryo Transfer 4:298
31. Yovich JL, Stanger JD (1984) The limitations of in vitro fertilization from males with severe oligospermia and abnormal sperm morphology. J Fertil Embryo Transfer 1:172

Other Specific Topics

Counselling the Infertile Couple

H. Kentenich, V.-S. Pastor, and D.E. Gagel

Introduction

Modern reproductive medicine offers a wide variety of invasive types of therapy such as insemination, in vitro fertilisation (IVF) and intracytoplasmatic sperm injection (ICSI). The problem which arises here is that the couple cannot easily understand the implications of each method. Diagnostic and treatment procedures involve many steps and each step requires the taking of blood samples, injections, ultrasound examinations, etc. The outcome of any of these stages can determine whether treatment should continue or should be stopped. These procedures are so complex that even trained doctors would be overtaxed withouth the aid of experts from other fields. From the other perspective, there is the couple, and the female patient in particular is the one suffering from being sterile. It is she who wants to become pregnant by entering into active therapy and to whom nearly everything can be offered.

This situation demonstrates that careful, psychosomatic oriented counselling is of utmost importance, otherwise the patient remains overwhelmed by the complexity of treatment.

Aims of Counselling

In the initial phase, it is essential to give the couple *information* about the different diagnostic steps and possibilities for treatment. This should occur during the first or second consulation. This information is essential because many patients have no idea what will happen during the various diagnostic and treatment procedures.

The second aim of counselling is to provide *emotional support* as it becomes necessary during treatment. The treatment phase, especially during hormonal stimulation, is a time of extreme tension accompanied by high expectations, and still a great number of treatment cycles fail. Emotional support should not just be given at its end, as in the event of failure, but should accompany the couple from the start.

In a wider sense, the aim of counselling is that patients *learn to discuss* their sterility crisis and mourning process. This implies not only talks between pa-

Table 1 Methods of counselling and psychotherapy

Information (film, video, brochure)	
Conversations with the patient	
Conversations with the couple	
Psychotherapy	- individual
	- couple
	- group
Self-help groups (e.g. Resolve, Nat. Ass. Childless)	
Supportive groups with a leader (discussion group)	

tient(s) and the doctor/psychologist/nurse (counsellor), but also open discussion within the partnership as well as with relatives and friends. Very often patients deal with their sterility by keeping their distress secret from others.

A further goal is that the couple learns to *accept alternatives.* Such alternatives might include a life without a child, and thereby the end of the therapy. Another possibility is adoption or use of donor semen/oocyte/embryo. However, this last alternative should be discussed very carefully with the couple because of the use of donor genetic material. For this reason, it is not always a viable alternative in every case.

Counselling should also help the couple to increase its *capacity for ambivalence.* Every couple has reasons and fantasies for wanting a child. Very often they say, "The most important thing in my life is to have a child. I would feel more comfortable with my own child." Yet in every patient there are also (unconscious) fears: "Will the child be healthy? Will it be handicapped? What about the changes in my body during the pregnancy? How will the relationship with my partner be when the child is born?" Through counselling, patients should be enabled to see both positive and negative sides of pregnancy and birth (happiness and burden).

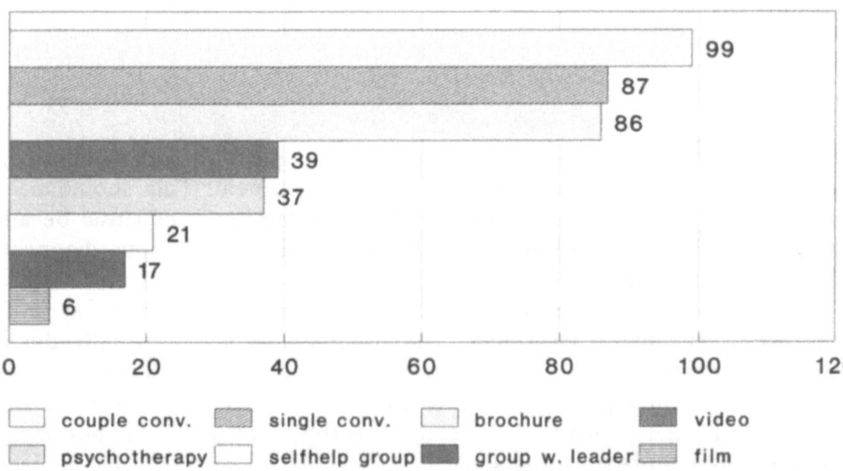

Fig. 1. Types of counselling offered in various European countries. Data are given as percentages ($n=78$ teams)

Table 1 shows the different methods of counselling. Of great significance are the self-help groups (e.g. RESOLVE in the United States, National Association of the Childless in the UK). These self-help groups can be very helpful to the couple and the patient. One disadvantage of these groups is that they have a high turnover rate among personnel and when a member becomes pregnant she leaves the self-help group in most instances.

Figure 1 gives an overview of the different kinds of counselling that have been offered in various European countries. In 1993 we carried out an investigation and surveyed nearly 150 different teams all over Europe. Seventy-eight teams responded to our inquiry. Figure 2 shows the programmes available to couples in the different European centres.

Information and Education

During the counselling process, information and education should cover:

1. *Reasons for sterility:* Very often the couple does not know the reason for sterility. It is quite common for men to deny their infertility and to project the cause of sterility onto their partner. Smaller disturbances (e.g. mild forms of hyperprolactinemia, corpus luteum insufficiency) are frequently discussed as the main reason for sterility, although they are not likely to be the primary cause.
2. *Different methods of treatment:* Modern types of treatment such as IVF are difficult for the couple to understand. For this reason, detailed information should be given on each step of the treatment.
3. *Success rate:* Many couples overestimate the success rate. They should be given the national statistics (AFS, national survey) so that the couple will be informed about the success rates of the different treatments.
4. *Stress of treatment:* The couple should know that the treatment alone brings with it medical and emotional problems. The medical aspects (hormonal treatment, ultrasound examinations, blood investigations, injections, IVF puncture, embryo transfer) are often well known after information. However, the emotional side (waiting for appropriate follicular development, waiting for fertilisation, waiting for pregnancy) is underestimated. During this time, the patient experiences a great deal of tension (Kentenich et al. 1987; Barma et al. 1988).
5. *Multiple/preterm deliveries:* When patients become pregnant during treatment (homologous insemination with stimulation, IVF, GIFT), nearly 20% of them have a multiple pregnancy, and preterm deliveries are quite common. Singleton pregnancies also frequently end in preterm delivery (Doyle et al. 1992; Rufat et al. 1994). The results are babies with higher rates of birth defects. Especially triplets can be an emotional and psychosocial burden for the mother (Bordt et al. 1994).
6. *Side-effect of drugs:* GNRH analogues are frequently used. It is well known that these drugs can produce a range of side-effects on the central nervous system (in connection with this side-effects due to the lack of estradiol or the presence of hot (flushes).

7. *Rate of complications:* Stimulation can end in a hyperstimulation syndrome. Although severe cases (OHSS III°) are rare, they can be life-threatening. A puncture during IVF has a complication rate of nearly 1 in a thousand (lesion of intestines, pelvic infection) (Schenker and Ezra 1994).

What Is Success?

There is no doubt that pregnancy and birth measure the success of the sterility treatment. Nevertheless, we should expand the definition of success. Success might also include:

1. *"Honest counselling":* The patient should know the chances of becoming pregnant as well as the risks and possible side-effects.
2. *Limitation of treatment to an acceptable level:* Very often patients demand therapy until they become pregnant. But pregnancy cannot be achieved in every case. We may consider it a success when we are able to limit the treatment to a level that is acceptable for the couple.
3. *Preventing multiple pregnancies:* Multiple pregnancies and preterm deliveries are a major problem in reproductive medicine. Pregnancies under 32 weeks of gestation have a handicapped rate of 28% (Ohrt 1994).
4. *Preventing medical risks:* In former times, useless operations (antefixation) were often performed. Nowadays, severe OHSS is one of the main risks of stimulation treatment.
5. *Satisfying sexual life:* Nearly one-third of all sterile couples have sexual disturbances (Möller and Fallström 1991; Golombok 1992). These problems are often aggravated by the treatment itself because the treatment works against a spontaneous sex life. When a couple is able to achieve a satisfying sexual life after a time of disturbances, the counselling and therapy can be seen as a success.
6. *Accepting one's own (the doctor's) limitations:* Reproductive medicine would lead us to believe that nearly everything is possible. And indeed for 15 years now, we have been able to treat severe cases of tubal sterility and nowadays the ICSI method appears to be able to treat severe cases of male infertility. However, not every case of sterility can be treated successfully. The doctors themselves have to learn to accept this limitation.
7. *Resolving the sterility crisis:* If after a long process of counselling (and treatment) the couple is able to end the therapy, even in the event of continued sterility, this can be viewed as a success. When the couple can accept sterility, this gives them a broader perspective on life and paves the way for a new direction in their future.

Who Should Counsel?

Figure 2 gives a survey of the counsellors throughout Europe. There are different types of counselling which can be carried out by doctors, nurses/so-

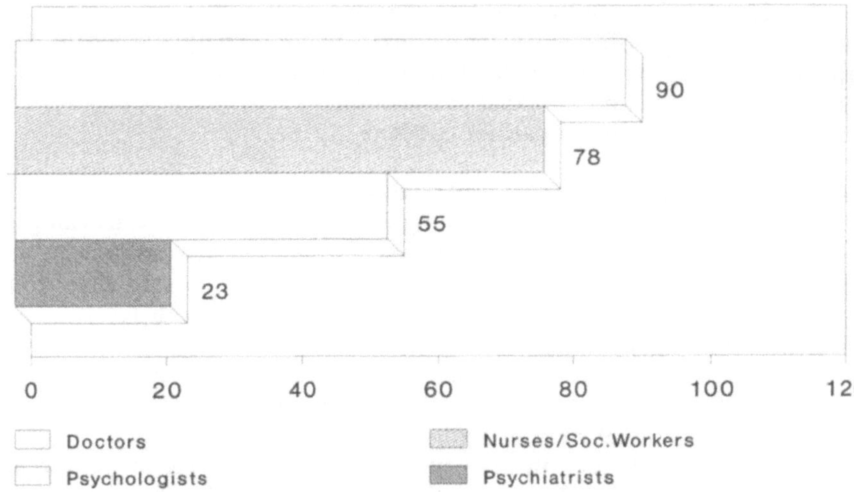

Fig. 2. Survey of counsellors throughout Europe. Data are given as percentages ($n=81$ teams)

cial workers, psychologists and psychiatrists. Each has advantages and disadvantages.

Counselling by a Doctor

In Germany, counselling is commonly provided by the gynaecologist. Its (possible) *advantage* is that medical and psychological counselling and treatment are administered by the same person .This means that personal talks on intimate subjects are held with only one person, which facilitates trust and a confidential relationship. If such rapport is achieved, the "psychosomatic approach" in the counselling process has been carried out successfully.

Possible *disadvantages* are:

1. Sufficient education and training are necessary. Not every doctor and gynaecologist is innately a good counsellor. During their university and postgraduate studies, they receive almost no training in counselling.
2. One possible danger arises when the doctor as "a good counsellor" is able to give adequate emotional support but provides "poor medical treatment", a situation which may occur since not every doctor can be highly specialised in both areas (emotional support, reproductive medicine).
3. If a single person takes on the responsibility for counselling and active treatment, this can lead to an uncritical attitude towards reproductive medicine. The doctor has no distance from his own actions, so he himself cannot see the possible disadvantages of his own treatment.

Even if the doctor is capable of performing the counselling, referral to a psychologist or psychiatrist may become necessary in certain cases:

1. In the case of psychogenic sterility
2. In the event of depressive/psychotic reactions during treatment

3. In the case of “never ending treatment”
4. For psychotherapy (due to severe neuroses, major anxiety, dysphoria, previous depression, depressive reaction during treatment)
5. For couple therapy due to sexual dysfunction
6. For couple therapy due to partner conflicts

Counselling by a Psychologist/Social worker/Nurse

The *advantage* of this form of counselling is that these professionals can provide a high quality of counselling based on their specialised training in this field for many years (Connolly et al. 1993). Such counselling can also be easily combined with short-term psychotherapy (Brandt and Zech 1991).
Possible *disadvantages* are:

1. The patient is torn in two directions (emotionally/physically). The doctor is responsible for the medical treatment and the psychologist/social worker/nurse for emotional counselling.
2. Intimate talks are held with the psychologist/social worker/nurse and are then avoided with the doctor. In this event, the doctor knows nothing about the patient’s feelings.
3. The patients feel they have been referred to the psychologist/social worker/nurse for “psychological screening”.
4. If the treatment is not successful, the patients may feel that they have been “passed on” to the psychologist because the doctor “failed”.

Combined Counselling by the Doctor and Psychologist

This type of counselling is described by Fiegl and Kemeter (1989) and Kemeter et al. (1992). The *advantages* are:

1. Two specialists work together.
2. Both can learn from each other. This is important because both doctor and psychologist can discuss and learn from the intentions and questions of one another.
3. The patient can talk about somatic and emotional problems at the same time.
4. In this situation the patient learns that somatic and emotional experiences are tied together.

One possible *disadvantage* is that this form of counselling requires a great deal of time, and the patient would prefer to express his emotions and feelings either to the doctor or to the psychologist only.

Problems in Counselling

Figure 3 gives a survey of how effective the European teams consider their counselling to be. The outcome is quite good, but it should be mentioned that only half of the teams are satisfied with their current state of counselling.

Thus, one is led to ask what problems occur during the counselling process.

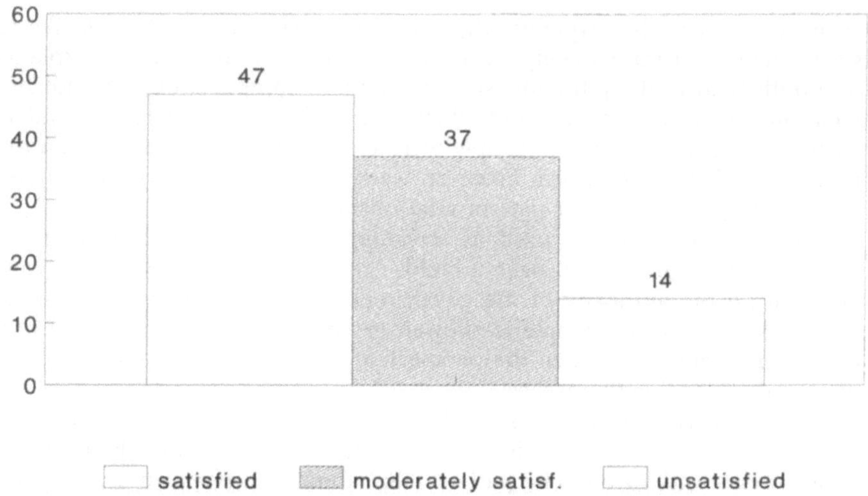

Fig. 3. Survey of satisfaction of European teams with their counselling ($n = 78$ teams)

1. *Coping with transference:* In every doctor-patient relationship transference becomes evident. The patient transfers her own feelings (resulting from her own personal history) onto the doctor. In this process, the doctor may come to represent important persons in the patient's history (i.e. her mother or father). In connection with the current conflict of sterility, this can lead to an idealisation of the doctor. Very often the patient feels that her doctor or reproductive centre is the best there is. The child and modern technical medicine are idealised as well, so that the patient believes the child will solve all of her personal problems and make life easier. Since technical medicine can help to overcome the sterility, it is also viewed as inherently good. These forms of idealisation imply that the patient denies the low succes rate of reproductive medicine.
2. *Coping with countertransference.* Every doctor and counsellor has his or her own traits and personal history and therefore he or she will react differently to certain patients. This often leads to the phenomenon of countertransference. Depending on the doctor's personality, the patient can be seen as "pleasant" or "unpleasant". If the doctor has compulsive tendencies, he may get along well with patients who arrive on time and take the medicine correctly, and he might have difficulties with "hysterical women" who forget to take their medicine at the proper time or come late to consultations.
3. An *unconscious understanding between the patient and doctor* is often observed in modern reproductive medicine: Both (doctor and patient) prefer active treatment (stimulation, IVF, micro-injection) because if they are actively engaged, no time remains for reflection, discussion, mourning or grief. This unconscious bond can be lead to defence against emotions since neither wants to accept failure (failed fertilisation, failed treatment

cycle, abortion). This explains why, after one cycle has failed, both like to start a new trial immediately. Such an emotional connection also explains why both tend to deny the low success rate and complications. We dot not mention this as a reproach to the doctor or patient, as we certainly understand that neither wishes to simply wait and let "the child come when the time is ripe". In this regard, however, we believe that an unconscious element underlies this doctor-patient relationship.

4. Counselling must not be used as *screening for parenthood.* In daily life every couple is allowed to have a child. Consequently, the counsellor cannot take on the authority of the government or medical services to make decisions as to which couple is allowed to have a baby and which is not. Counselling can only widen the perspective of the couple so that they can make a decision for themselves.
5. *Everyone is a counsellor.* We should be aware that the patient has contact to other patients, relatives, friends, the porter and cleaners of the hospital, other nurses and so on. The patient talks about her problem and experiences in sterility treatment, and she receives a great many answers. Every one of these contacts has formed his or her own opinions or even had similar experiences.
6. *"Bombarding" with psychological questions:* Since sterility and sexuality are closely linked, the question of sex is an important one. But if we ask the patient or couple questions which they feel to be too intimate, emotional or confusing, this will provoke defence reactions. This may ruin future opportunities. As such, it is important to know which questions should be asked and at what time.
7. *Technology can intimidate or arouse emotions:* Modern reproductive medicine implements highly technical equipment. By using ultrasound machines, the patient can see how the follicles are growing during the phase of stimulation. A normal growing process shows 2 mm of follicular development each day. The patient sees this on the machine, and the doctor and patient discuss this growing process, but they do not talk about emotions. On the other hand, this machine can provoke many different types of emotions, such as when one woman compares her own follicular growth with another patient's (i.e. in the waiting-room). The patient with poor follicular development may feel herself to be "inadequate".
8. *Total submission of the body to the doctor:* IVF and related types of treatment demand that the body react in a predefined manner. Normal treatment should lead to multiple follicular growth, the oocyte should be of good quality, the embryos should "look good" and the hormonal patterns should react in a "certain" way. The patient herself carries little responsibility for what is done during this process. The doctor, along with modern reproductive medicine, "manipulates" her body. Consequently, it is our understanding that the patient relinquishes responsibility for her body, thus losing her body competence.

Who Counsels the Counsellor?

Not every doctor/psychologist/nurse/social worker is born to be a counsellor. Adequate training is necessary. Some countries have a national organisaton for counsellors (UK) which develops guidelines for professional counselling. Such organisations provide many advantages, but they cannot solve all the problems. Because counselling is conducted by a team of reproductive medical workers, it leads to the impression that the counsellor or team (especially when done by doctors) receives external supervision. Psychologists and psychotherapists should join team sessions to try do discover "blind spots" in a team. Their external standpoint can help the team resolve its conflicts and find its own path.

Doctors frequently make use of Balint groups since they provide an arena in which doctors can discuss difficult cases, treatments and doctor-patients relationships. These Balint groups focus on the interaction between the doctor/counsellor and the patient. Since difficulties in the doctor-patient relationship are always specific to the persons involved and are determined by the particular qualities of the patient, the doctor and their interaction, discussion in a group (with a supportive atmosphere) takes on valuable meaning. In many European countries, gynaecologists have extensive experience with Balint groups.

In conclusion, Table 2 lists some key practical questions, including a few remarks:

1. *How long have you been trying to get pregnant?* It sometimes happens that the patient has just stopped taking the pill and already comes in for consultation. Occasionally one can observe a compulsive approach in such behaviour since the patient believes that her body should behave like a machine to fit in with the usual predictability of her lifestyle.
2. *Who suffers most from the sterility?* In most cases, the woman suffers more than her partner. This is understandable since the man could never become pregnant or have a child. On the other hand, the suffering can be much greater for the husband if the female patient has children from an

Table 2 Key questions?

How long have you been trying to get pregnant?
How long have you been in treatment?
What is the reason for sterility?
Who suffers most from the sterility?
Why do you want the child now?
Sexual life (frequency, anorgasm, dyspareunia)?
What has changed in your life since you found out about the sterility?
Psychosomatic complaints (asthma, ulcer, Crohn's disease)?
Psychiatric/psychotherapeutic (pretreatment-)?
When you consider your own childhood, what would you pass on to your child and what would you do differently?
What about alternatives (adoption, foster child)?
What are your limits for treatment?
How long will you continue the treatment?
What about living without a child?

earlier relationship, for example, or if the source of this suffering stems from male sterility. In this situation, the sterility is also his "fault", as far as his subjective feelings are concerned.

3. *Why do you want the child now?* The desire for a child arises at certain times in a partnership. Frequently we observe that the desire for a child takes on great significance when a family member has recently died or when another sort of heavy loss can be observed. In these cases, the relevancy of the desire for a child is determined by the point in time. As counsellors, we have to be able to trace the time-frame of the sterility and the relevance of the desire for a child.
4. *What has changed in your life since you found out about the sterility?* Many couples have completely altered their daily lives after finding out about their sterility. The sexuality is frequently perceived exclusively as goal-oriented. In some instances, the patient believes that she will become pregnant faster if she gives up her occupation because then she can devote herself entirely to the sterility diagnostics and therapy. This, however, leads in most cases to greater focus on the desire for a child and fixation on the sterility, which ultimately becomes counterproductive.
5. *Psychosomatic complaints?* We also have to ask the patient about psychosomatic complaints such as asthma, pelvic pain, intestinal troubles, skin disorders, dysmenorrhea, etc. And the question of previous or current psychiatric or psychotherapeutic treatment is essential. By focusing on purely anatomical findings, a person cannot be grasped in his or her entirety. Many patients report a series of psychosomatic complaints which cause them additional strain. The counsellor should be aware of these troubles.
6. *When you consider your own childhood, what would you pass on to your child and what would you want to do differently?* This question is not always suitable for the first consultation. It is important to know, however (particularly with "complicated" couples), how the partners were moulded during their own childhood. Many patients have had an impoverished childhood or they idealise their childhood (or their father or mother) because this helps them maintain the fantasy of a happy childhood. Here the danger may exist that the couple has a fixed idea of how the child will be, the child that is to be conceived through sterility therapy. The ensuing childhood is to be the same as their own or it should be exactly the opposite in order to spare the child the worry and suffering that the partners experienced in their own childhood. The child that is to be conceived can thus be instrumentalised in this situation.
7. *What about alternatives?* The question as to alternatives, length of treatment and possible conclusion and the question about how they would imagine a life without a child have to be discussed at some point during the course of the counselling process. These questions do not have to be asked at the outset. Sterility therapy alone is not sufficient if the question of alternatives first appears at the end of a frustrated therapy. If this occurs, the couple will interpret any reference to alternatives as punishment for an unsuccessful therapy.

In summary, counselling means giving the couple the opportunity to place this particularly painful experience in relation to the greater context of their lives at the time of the sterility crisis. Counselling is not formal psychotherapy. Counselling should, on a professional basis, however, point the way out of this crisis.

References

Baram D, Tourtelot E, Muechler E, Huang KE (1988) Psychosocial adjustment following unsuccessful IVF. J Psychosom Obstet Gynaecol 9:181–190

Bordt J, Jager J, Grutzner H (1994) Parenting problems raising complete triplets and quadruplets. Human Reprod 9 (Suppl 3):10 (Abstract)

Brandt KH, Zech H (1991) Entwicklung von Prognosekriterien für IVF nach Kurzzeit-Psychotherapie. Fertilität 7:98–100

Connolly KJ, Edelmann RJ, Bartlett H, Cooke ID, Lenton E, Pike S (1993) An evaluation of counselling for couples undergoing treatment for in-vitro fertilization. Hum Reprod 8:1332–1338

Doyle P, Beral V, Maconochie N (1992) Preterm delivery, low birth weight and small-for-gestational-age in liveborn single babies resulting from in vitro fertilization. Human Reprod 7:425–428

Fiegl J, Kemeter P (1989) Die in-vitro-Fertilisation aus der Sicht einer gynäkologisch-psychologischen Zusammenarbeit. Fertilität 5:156–161

Golombok S (1992) Psychological functioning in infertility patients. Hum Reprod 7:208-212

Kemeter P, Fiegl J, Bydowski ML (1992) A psychosomatic approach to infertility and assisted reproduction. In: Wijma K, von Schoultz B (eds) Reproductive life. Parthenon, Carnforth, pp 572–577

Kentenich H, Hölzle C, Schmiady H, Stauber M (1987) "Am schlimmsten ist das Warten!" Wie Paare die in-vitro-Fertilisation erleben. Sexualmedizin 16:364–370

Kentenich H (1989) Psychological guidance of IVF patients. Hum Reprod 4 (Suppl) 17–22

Möller A, Fallström K (1991) Psychological consequences of infertility: a longitudinal study. J Psychosom Obstet Gynaecol 12:27–45

Ohrt B (1994) Langzeitprognosen von Frühgeburten. 50 Kongreß der Deutschen Gesellschaft für Gynäkologie und Geburtshilfe. Munich, Aug 23.–27th, 1994

Rufat P, Olivennes F, De Mouzon J, Dehan M, Frydman R (1994) Task force report on the outcome of pregnancies and children conceived by in vitro fertilization (France: 1987 to 1989), Fertil Steril 61:324–330

Schenker JG, Ezra Y (1994) Complications of assisted reproductive techniques. Fertil Steril 61:411-422

Ethical and Psychological Problems in Sterility Treatment

P. Bielfeld and L. Beck

Introduction

Immense technological progress during the past few years has encouraged further development of manipulation in various fields of medicine. Likewise it has promoted the medical challenge of influencing processes of human procreation, birth, life and death.

In 1978 the first child who owed its existence to extracorporeal fertilisation followed by embryo transfer to the maternal uterus was born in Great Britain. Ever since, technically assisted reproduction of human life has given rise to questions demanding more than just answers based on medical facts. In order to make decisions in these fields in a pluralistic society, such as the Federal Republic of Germany, judgements as to the values, wishes and objectives expressed by adherents of different attitudes and orientations must be considered. It would not be correct to request new ethics as a consequence of technical progress in diagnosis and therapeutics; however, the doctor's scope of responsibility, having been augmented by the development of new techniques, requires more profound reflection regarding traditional medical morals and their transformation and translation into new situations. Moreover, a more intense moral differentiation between what is technically feasible, medically indicated and morally justified is required [9]. From life's experience we each gain a personal perception of values. Such *judgements as to values* serve as a prism for the reflection of information before interpretation and monitoring in decisions relevant to life. *Morals* can be defined as generally adopted attitudes towards right and wrong, what should and what should not be done [1]. *Ethics* is the science of moral behaviour. Ethical behaviour is practised on the basis of education, development, and formation of opinions on the world and people from which are derived points of view towards values and attitudes [5].

Psychosocial Aspects of Assisted Human Reproduction

Independent of which kind of infertility therapy is applied, there is an ethical commitment to act for the well-being and rights of the child. Further to correct definition of the indication, a conversation with the couple is desirable, taking into consideration psychosomatic aspects. Does the request for therapy in fact aim at fulfilling the couple's joint desire for a child as opposed to simply restoring the self-reliance of the infertile couple or of one of the partners. Desires for a child repeatedly put forward with emphasis conceal problems closely connected with desires of the persons that have almost nothing to do with the child desired [8]. While giving full acknowledgement to the partner's sufferings, treatment must nevertheless primarily focus on the future well-being of the longed for child: otherwise the child would be a subject, misused as a means to serve a purpose [4].

Ethical Aspects of Assisted Human Reproduction

Current methods of assisted reproduction medicine comprise:

1. Insemination introducing sperm into the woman's genital tract (pericervically, intracervically, intrauterine, intratubal) or into the peritoneum (intraperitoneally) at the peak of ovulation.
2. Retrieval of oocytes from the ovary and transfer of the oocyte together with sperm into the fallopian tube (GIFT = gamete intrafallopian transfer).
3. Retrieval of oocytes from the ovary and fertilisation by sperms in vitro followed by zygote or embryo transfer into the fallopian tube (ZIFT = zygote intrafallopian transfer; EIFT = embryo intrafallopian transfer) or the uterus (IVF-ET = in vitro fertilisation and embryo transfer).

Application of the above-mentioned methods in a homologous system, i.e. using the gametes of the couple concerned within infertility therapy that represents a last resort, is nowadays not questioned by the majority of physicians and society, as far as either ethical or legal aspects are concerned. The identity of genetic and social parenthood is guaranteed as in families without infertility problems.

In the heterologous system the scope of implementation of the aforementioned methods of assisted reproduction is wide and frequently burdened by ethical (and legal) problems: what predominates in the discussion is the annulment of identity of genetic and social parenthood. Ensuing problems may prove to be a great burden to the procreated child, who is entitled to information on its identity and parental relationship, as well as to the partnership itself. Conveyance of natural descent and social environment essential for the self-comprehension of our society must not be denied to a child. It might be fateful for a child to be ignorant of its descent [7, 8]. Discussions on the question of the personal finding of identity of a man procreated in such a way have, above all in the Federal Republic of Germany, been ethically closely linked to the person's right to know the genetic father or mother [2].

Heterologous inseminations inevitably provoke a separation between social and genetic fatherhood. The fact that the donor of the semen invades matrimony as a third person might be harmful to the child's well-being and to the partnership as well. Difficulties are likely to arise in cases where the child's development differs from the expectations its parents cherish. The adoption of strict criteria for indications (considerably disturbed fertility of the husband, auto-gonosomal hereditary disease), unequivocal documentation of a healthy semen donor (no mixture of semen) and absence of commercialisation (voluntary and free donation of semen) should become preconditions. Procedures aimed at sperm selection for sex determination should only be implemented to avoid severe hereditary diseases which are sex-specific.

The utilisation of donor oocytes generates problems as described above. Furthermore, there are problems from a medical point of view since the follicles can only be retrieved by an invasive operation that generally requires preliminary treatment of the donor with hormones. This procedure involves a separation of genetic and social motherhood. Since in vitro fertilisation allows the procreation of human life in a laboratory it ought ot be ensured, given the ethical and legal considerations, that as few embryos are procreated as are required and appropriate. These embryos should not be manipulated except for the child's benefit.

The procedure of *embryo donation* comprises the transfer of an embryo into the uterus of a woman, an embryo who is genetically native to neither her nor her husband. The central argument against oocyte and embryo donation is the fact that these techniques will tear apart the unity of descent and birth which have so far been inseparable [5]. Moreover, the doctors' ethical conflict lies in the role that indirectly compels him to act as a grower of man since he decides on the donor of semen and/or the donor of the oocyte, thus making a selection [4]. A comparison between the donation of an oocyte and a prenatal adoption neglects that an adoption is primarily focused on caring for children without parents and not for childless couples.

The term *surrogate motherhood* encompasses two forms:

1. Artificial fertilisation of the lender mother with semen of the "orderer", carrying the pregnancy to full term and handing over the child after its birth.
2. Introduction of a generally extracorporeally fertilised oocyte into the uterus of a women who carries the child to full term for the "orderers".

These different forms of surrogate motherhood involve the separation of motherhood similar to oocyte and embryo donation. A commercialised application makes the woman an instrument, degrading her to a birth machine and thus violating the dignity of man.

Artificial inseminations in single women deliberately deprive the child of its father.

The following methods cannot be accepted ethically:

1. *Cloning:* creation of genetically identical multiple fetuses
2. *Creation of chimeras:* insertion of alien genetic information into a fertilised oocyte
3. *Creation of hybrids:* crossing of two genetically different individuals (e.g. man-animal).

These techniques vigorously infringe the value and dignity of man and are explicitly prohibited in the German Act on the Protection of Embryos.

Conclusion

The procedures used in reproductive medicine and the future possibilities to be anticipated from genetic techniques raise fundamental ethical questions. In a situation of conflict with the patient's wish for a child on the one hand and the wide range of objections against certain procedures of assisted reproductive medicine on the other, the doctor is attributed a key role: to repress the greed of man and the imaginary right to try anything that is feasible, and to fasten the understanding that human medicine may also mean renunciation.

Research in medicine strongly needs to be accompanied by ethics that are open towards new procedures, leaving to the doctor his share of responsibility for what he does. Our society rightly claims that ethical aspects of medicine should be discussed so as to continuously redefine the ethical limits of medical action. Ethical responsbility applies to the doctor/scientist as well as to the society requesting research and medical progress.

References

1. American College of Obstetricians and Gynecologists (1989) ACOG technical bulletin no. 136/1989. ACOG Washington, DC
2. Arbeitsgruppe BMJ/BMFT (Benda-Kommission) (1985) (eds): In-vitro-fertilisation. Schweitzer, Munich (Gentechnologie vol 6)
3. Gesetz zum Schutz von Embryonen (Embryonenschutzgesetz-ESchG) (1990) Bundesgesetzblatt, Part 1, p 2746
4. Hepp H (1988) Reproduktionsmedizin im Spannungsfeld von Ethik und Recht. Gynäkologe 21:1–12
5. Hirsch GE (1989) Juristische Aspekte in der Reproduktionsmedizin. In: Schirren C (ed) Unerfüllter Kinderwunsch. Deutscher Ärzteverlag, Cologne
7. Kluxen W (1985) Manipulierte Menschenordnung. In: Genforschung – Fluch oder Segen? Schweitzer, Munich (Gentechnologie. Chancen und Risiken)
8. Petersen P, Teichmann A Machen oder kommen lassen. Unsere Beziehung zur Kindesankunft. Dtsch Ärzteblatt 80:62
9. Sass HM (1989) Menschliche Fortpflanzung unter ethischen Aspekten. In: Schneider HPG (ed) Sexualmedizin, Infertilität, Familienplanung. Urban and Schwarzenberg, Munich

Springer-Verlag and the Environment

We at Springer-Verlag firmly believe that an international science publisher has a special obligation to the environment, and our corporate policies consistently reflect this conviction.

We also expect our business partners – paper mills, printers, packaging manufacturers, etc. – to commit themselves to using environmentally friendly materials and production processes.

The paper in this book is made from low- or no-chlorine pulp and is acid free, in conformance with international standards for paper permanency.

MIX
Papier aus verantwortungsvollen Quellen
Paper from responsible sources
FSC® C105338

FSC
www.fsc.org

If you have any concerns about our products, you can contact us on
ProductSafety@springernature.com

In case Publisher is established outside the EU, the EU authorized representative is:
Springer Nature Customer Service Center GmbH
Europaplatz 3, 69115 Heidelberg, Germany

Printed by Libri Plureos GmbH
in Hamburg, Germany